THE DEGENERATIVE CERVICAL SPINE

THE DEGENERATIVE CERVICAL SPINE

Editors

Marek Szpalski, M.D.
Senior Consultant and Associate Professor
Department of Orthopaedics
Centre Hospitalier Molière Longchamp
Teaching Hospital of the Free University of Brussels
Brussels, Belgium

Robert Gunzburg, M.D., Ph.D.
Senior Consultant
Department of Orthopaedics
Centenary Clinic
Antwerp, Belgium

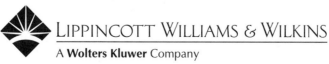

LIPPINCOTT WILLIAMS & WILKINS
A **Wolters Kluwer** Company
Philadelphia • Baltimore • New York • London
Buenos Aires • Hong Kong • Sydney • Tokyo

Acquisitions Editor: Robert Hurley
Developmental Editor: Brigitte Wilke
Manufacturing Manager: Colin Warnock
Production Manager: Toni Ann Scaramuzzo
Production Editor: Michael Mallard
Cover Designer: Patricia Gast
Compositor: Lippincott Williams & Wilkins Desktop Division
Printer: Edwards Brothers

© 2001 by LIPPINCOTT WILLIAMS & WILKINS
530 Walnut Street
Philadelphia, PA 19106 USA
LWW.com

Printed in the USA

Library of Congress Cataloging-in-Publication Data
The degenerative cervical spine / editors, Marek Szpalski, Robert Gunsburg.
    p. ; cm.
Includes bibliographical references and index.
ISBN 0-7817-3037-6 (hardcover)
    1. Cervical vertebrae—Diseases.   2. Cervical vertebrae—Abnormalities.
3. Spine—Abnormalities. I. Szpalski, Marek. II. Gunzburg, Robert.
[DNLM: 1. Cervical Vertebrae. 2. Spinal Diseases—therapy. 3. Neck Pain—therapy.
4. Orthopedic Procedures. 5. Spinal Diseases—diagnosis. WE 725 D3167 2001]
RD531.D44 2001
617.5′6—dc21

00-063998

Care has been taken to confirm the accuracy of the information presented and to describe generally accepted practices. However, the authors, editors, and publisher are not responsible for errors or omissions or for any consequences from application of the information in this book and make no warranty, expressed or implied, with respect to the currency, completeness, or accuracy of the contents of the publication. Application of this information in a particular situation remains the professional responsibility of the practitioner.

The authors, editors, and publisher have exerted every effort to ensure that drug selection and dosage set forth in this text are in accordance with current recommendations and practice at the time of publication. However, in view of ongoing research, changes in government regulations, and the constant flow of information relating to drug therapy and drug reactions, the reader is urged to check the package insert for each drug for any change in indications and dosage and for added warnings and precautions. This is particularly important when the recommended agent is a new or infrequently employed drug.

Some drugs and medical devices presented in this publication have Food and Drug Administration (FDA) clearance for limited use in restricted research settings. It is the responsibility of the health care provider to ascertain the FDA status of each drug or device planned for use in their clinical practice.

10 9 8 7 6 5 4 3 2 1

Contents

v

Section 5. Surgical Treatment Modalities Section

Contributing Authors

Federico Balague, M.D.   *Médecin-Chef Adjoint, Service de Rhumatologie, Médecine Physique, and Rééducation, Hôpital Cantonal,1708 Fribourg, Switzerland*

Erik J. Barbaix, M.D.   *Department of Manual Therapy, Vrije Universiteit Brussel, B-1090 Brussels, Belgium*

Jacques Benezech, M.D.   *Service de Neurochirurgie, Clinique Rech, 34000 Montpellier, France*

Michel Benoist, M.D.   *Consultant Rheumatologist of Paris Hospitals, University of Paris VII, 75116 Paris, France*

Helena Brisby, M.D.   *Research Associate, Department of Orthopaedics, Göteborg University, Sahlgrenska University Hospital, SE-413 45 Göteborg, Sweden*

A. Kim Burton, Ph.D., D.O.   *Spinal Research Unit, University of Huddersfield, Huddersfield HD1 2SP, United Kingdom*

Wolfhard Caspar, M.D., Ph.D.   *Neurosurgical Department, University of Saarland, D-66421 Homburg, Germany*

Eric Chamberlin, M.D.   *Department of Orthopaedic Surgery, Carolinas Medical Center, Charlotte, North Carolina 28232*

Jan Pieter Clarijs, Ph.D.   *Professor, Department of Experimental Anatomy, Dean, Faculty of Physical Education and Physical Therapy, Vrije Universiteit Brussel, B-1090 Brussels, Belgium*

Lutz Claes, Ph.D.   *Director, Institute for Orthopaedic Research and Biomechanics, University of Ulm, D-89081 Ulm, Germany*

Henry Vernon Crock, M.D., F.R.C.S., F.R.A.C.S.   *Spinal Dirorders Unit, Cromwell Hospital, London SW5 0TU, United Kingdom*

Valère Debois, M.D.   *Department of Neurosurgery, St. Maartens Zickenhuis, B-2570 Duffel, Belgium*

Peter Donceel, M.D., Ph.D.   *Department of Occupational and Insurance Medicine, School of Publick Health, Katholieke Universiteit Leuven, B-3000 Leuven, Belgium*

Marc G. Du Bois, M.D.   *Research Fellow, Department of Occupational and Insurance Medicine, School of Public Health, Katholieke Universiteit Leuven, B-3000 Leuven, Belgium*

Jean Dudler, M.D.   *Service de Rhumatologie, Hôpital Cantonal, CHUV 1011 Lausanne, Switzerland*

Jiri Dvorak, M.D.   *Chief, Spine Unit, Department of Neurology, Schulthess Clinic, CH-8008 Zurich, Switzerland*

Maurice D. Gosby   *Columbia Union College, Takoma Park, Maryland 20912*

Anukul Kumar Deb Goswami, M.S., M.Ch., F.R.C.S.(Orth), D.N.B.   *Honorary Lecturer, Faculty of Health, University of Central Lancaster, Preston PR1 2HE; Department of Spinal Surgery, The Spinal Foundation, The Arbury Centre, Rochdale 0L11 4LZ, United Kingdom*

Charles G. Greenough, M.D., M.Chir., F.R.C.S.   *Consultant Orthopedic Surgeon, Middlesborough General Hospital, Middlesborough TS5 5AZ, United Kingdom*

Pierre Guigui, M.D.   *Department of Orthopedic Surgery, Hôpital Beaujon, 92110 Clichy, France*

Philippe Gutwirth, M.D.   *Surgeon, Department of Vascular Surgery, Antwerp Blood Vessel Centre, Centenary Clinic, B-2018 Antwerp, Belgium*

Robert Gunzburg, M.D., Ph.D.   *Senior Consultant, Department of Orthopaedics, Centenary Clinic, B-2018 Antwerp, Belgium*

Manny Halpern, Ph.D., C.P.E.   *Adjunct Clinical Assistant Professor, Department of Occupational Therapy, New York University; Associate Director for Ergonomic Services, Occupational and Industrial Orthopaedic Center, Hospital for Joint Diseases, Mount Sinai NYU Heath, New York, New York 10014*

Edward N. Hanley, Jr., M.D.   *Department of Orthopaedic Surgery, Carolinas Medical Center, Charlotte, North Carolina 28232*

Bernard Jeanneret, M.D.   *Professor, Department of Orthopaedic Surgery, University of Basel, CH-4012 Basel, Switzerland*

Peter M. Klara, M.D., Ph.D.   *Associate Professor, Department of Neurosurgery, Eastern Virginia Medical School, Norfolk, Virginia 23507*

Martin T. N. Knight, M.D., F.R.C.S.   *The Spinal Foundation, The Arbury Centre, Rochdale 0L11 4LZ, United Kingdom*

Bengt I. Lind, M.D., Ph.D.   *Associate Professor, Department of Orthopedics, University of Göteborg, Sahlgrenska University Hospital, S-413 45 Göteborg, Sweden*

Guy Matgé, M.D.   *Department of Neurosurgery, Centre Hospitalier, L-1210 Luxembourg, Luxembourg*

Christian Melot, M.D., Ph.D., MSciBiostat, MsciHealthEconomics   *Professor, Faculty of Medicine, Free University of Brussels; Department of Intensive Care, Erasme University Hospital, B-1070 Brussels, Belgium*

Tim McClune, D.O.   *Research Associate, Spinal Research Unit, University of Huddersfield, Huddersfield HD1 2SP, United Kingdom*

B. P. Mortele   *Department of Radiology-Magnetic Resonance Unit, Cazk Groeninghe, B-8500 Kortrijk, Belgium*

A. Muller   *Spine Unit, Department of Neurology, Schulthess Clinic, CH-8008 Zurich, Switzerland*

Margareta Nordin, Dr.Sci.   *Director, Occupational and Industrial Orthopaedic Center, Hospital for Joint Diseases, Mount Sinai NYU Health; Research Professor, Department of Orthopaedic Surgery and Department of Environmental Medicine, School of Medicine, New York University, New York, New York 10014*

Claes Olerund, M.D., Ph.D.   *Associate Professor, Department of Orthopedics; Head, Section for Spinal Surgery, Uppsala University Hospital, SE-75185 Uppsala, Sweden*

Kjell Olmarker, M.D., Ph.D.   *Associate Research Professor, Department of Orthopaedics, Göteborg University, Sahlgrenska University Hospital, SE-413 45 Göteborg, Sweden*

Janos T. Patko, M.D.   *The Spinal Foundation, The Arbury Centre, Rochdale 0L11 4LZ, United Kingdom*

Markus Pietrek, M.D.   *Research Fellow, Occupational and Industrial Orthopaedic Center, Hospital for Joint Diseases Orthopaedic Institute, Mount Sinai NYU Health; Instructor, Program of Ergonomics and Biomechanics, New York University, New York, New York 10014*

Tim Pigott, D.M., F.R.C.S.   *Consultant Neurosurgeon, Department of Neurosurgery, Walton Centre for Neurology and Neurosurgery, Liverpool L9 7LJ, United Kingdom*

Charles Pither, M.B.B.S., F.R.C.A.   *Consultant, Pain Management Unit, St. Thomas' Hospital, London SE1 7EH, United Kingdom*

Tobias R. Pitzen, M.D.   *Research Fellow, Neurosurgical Department, University of Saarland, D-66421 Homburg, Germany*

Malcolm H. Pope, Dr.Med.Sc., Ph.D.   *Chair of Safety and Health, Liberty Safework Research Center, University of Aberdeen, Aberdeen AB9 2ZD, United Kingdom*

Bjorn Rydevik, M.D., Ph.D.   *Professor and Chairman, Department of Orthopaedics, Göteborg University, Sahlgrenska University Hospital, SE-413 45 Göteborg, Sweden*

P.C. Seynaeve   *Department of Radiology-Magnetic Resonance Unit, Cazk Groeninghe, B-8500 Kortrijk, Belgium*

Dan M. Spengler, M.D.   *Professor and Chairman, Department of Orthopaedics and Rehabilitation, Vanderbilt University Medical Center, Nashville, Tennessee 37232*

Wolf-Ingo Steudel, M.D., Ph.D.   *Neurosurgical Department, University of Saarland, D-66421 Homburg, Germany*

Marek Szpalski, M.D.   *Senior Consultant and Associate Professor, Department of Orthopaedics, Centre Hospitalier Molière Longchamp, Teaching Hospital of the Free University of Brussels, B-1180 Brussels, Belgium*

Jean Pierre Van Buyten, M.D.   *Department of Anesthesia and Pain Management, Maria Middelares Hospital, B-9100 St. Niklaas, Belgium*

Peter Van Roy, M.D.   *Professor, Department of Experimental Anatomy, Vrije Universiteit Brussels, B-1090 Brussel, Brussels*

Dirk Vandevelde, M.D.   *Department of Orthopaedic Surgery, University Hospital Antwerp, B-2650 Edegem, Belgium*

Heiko Visarius, Ph.D.   *Director, Medivision Institute, CH-4436 Oberdorf, Switzerland*

Hans-Joachim Wilke, Ph.D.   *Department of Orthopaedic Research and Biomechanics, University of Ulm, D-89081 Ulm, Germany*

Jan T. Wilmink, M.D., Ph.D.   *Professor of Neuroradiology, Academisch Ziekenhuis Maastricht, 6202 AZ Maastricht, The Netherlands*

Björn Zoëga, M.D., Ph.D.   *Assistant Professor, Department of Orthopedics, University of Göteborg, Sahlgrenska University Hospital, S-413 45 Göteborg, Sweden*

Preface

Degenerative cervical spine disorders may have various etiologies and a diversified clinical presentation. They are among the most common spinal problems encountered in everyday practice. This book covers this important topic from anatomy to economic considerations through physiopathology, clinical presentation, diagnosis, conservative and surgical treatment.

Although inflammatory cervical disorders such as rheumatoid arthritis are not the subject of this book, have different origins, characteristics and specific medical treatments, their mechanical consequences may often be similar to those of degenerative disorders and will justify similar techniques in surgical handling. They are therefore covered in some surgical chapters.

The review of the degenerative spine presented in this book will familiarize the reader with all the areas of degenerative cervical disorders, with some of which he might be less familiar because of a different field of expertise.

The basic science section covers the anatomy and biomechanics of the cervical segment as well as the actual theories and hypothesis explaining the origin of cervical pain.

The second section deals with clinical presentation, natural history, and the important vascular consequences of cervical degeneration. Differentiation between congenital and degenerative stenosis is also discussed here.

The diagnosis section deals with the latest possibilities of imaging and electrophysiological technologies in the evaluation of cervical disorders. The different imaging techniques are extensively covered and the true clinical significance of many findings is thoroughly discussed.

The treatment section deals first with conservative treatment, it covers rheumatological and physical medicine treatments. The numerous questions about the use of manipulation as well as the true efficacy of orthoses are also treated in this section. An important topic in conservative treatment is pain therapy and a chapter is dedicated to the new techniques of spinal cord stimulation and pain control through radiofrequency application.

Many different surgical techniques have been described in the treatment of cervical disorders. This book summarizes the different approaches, techniques and instrumentations with results and cost considerations. Chapters focus on the complex topics of laminoplasties and cervico-occipital fusions, often required in rheumatoid arthritis.

Finally, the very important questions of costs and quality assessment are extensively treated. This is a major subject that will become increasingly important as the concept of "Evidence Based Medicine" becomes the gold standard of treatment acceptance and reimbursement. The cost of surgical management and the cost-utility ratios of different treatments are discussed. The effective outcome assessment needed to assess results is also discussed and a handling algorithm is proposed.

This book helps the reader find his way in the often complex issues surrounding the degenerative cervical spine. The thorough discussions by opinion leaders in this field make this book a welcome addition to the library of many professionals, clinicians as well as scientists dealing with cervical spine pathologies.

Marek Szpalski, M.D.
Robert Gunzburg, M.D., Ph.D.

SECTION 1

Basics

The Degenerative Cervical Spine,
edited by Marek Szpalski and Robert Gunzburg
Lippincott Williams & Wilkins, Philadelphia © 2001.

1

Functional Anatomy of the Cervical Spine

Peter Van Roy, Erik Barbaix, Jan P. Clarijs

*Department of Experimental Anatomy, Vrije Universiteit Brussel,
1090 Brussels, Belgium*

FUNCTIONAL ANATOMY OF THE UPPER CERVICAL SPINE
  The Atlantooccipital Junction • The Atlantoaxial Joint • Motion in the Upper Cervical Spine
FUNCTIONAL ANATOMY OF THE MIDDLE AND THE LOWER CERVICAL SPINE
  Zygapophyseal Joints • Uncinate Processes and Intervertebral Discs • Ligaments • Developmental and Secondary Anomalies • Global Cervical Motion
THE COURSE OF THE VERTEBRAL ARTERY
  First Segment of the Vertebral Artery • Variations of the Second Segment and Its Bony Canal • Third Segment • Fourth Segment
MUSCULAR VARIANTS
DISCUSSION

The cervical spine is a lordotic spinal section composed of seven vertebrae. Variations in the number of cervical vertebrae probably do not occur (13). The first two vertebrae, the atlas and the axis, have particular morphologic features. The other five cervical vertebrae typically, have bifurcated spinous and transverse processes and uncinate processes at the craniolateral side of the corpora. The transverse processes have foramina for the vertebral artery. The anteroposterior diameter of the cervical vertebral bodies gradually increases from an average of 16.5 mm at C3 to 19.3 mm at C7. The anteroposterior depth at the endplates is greater by approximately 2 mm. The superior end plate always is larger than the inferior endplate. The mean depths of the inferior end plate vary, but the depth generally increases from C2 to C6 then decreases to C7 (20,50). The mean height of disc space is about 4 mm near the anterior edge and is between 2.5 and 3 mm near the posterior edge (50). The cervical spinal canal has an anteroposterior diameter of at least 14 mm at the level of the foramen magnum, 13 mm at C1 and C2, and 12 mm below C2 (115). Morphologic variants, not to be confused with anomalies, appear in both the skeletal and soft-tissue components. This anatomic variability has several functional consequences and hampers determination of true diameters of the spinal canal with ratios obtained from measurements of bony dimensions on radiographs or computed tomographic (CT) scans.

FUNCTIONAL ANATOMY OF THE UPPER CERVICAL SPINE

The Atlantooccipital Junction

Frequent Site of Articular Tropism

The craniocervical junction is characterized by a typical joint configuration between the occipital condyles and the large bean-, kidney-, or slipper-shaped facets on the superior aspect of the lateral masses of C1. The morphologic features of the atlantooccipital (C0-1) joint are highly variable. The joint often has articular tropism, which may be caused by differences in the inclination, curvature, dimensions, or shape of the left and right facets (33,63,80,90,104,107). Unequal constrictions or marked grooves may divide the articular surfaces into two so-called pressure facets (facies articularis bipartita) (Fig. 1.1A,D) (80,90). Left-right asymmetry can be caused by asymmetric implantation on the lateral mass.

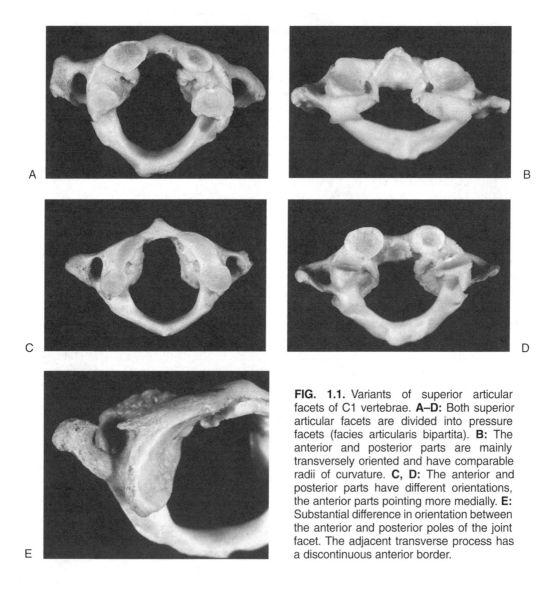

FIG. 1.1. Variants of superior articular facets of C1 vertebrae. **A–D:** Both superior articular facets are divided into pressure facets (facies articularis bipartita). **B:** The anterior and posterior parts are mainly transversely oriented and have comparable radii of curvature. **C, D:** The anterior and posterior parts have different orientations, the anterior parts pointing more medially. **E:** Substantial difference in orientation between the anterior and posterior poles of the joint facet. The adjacent transverse process has a discontinuous anterior border.

Ball and Socket or Ellipsoid Joint?

The atlantooccipital junction comprises two distinct articular compartments that have convergent anterior poles. This structure contributes to flexion, extension, and lateral bending of the neck. Panjabi et al. (73) drew attention to controversy about axial rotation at this level. It is generally believed that the C0-1 junction does not provide axial rotation. However, a reduced amount of axial rotation has been found at C0-1 on functional CT images and during in vitro radiographic stereo photogrammetric experiments (73,79). The controversy about axial rotation can be explained not only by different research methods (e.g., use of two-dimensional versus three-dimensional motion analysis, the presence of variable loading conditions, and greater or less sensitivity of the measuring instruments) but also by anatomic variation. If the anterior and posterior parts of the articular facets have comparable radii of curvature and if they can be considered to belong to a common, slightly curved and mainly transversely oriented surface, then both resulting articular configurations can be regarded as parts of an irregular ball and socket joint, which allows a certain amount of axial rotation (Fig. 1.1B). Frequently, however, the anterior parts of the joint facets (sometimes the anterior pressure facets) strongly point medially and reach a definitely more oblique orientation than the posterior parts by tilting about their longitudinal axes (Fig. 1.1C–E). In this case the resulting configuration can be regarded as part of a modified ellipsoid joint capable of no or only slight axial rotation. A double C–shaped configuration is depicted in axial sections through the atlantooccipital joint (see Fig. 1.5.A,B). Shape, curvature, and orientation of the articular facets but also deformation of the articular cartilage and steering by articular capsules and ligaments may account for differences in joint motion.

Bony Anomalies

The frequency of occipitalization of the atlas found in large series is estimated at 0.1% to 1% (7,8; data of Macalister cited in 80; data of von Torklus cited in 93). Higher frequencies have been reported in smaller series (60). However, it cannot be excluded that some specimens were kept precisely because of the presence of occipitalization (1.95% in the collection of the Faculty of Medicine of Porto, 2% in Lisbon, and as high as 4.2% in Coimbra).

Different degrees of aplasia and gaps in the posterior arch of the atlas, erroneously called spina bifida, have been described. They are frequent in cases of occipitalization (7). An isolated median ossified fragment between bilateral areas of aplasia occasionally is found to represent the posterior tubercle. Gaps and aplasia of the anterior arch are much more exceptional (0.1 versus 4%). Considerable instability as a consequence of simultaneous existence of gaps in both the posterior and anterior arches has been found to cause a so-called *atlas bipartitus*. A supernumerary articular facet on the anterior arch may articulate with a condylus tertius of the occipital bone. An additional joint facet for the occipital bone at the superior aspect of a transverse process represents an epitransverse process (80,104).

The Atlantoaxial Joint

A Unique Spinal Joint Complex

The C1-2 junction displays a unique spinal joint complex. It functions without an intervertebral disc. Flexion, extension, and axial rotation take place between the lateral

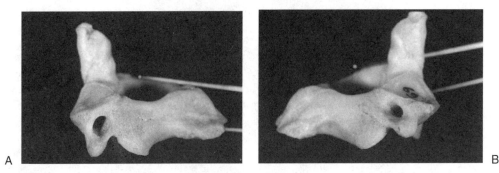

A   B

FIG. 1.2. Left and right superior articular facets and transverse process of C2. Obliterated anteroposterior (AP) convexity of the superior articular facets has changed into a slight AP concavity on the right side **(B)**. The left transverse foramen **(A)** has a larger transverse foramen. Crowned dens is visible.

joint facets, operating in a convex to convex configuration. Movement simultaneously appears in the pivot joint between the odontoid process, its corresponding facet on the anterior arch, and the transverse ligament of the atlas. The transverse atlantal ligament, part of the cruciform ligament, has a key function in stability of the C1-2 junction (24). The anteroposterior convexity of both articular surfaces of the lateral C1-2 joints is partially composed of the articular cartilage and may disappear as a result of degeneration (Fig. 1.2, compare with Fig. 1.6A). The superior articular facets of C2 normally are the largest facets in the spine (75). This general statement may be overruled by the presence of pancake-shaped facets caused by degenerative enlargement at lower levels (Fig. 1.3). An axial section through the atlantoaxial joint in about 40 degrees of rotation to the right illustrates how the left inferior facet of the atlas moves forward on the left superior facet of the axis, whereas the right inferior facet of the atlas moves backward on its counterpart on the axis (Fig. 1.4). Loose capsules are needed to allow such large excursions.

    The C1-2 junction provides nearly one half of the axial rotation capability of the cervical spine. Successive axial sections through the upper cervical spine depict the three

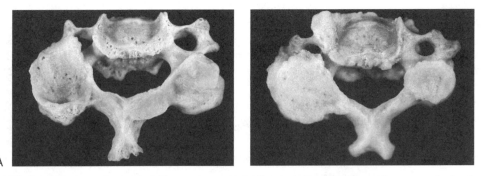

A   B

FIG. 1.3. Tropism of superior zygapophyseal joint facets in the middle and lower cervical spine caused by degenerative enlargement. **A:** Nearthrotic facet on the right lamina. **B:** Degenerative changes of uncinate processes accentuate possible encroaching effects on the intervertebral foramen and vertebral artery.

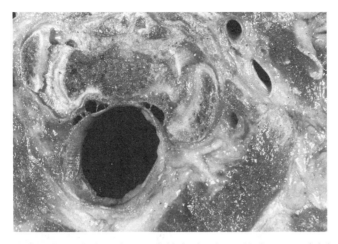

FIG. 1.4. Axial section through the atlantoaxial joint in about 40 degrees of right axial rotation. The left inferior facet of the atlas has moved forward on the left superior facet of the axis, whereas the right inferior facet of the atlas has moved backward on its counterpart on the axis. The C2 ganglion is present behind the right lateral C1-2 joint. It appears slightly darker (reddish) than the anterior and posterior rami.

possible cranial insertions of the alar ligaments (Fig. 1.5). The alar ligaments connect the odontoid process and the occipital bone. They may send additional attachments to the lateral mass and sometimes also to the anterior arch of the atlas (17). The alar ligaments play an important role in the control of axial rotation and lateral bending in the upper cervical spine. In Fig. 1.5B, an alar ligament is partially wound around the dens.

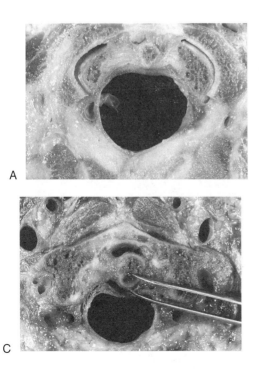

A

B

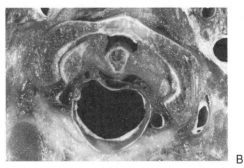

C

FIG. 1.5. Axial sections through the atlanto-occipital joint depict the connections of the alar ligaments to the occipital bone and atlas. **A:** Transverse section through the apex of the odontoid process shows dense connective tissue near the occipital condyles. **B:** Lower section through the occipital condyles depicts the alar connections to the anterior arch. The alar ligament is partially wound around the dens. **C:** Axial section below the occipital condyles shows the alar connections to the lateral mass of the atlas.

Bony Anomalies of C2

Aplasia (Fig. 1.6B), gaps, and true spina bifida can occur in the axis. Diagnostic problems can result from the finding of a persistent ossiculum terminale (Bergman ossicle) or os odontoideum. The ossiculum terminale represents a secondary ossification center (68). It occurs among 26% of healthy children between 5 and 11 years of age (31). In most cases fusion with the odontoid process follows between 10 and 13 years of age (68). Persistent ossiculum terminale is caused by failure of fusion of the terminal ossicle to the remainder of the odontoid process (92,93). It is not to be confused with calcification or ossification of ligaments. Agenesis of the terminal ossification center causes dens bicornis.

The os odontoideum is an independent osseous structure located cephalad to the body of C2 (92,93). A distinction should be made between stable and unstable forms. Fractures of the dens should be taken into account in the etiology of os odontoideum (31,68). The anterior aspect of the odontoid process may have an irregular or flat, straight or slightly retrograde curved profile. The anterior arch sometimes fits into a small anterior groove on the dens (110). The anterior facet of normal odontoid processes has a posterior inclination between 1 degrees and 29 degrees, whereas the odontoid process itself may have a posterior tilt angle as great as 45 degrees (55). Variations in the shape of the dens can be accentuated by considerable osteophytic enlargement of the anterior articular surface, which is common. The corresponding facet for the dens on the anterior arch of the atlas also may have secondary enlargement, which often causes left-right asymmetry (107). Ossification and calcification can develop in the ligaments at the tip of the dens and give rise to a so-called crowned odontoid process (Fig. 1.6A) or spiked helmet dens. Ossifi-

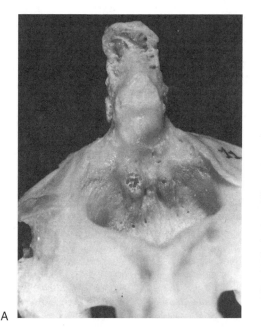
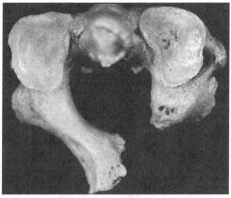

A   B

FIG. 1.6. Secondary change as opposed to anomaly of C2. **A:** Crowned dens. **B:** Aplasia of the right lamina.

cation and calcification that develop in the anterior atlantooccipital membrane give rise to a peridental aureole (80).

Motion in the Upper Cervical Spine

Head Retraction and Protrusion versus Cervical Flexion and Extension

The full end range of flexion at C0-1 and C1-2 is reached in head retraction rather than in full flexion of the cervical spine. The full range of extension at C0-1 and C1-2 is rather achieved in head protrusion (70).

Joint Configurations That Cause Deviating Patterns of Coupled Motion

The joint configurations in the upper cervical spine produce local mechanisms of coupled motion. Panjabi et al. (74) conducted a detailed in vitro study of the postural dependency of segmental coupling patterns in the upper cervical spine. At C0-1 and C1-2, the main motion of axial rotation induces lateral bending to the opposite side. However, only a restrained amount of lateral bending is possible at C1-2. In the neutral position, the main motion of lateral bending induces axial rotation to the ipsilateral side at C0-1 and to the opposite side at C1-2. The amount of coupled axial rotation in lateral bending at C1-2 is larger than the main motion component as long as lateral bending starts from the neutral position. When performed in full flexion, the main motion of lateral bending produces much less ipsilateral axial rotation. The flexion posture also strongly reduces the lateral bending component itself.

When the principal motions of axial rotation and lateral bending are applied in the neutral position, the accompanying coupled motion in the sagittal plane is extension at C0-1 and flexion at C1-2. In full extension, however, an accompanying extension component was recorded at both levels (74). A flexion component likewise became obvious when axial or lateral bending torques were introduced in the full flexion posture. Thus the coupled patterns of extension at C0-1 were accentuated in the extension posture and switched into a flexion component when the full flexion posture was adopted. Coupled patterns of flexion at C1-2, however, were enhanced in full flexion but switched into an extension component when the main motion was applied in a full extension posture (74).

Topographic Consequences of Anterolateral Articular Pillars

The articular pillars of the upper cervical spine are located more anterolaterally along the spinal canal than those in the middle and lower parts of the cervical spine. As a consequence C1 and C2 nerve roots emerge behind these articular processes. Unlike in the lower levels, in the upper cervical spine the zygapophyseal joints are innervated by ventral rami (10). Degenerative enlargements are more frequent in the superior than in the inferior articular facets of C1. This may endanger the C2 nerve root ganglion, which is situated directly behind the atlantoaxial joint between the posterior arch of the atlas and the lamina of C2, where it can be crushed (47). Figure 1.4 shows the position of the C2 ganglion directly behind the right compartment of the C1-2 junction. Carefully freed from the surrounding tissues, the ganglion appears more reddish than the nerve bundles of the C2 nerve root. This is indicative of the rich blood supply of spinal ganglia (14,85), probably in response to high local metabolic demand (87). Along its anterolateral course, the ventral ramus passes the vascular plexus of the vertebral artery and veins, to which it is tightly attached. The dorsal ramus can be followed on its course through the posterior cervical muscles, where it continues as the major occipital nerve.

FUNCTIONAL ANATOMY OF THE MIDDLE AND THE LOWER CERVICAL SPINE

Zygapophyseal Joints

Weight-bearing Joint Facets

The successive articular processes of the middle and lower cervical spine constitute two highly mobile dorsolateral columns with slightly dorsocranially oriented upper and slightly ventrocaudally oriented inferior articular facets. The oblique orientation between a coronal and a transverse plane indicates an important weight-bearing function. This function decreases at the cervicothoracic transitional level, where there are steeper inclinations of articular facets and where the vertebral bodies carry a relatively higher percentage of the load. The inclination of the articular surfaces relative to the coronal plane tends to be larger in women than in men. At C6 and C7, the lateral mass is markedly thinner than in the rest of the cervical spine (27). At C5, C6, and C7, the values of the interfacet angles of the superior articular facets are close to 180 degrees, whereas at C3 and C4, the interfacet angles are smaller (58).

Joints Acting Near Neurovascular Bundles

Because of the compact architecture of cervical vertebrae, the facet joints lie close to the exiting nerve roots and vessels that connect the central spinal canal to the longitudinal channel of the vertebral artery. From C3 to C7, nerve roots emerge in the anterolateral direction. They usually are situated in the lower part of a cervical intervertebral foramen (26,76) lying on top of the transverse process in the groove formed by unification of the real transverse process and the rib homologue. The segmental artery usually runs through the upper part of the intervertebral foramen with its corresponding veins and the sinuvertebral nerve(s). The vertebral artery is situated in front of the emerging nerve roots. During its posterior course, the dorsal ramus curves along the lateral aspect of the superior articular process (21).

On average the dimensions of the intervertebral foramina increase from the cephalic to the caudal aspect, but the dimensions of the C2-3 foramen are larger than those of the more caudal ones. Together with the existence of larger uncinate processes at C4-6, this phenomenon may partially explain the frequent involvement of these levels in root damage by osteophytes (19,22).

The size of the intervertebral increases in flexion and decreases in extension and in ipsilateral rotation. This change is most pronounced in the lower segments, resulting in 10% enlargement at 30 degrees of flexion and decrease in size up to 13% in 30 degrees of extension (113).

The size and surface area of the neural foramina tend to decrease in the degenerative cervical spine. Degenerative enlargement of the inferior facets especially may reduce the width in the middle of the foramina, forcing the nerve roots to use the upper part of the reduced neural canal (38). Disc height also largely influences the dimensions of the intervertebral foramina. In an experimental in vitro study, 1-mm reduction in available disc height decreased foraminal area by 20% to 30%. After 3-mm reduction, the foraminal area decreased 35% to 45% (48).

Uncinate Processes and Intervertebral Discs

Uncovertebral Joints: Secondhand Anatomy?

Cervical vertebral bodies including the uncinate processes develop from three ossification centers—one central and two lateral. The lateral ossification centers, also developing into the posterior arch, are slightly cephalad to the central ossification center developing into the main part of the body. This explains the presence of uncinate processes in the boundary zone at the craniolateral aspect of the vertebral body and corresponding lateral recesses at its caudal aspect. Uncovertebral joints subsequently develop within the areolar connective tissue that is originally situated along the lateral aspect of the intervertebral discs (37,101). A remnant of this tissue band develops into the fibroligamentous tissues that encase the vertebral artery and nerve roots (23). Uncinate processes are unique to mammals with a bipedal gait (78).

Within a cervical motion segment, the uncinate processes of the vertebral body below give the upper vertebral end plate a slight concavity in the left-right direction (Fig. 1.3A), whereas this end plate has a slight convexity in the anteroposterior direction. The corresponding lower end plate of the upper vertebral body has the opposite curvatures (46). Uncinate processes guide flexion and extension. The posterior foraminal part limits posterior translation and lateral bending and plays a role in the coupling motion between axial rotation and lateral bending (79,110). This structure contributes substantially to stability of the motion segment; the greatest stabilizing effect occurs in extension (45).

The periarticular nervous plexus of the vertebral artery is in close contact with the posterior edge of the uncinate process. Uncinate osteophytes consequently can endanger the vertebral artery and its surrounding sympathetic plexus, particularly at high levels, where the distance between the apex of the uncinate process and the medial border of the transverse foramen may be less than 2 mm (22,45). Composing the anterior wall of the intervertebral foramen, the posterior part of the uncinate process also may encroach on the emerging nerve roots (Fig. 1.3B).

The tip of the uncinate processes is 1 or 2 mm medial to the superior zygapophyseal joint (26) and about 1 mm from the body of the vertebra above (49,71). The dimension of the base of the uncinate process and the interuncinate distance steadily increase from C3 to C7. The highest uncinate processes are those at C4-6. In the lower cervical spine, the uncinate processes are located more dorsolaterally (32,84), and the height decreases gradually. Individual differences are common, and secondary enlargements often cause left-right asymmetry (Fig. 1.3B).

Intervertebral Discs

Microscopic dissection of cervical intervertebral discs has shown that the morphologic features of cervical intervertebral discs differ substantially from the traditional description, in which the nucleus pulposus is surrounded by a continuous anulus fibrosus composed of crossing collagen fibers in successive concentric lamellae (57). In the cervical spine, the relatively small nucleus pulposus is embedded in a central core of fibrocartilaginous material. The anulus fibrosus is divided into an anterior and a posterior part. The anterior part of the anulus is crescentic with a thick part in front of the central fibrocartilaginous core and tapering lateral extensions directed toward the uncinate region. Anterior anulus fibers are slightly oblique and partially interwoven near the midline. This anterior part of the anulus is moon shaped on axial sections, and the anteroposterior dimensions decrease from the midline toward the lateral sides of the disc. The much smaller and thinner posterior part is composed of longitudinally oriented collagen fibers that cover only the central part of the fibrocartilaginous core.

In the nucleus pulposus of the cervical discs of adolescents and adults, high rates of cell activity have been found near the cartilaginous end plates, suggesting the presence of regeneration. Thus the end plate might play an important role in maintenance of the nucleus pulposus. Calcification, ossification, and detachment of the end plate may trigger obliteration of the disc (67).

During the first decades of life, the structure of cervical intervertebral discs undergoes important changes, which occur in relation to different phases in the secondary development of the uncovertebral joints. The onset of horizontal clefts in the lateral aspects of the disc has even been found in a 9-year-old child (101). Early regression of the nucleus may lead progressively to the disappearance of nuclear material. Partial clefts probably develop as a functional adaptation to maintain rotational capability when the elastic properties of the anulus decrease. This hypothesis is heightened by the fact that the clefts occur predominantly in the posterior anulus, where the disc material undergoes the largest excursion around the axes of motion (78). Several originally separate clefts may extend progressively toward each other, and horizontal splitting of the disc into two layers of connective tissue may occur. This may be important from the third decade on, especially in the uppermost intervertebral discs (57,98,101). Among 135 cervical discs from autopsy specimens of persons 20 to 85 years of age, 61% had horizontal clefts and 49% had vertical clefts extending to the end plate; in 15% of instances this was associated with herniation of the end plate. In 21 specimens from surgical discectomy among patients 37 to 68 years of age, all the end plates were fragmented through vertical clefts. The frequency of clefts was age related (44). Although such cleavage of the intervertebral disc may not be generalized, it corresponds well with the functional model of concentric movement of the end plates and zygapophyseal joints presented by Penning (77).

Ligaments

The anterior longitudinal ligament (ALL) is composed of four layers. The superficial layer covers several motion segments. The intermediate layer covers only one motion segment and inserts on the anterior aspect of successive vertebral bodies. The deep layer runs between adjacent end plates and covers the intervertebral disc. The fourth layer consists of alar expansions and courses downward and laterally to attach on the lateral border of the vertebra immediately below to form a thin curtain over the lateral aspect of each disc. The most cranial and lateral of its fibers reach the summit of the uncinate process. The posterior longitudinal ligament (PLL) consists of three layers. The superficial layer has a central longitudinal part and lateral expansions that sweep out to the basis of the pedicles one or two segments below. The intermediate and deep layers span only one motion segment (57,82).

Stress-strain curves for the ALL and PLL show a trend toward less stiffness and more energy at failure for the ALL that for the PLL (81). Calcification and ossification of the PLL and to a lesser extent of the ALL are present in the "Japanese disease" (ossification of the PLL) and in rheumatic conditions, such as Bechterew disease, Forestier disease, and Reiter syndrome, and in psoriatic arthritis (39,64). Osteophytes are extremely frequent in osteoarthritis.

The distance between laminae is only 1 to 3 mm. The inferior border of the lamina is below the inferior border of the disc under the corresponding vertebra (26). As a consequence, in the cervical spine the ligamenta flava are extremely short. This probably explains the ossification of these ligaments in degenerative synostosis (Fig. 1.7). Through loss of disc height, the distance between successive laminae can be further reduced, leading to devel-

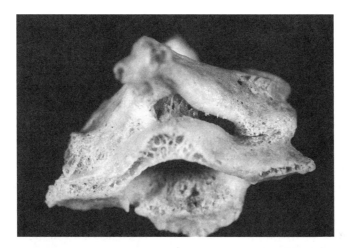

FIG. 1.7. Posterior view shows synostosis between C2 and C3, complete on the left side and incomplete on the right. Ossification of the right ligamemtum flavum is evident.

opment of neoarthrosis between laminae (Fig. 1.3A). In a study of the trabecular patterns of the laminae combined with morphometric observations, investigators concluded that the laminae of C2 and C7 are heavily loaded and probably play a role in stability of the cervical spine, whereas the laminae of the other vertebrae probably do not (72).

Between the posterior arches of C1 and C2, connections between the nuchal ligament and the dural sac have been described (59). The existence of connections between the dural sac and the posterior atlantooccipital membrane and between the dural sac and the rectus capitis posterior minor muscle has been confirmed (35).

Developmental and Secondary Anomalies

Because of a lack of ossification of the spinous process, spina bifida can occur in all cervical vertebrae, but it is less frequent than in the lumbar spine. In C3-7, agenesis of a pedicle can be caused by failure of a ventral ossification center. The lower cervical vertebrae are most often affected. Absence of a pedicle often is associated with abnormality of a transverse process and displacement of the articular process, resulting in enlargement of the intervertebral foramen (89). Anomalous development may produce hemivertebrae. Another type of segmentation anomaly is known as *isolated block vertebrae,* but these are more frequently associated with other congenital disorders. Fusion of vertebrae can occur as a consequence of degenerative disease with secondary arthrodesis of uncovertebral or zygapophyseal joints (Fig. 1.7). Ossification of the PLL and ligamenta flava is a well-known cause of progressive cervical myelopathy. It has a much higher incidence among Japanese and other Asians (more than 2%) than among non-Asians (0.16%) (36,56,64).

The bifurcate aspect of the transverse processes of the cervical vertebrae is the result of fusion between a true transverse process and a vestige of a cervical rib. The anterior tubercle of a cervical transverse process represents the rib homologue. This may be discontinuous, leading to an incomplete foramen (Fig. 1.1E) (99,107). The closing bar at the lateral end of the transverse foramen corresponds to an ossified costotransverse ligament or joint. Its upper side is concave. The dimension of the anterior tubercle of the transverse processes is highly variable. Different stages of elongation of this tubercle mimic a cervical rib (8,34). True cervical ribs of variable dimension may exist at the level of C7. They sometimes are reduced to fibrous strings between the transverse process and the first rib. Their role in thoracic outlet syndrome is well known.

Global Cervical Motion

Finite Centers of Rotation

To differentiate spinal instability, qualitative study of cervical motion in which centers of rotation are determined from CT scans (79), cineradiographs (106), or conventional radiographs (2–4,18,66) has been substantially investigated. From a methodologic point of view, the expression *instantaneous center of rotation* (ICR) can be used if a large number of succeeding motion steps (or steps of motion) are evaluated and if the time between each step is minimized. These conditions can be met with x-ray cinematography. When only one or a few positions in flexion and extension are compared, the expression *finite center of rotation* (FCR) is more appropriate (111). The path followed by succeeding ICRs or FCRs is called the *centrode*. ICR, FCR, and centrode are typical expressions in two-dimensional joint kinematics. Thus this method is valid only as long as the succeeding axes around which motion occurs remain parallel to each other and perpendicular to the plane of motion. Increasing the number of succeeding stages of motion to be compared improves the amount of information about the path of motion. Thus an ICR approach will generally be more informative than an FCR approach, but the latter often is the choice to avoid the risks of radiation exposure through multiple radiographs.

Allowing for the effect of technical errors, normal distributions of FCRs for sagittal motion of the cervical spine have been presented (4). In flexion and extension, FCRs are situated in the lower vertebral body of a motion segment. Higher motion segments allow more translation, which places these centers of rotation in a more caudal position. In the lower cervical spine, FCRs tend to lie closer to the vertebral endplate. Taller superior articular processes may account for a decrease in the amount of translation in the caudal motion segments and for a higher and more anterior location of the FCRs at these levels (66). Abnormal FCRs have been recorded for patients with neck pain (2). In the degenerative cervical spine, FCRs tend to display a shift in the anterior and caudal direction and a tendency toward hypomobility (18).

Segmental versus Regional Coupled Motion

Axial rotation of the middle and lower cervical spine induces coupled ipsilateral lateral bending; lateral bending induces coupled ipsilateral rotation. This coupled motion is provoked by the bony configuration of the joint facets and uncinate processes. Coupled motion is more pronounced in the middle than in the lower cervical spine (52,69) and may partially be counteracted in the upper cervical spine, where the amount and direction of coupled motion depend on posture (74). Patterns of coupled motion of the entire cervical spine are produced by additional but sometimes counteracting components of coupling motion in each of the constituent motion segments. Influenced by left-right differences or local degenerative features, these motion effects necessitate three-dimensional assessment. Modern equipment for real-time measurement of global coupled motion includes computerized electrogoniometers (30) and electromagnetic tracking devices (103,108). These tools become particularly attractive when simultaneous graphic display of three-dimensional motion components provides time-dependent mapping of coupled motion. Examples of interindividual and left-right differences of coupled motion in the frontal and sagittal planes during axial rotation are shown in Fig. 1.8A,B. Individual par-

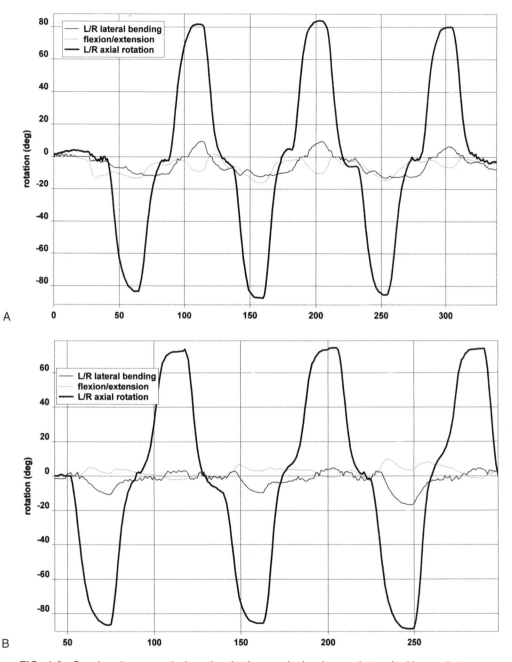

FIG. 1.8. Graphs show coupled motion in the cervical spine registered with an electromagnetic tracking device. The main motion is axial rotation. Negative values are for left rotation, left lateral bending, and flexion. Positive values are for right right axial rotation, right lateral bending, and extension. **A:** Healthy female volunteer, 24 years of age. Different left and right patterns of ipsilateral lateral bending. Axial rotations to the left and to the right are accompanied by flexion components. **B:** Healthy male volunteer, 34 years of age. Different left and right patterns of ipsilateral lateral bending. Axial rotation to the left is accompanied by an extension component, which does not occur in axial rotation to the right.

(continued on next page)

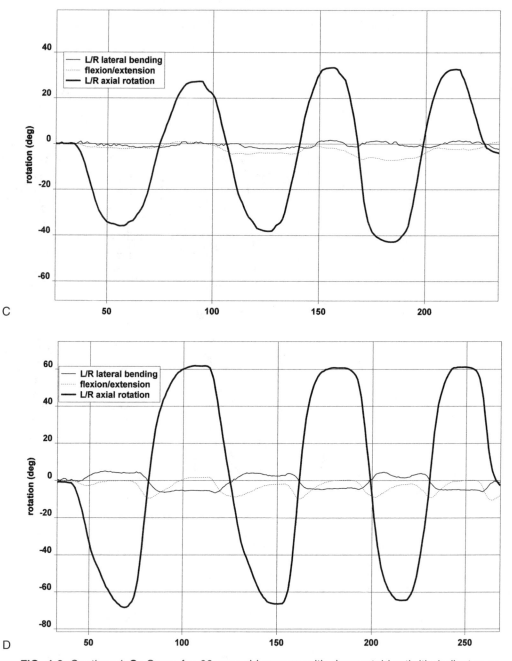

FIG. 1.8 *Continued.* **C:** Curve for 66-year-old woman with rheumatoid arthritis indicates reduced range of axial rotation. The ipsilateral lateral bending component tends to vanish. **D:** Curve for 74-year-old woman with rheumatoid arthritis patient indicates obvious coupled lateral bending to the opposite side.

ticularities of the motion patterns probably reflect individual morphologic characteristics of the cervical vertebrae, such as tropism of the zygapophyseal joint facets, variability of the uncinate processes, status of intervertebral discs, and slight asymmetry of the bony lever arms for the steering muscles. Flattened curves of coupled motion and in some cases reverse patterns may be found in rheumatoid arthritis (Fig. 1.8C,D).

Effect of Age and Sex on Cervical Motion

A metaanalysis of normative cervical motion showed greater passive than active range of motion (ROM) and decreasing ROM with age among all subjects, and larger ROM among women than among men (12). The outcomes obtained with the nine different measurement techniques in the studies analyzed showed considerable differences within and between the different methods and setups for measuring ROM. In the middle and lower cervical spine, stability is provided mainly by the intervertebral disc, the uncinate processes, and the posterior elements. Loss of stability often follows a stage of disc degeneration and is followed by restabilization through secondary adaptation of the facet joints and uncinate processes, spur formation at the vertebral bodies, and secondary changes in the spinal ligaments (16). Important secondary changes in the motion segments may explain why older persons have larger ranges of axial rotation starting from protraction, retraction, or flexion (109). Younger persons have larger ranges of axial rotation starting at the neutral or extension position. Although the ROM of axial rotation may be substantially less among men than among women during the fourth and the fifth decades of life, the decrease in coupled motion in axial rotation through aging is similar for both sexes (30,103).

Influence of Motion on the Dimensions of the Spinal Canal

The cervical spinal canal requires an anteroposterior diameter of at least 14 mm at the level of the foramen magnum, 13 mm at C1 and C2, and 12 mm below C2 (115). Sagittal diameters tend to be slightly smaller among Japanese than among European adults (62). Degenerative enlargements of the zygapophyseal joints and end plates may cause asymmetry of the bony spinal canal (Fig. 1.3), which may cause focal encroachment on neural tissue. The space available for the spinal cord is determined by the sagittal diameters of the vertebral foramina and the amount of protrusion of disc material and ligamenta flava. It is worthwhile to differentiate the subarachnoid space from the epidural spaces containing wide venous plexuses (24,84,85). The blood vessels and cerebrospinal fluid in the subarachnoid space and the blood vessels in the epidural space are of physiologic importance to the spinal cord (14). Because the cervical spine is composed of a number of synovial joints, symphyses, and syndesmoses arranged in parallel within one single motion segment and acting in a serial arrangement throughout the entire cervical spine, the spinal canal is continuously trimmed by muscular action that allows movement and deformation without loss of the main configuration.

Flexion of the cervical spine causes elongation of the ligamenta flava and widens the sagittal diameter of the spinal canal (11,85). Flexion causes substantial narrowing of the anterior subarachnoid space, particularly at C4-7, and considerable widening of the posterior subarachnoid space (61). Flexion causes displacement of 1.5 cm of dura relative to the pedicles (flexion of the entire spine produces displacement of 2.5 cm) (43). The spinal cord also elongates, the posterior surface being more stretched than the anterior surface. Accordingly the diameter of the spinal cord decreases. The lower part of the cervical spinal cord moves cephalad relative to the vertebrae, whereas the upper cord moves in the caudal direction (114).

The sagittal diameter of the spinal canal decreases in extension. Shortening of the spinal cord and dura coincides with some bulging of the intervertebral discs and a great deal of folding of the ligamenta flava (11,61,85). Therefore only a small increase in the diameter of the anterior subarachnoid space is noticed (61), and all the subarachnoid and epidural spaces reach their smallest size. The attachments between the dural sac and the nuchal ligaments, posterior atlantooccipital membrane, and rectus capitis posterior minor muscle probably also play a role in maintaining a certain degree of stretching of the dural sac (35,59).

THE COURSE OF THE VERTEBRAL ARTERY

First Segment of the Vertebral Artery

The first segment of the vertebral artery is situated between its origin at the subclavian artery and its entry into the transverse foramen, generally of C6. The vertebral artery usually represents the first branch of the subclavian artery. In most instances the vertebral artery has a cranial (47%) or dorsal (44%) origin on the circumference of the subclavian artery. High percentages of tortuosity of this first segment of the vertebral artery (39%) have been found in radiologic and sonographic studies involving a predominantly elderly population and in studies of anatomic preparations (54,102). The vertebral artery has a tortuous origin on both the left and the right subclavian artery in Fig. 1.9A).

In 3.5% to 6% of instances, the vertebral artery originates from another artery—the aortic arch (Fig. 1.9B), the thyrocervical trunk, the brachiocephalic trunk, the common carotid artery, the internal carotid artery, or the superficial cervical artery. Sometimes it has two origins (8,51,54,65,91).

In 88% to 90% of instances, the artery reaches its intraforaminal course at the level of C6 (8,105). In the other instances, the artery enters at C5 or to a lesser extent at C7 and seldom at C3 or C4 (91). If the vertebral artery has a bifid origin of, one vertebral artery originating from the subclavian artery usually enters the transverse foramen of C6. The other usually originates directly from the aortic arch or from the subclavian artery and enters the transverse foramen of C5 or C4 (29,97).

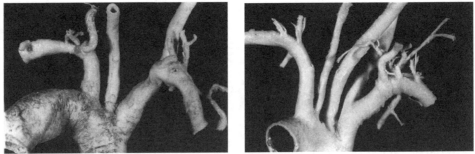

A   B

FIG. 1.9. Variants of the origin of the vertebral artery. **A:** Tortuous origin of the vertebral artery from both the left and the right subclavian arteries. **B:** Direct origin of the left vertebral artery from the aortic arch.

Variations in the Second Segment and Its Bony Canal

The second segment is situated in the bony canal, made by the succeeding transverse foramina. It ends at the laterally oriented exit of the transverse foramen of C2. A plexus of vertebral veins and sympathetic nerve fibers originating from the stellate, middle, and inferior cervical ganglia surround the artery in this second section (100,112). In the rare case of a double origin without later fusion, one artery runs through the transverse foramina, and the other follows a partial course in front of the transverse processes. Fenestration also may occur within the second section proper.

In normal circumstances, the artery follows a straight course from C6 to C2 through the successive transverse foramina. However, a tortuous course may result from spondylosis and degenerative changes in the uncinate processes (85). The transverse foramina of C5 and C6 are most frequently affected (96).

The shape and dimensions of the succeeding transverse foramina and the morphologic features of the tunnel through the C2 transverse process may have important interindividual differences. Rounded transverse foramina are predominantly present at C6 and at the lateral exit of the C2 transverse foramen. Mostly ovoid transverse foramina are encountered at other levels (96).

The transverse foramen of C7 contains sympathetic nerve branches originating from the stellate ganglion, arterial branches emerging from the ascending or the deep cervical artery and the accompanying veins, areolar connective tissue, and adipose tissue (40). This transverse foramen may be small or subdivided into two or more compartments, but it is seldom absent.

At the level of the intertransverse space, the vertebral artery and nerve root are encased in a fibroligamentous band attached to the lateral aspect of the uncinate process and uncovertebral joint, which combines the vertebral artery, nerve root, and uncinate process to form a complex or unit (23). The artery is in contact with or even compresses the dorsal ganglion of C3 to C6 in most spines, especially at the level of the C5 dorsal root ganglion. This could at least partly explain the disconcerting frequency of "dissociated motor loss" of the deltoid muscle after cervical spinal surgery (1).

Degenerative processes may influence the angular course through the transverse processes of C2, such as deformation of the openings of the transverse processes at the site of tortuosity of the vertebral artery (95). This illustrates the influence of blood vessels on bone tissue. Erosion of the canal for the vertebral artery at the transverse foramen of C2 is more common when the angle between the vertical and horizontal parts is less than 50 degrees. These erosions sometimes reduce the height of the lateral mass to less than 2 mm, occasionally with perforation into the vertebral foramen (53,94). Erosion is predominantly left-sided, possibly because of a larger diameter of the left vertebral artery (Fig. 1.10) (116). This is in accordance with considerably larger left caudal and lateral diameters of the C2 transverse foramen found in an osteometric study (41). The difference between the diameters of left and right transverse foramina is clear in Fig. 1.2.

The variation of the size of the foramen and the pedicle width between sexes and between sides is remarkable. CT scans have shown that the lateral wall of the pedicle is much thinner than the medial wall. Screw placement as close as possible to the mediosuperior cortex is recommended to avoid violation of the transverse foramen if transpedicular screw fixation in C2 is intended (28).

Three parallel columns of arterial supply make longitudinal vascular axes in and around the cervical spine (105). The vertebral artery represents the longitudinal axis in the center. Anastomoses to the anterior column are made by the ascending cervical and

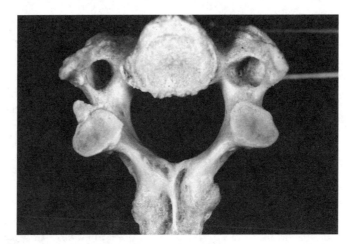

FIG. 1.10. Bony erosion at the left pedicle of C2 (inferior view) caused by the vertebral artery.

pharyngeal arteries. A second anastomotic network connects the vertebral artery to the deep cervical artery and the occipital artery, which constitute the dorsal column. Branches from the thyrocervical trunk and from ascending intercostal arteries of the thoracic aorta (15) as well as anastomoses with the deep cervical artery (100,105) contribute to the segmental blood supply in the lower cervical spine. Vessels originating from the ascending pharyngeal and occipital branches of the external carotid artery contribute to the blood supply of the upper cervical spine (15,100).

Third Segment

The third segment of the vertebral artery starts at the lateral exit of the C2 transverse foramen, develops a loop toward the broader transverse process of C1, passes through the transverse process of C1, and curves posteriorly to follow the groove at the upper aspect of the posterior arch of the atlas. This segment turns medially around the posterior aspect of upper articular process and finally pierces the dura mater. Various loop formations in this segment have been described. In some instances the vertebral artery may not pass through the transverse process but may reach the spinal canal along the anterior arch of the atlas. Fenestration of the vertebral artery and an early origin of the posterior inferior cerebellar artery also can occur in this segment (88).

The groove for the vertebral artery may have three types of ponticuli—the ponticulus posterior, the ponticulus lateralis, and the ponticulus posterolateralis. The reported frequency of a complete ponticulus posterior (Fig. 1.12A) or foramen retroarticulare bridging from the dorsal edge of the lateral mass over the groove of the vertebral artery to the posterior arch varies between 1.2% (25) and 13.4% (42). The presence of this structure has been positively correlated with migraine without aura, and removal has been recommended. In case of incomplete bridging (Fig. 1.12B,C), the groove and two convergent spinules form 75% of a bony ring, sometimes a nearly closed ring (Fig. 1.12D), that encircles the neurovascular bundle. The frequency of occurrence of a ponticulus lateralis that expands from the lateral mass over the transverse foramen to the tip of the transverse process (Fig. 1.12E) is about 2% to 3%. Sometimes complete bridging is found between

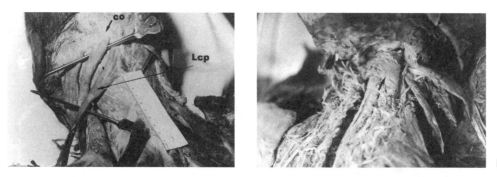

FIG. 1.11. Muscular variants in the neck region. **A:** Cleidooccipitalis muscle (*co*) from the sternocleidomastoid and levator claviclulae posterior (*Lcp*). **B:** Digastricus nuchae muscle (*arrow*) at C2.

both types of ponticuli that covers the entire pars atlantica of the vertebral artery to form a ponticulus posterolateralis.

Fourth Segment

The fourth segment of the vertebral artery extends from the transition through the dura (Fig. 1.5A) to the junction with the contralateral vertebral artery to form the basilar artery. In this segment, the artery enters the foramen magnum and mainly travels an intracranial course on the clivus in front of the medulla oblongata.

MUSCULAR VARIANTS

Although the medial border of the longus colli muscle has been used as a reference line to define the position of the vertebral artery (71), myologic variations are frequent in the neck region (8,99). Among the prevertebral muscles, there is variation in the number of bellies of the longus colli and longus capitis muscles. The longus capitis muscle sometimes crosses the midline or may be partially fused with the anterior scalene muscle, some belly passing between branches of the cervical plexus. Supernumerary muscles can be present between the occipital bone and the anterior tubercle of C1 (rectus capitis anterior internus muscle in 5% of bodies) or the lateral mass of C1 (rectus capitis intermedius muscle) or C2 (epistropheobasilaris muscle). These muscles may coexist with or replace an absent rectus capitis anterior muscle.

The rectus capitis lateralis muscle may originate from C2 or even C3. A rectus lateralis accessorius muscle may originate from the lateral process of C1 and insert onto the mastoid process. The rectus capitis posterior muscles can be fused or doubled by bellies originating from the nuchal ligament between C3 and C6.

The cervical parts of iliocostalis and longissimus muscles also have variations in number of bellies. An iliocostalis pars capitis may be present, and the longissimus cervicis muscle may detach a well-individualized belly either from T7, called the mastoideus lateralis muscle or from C1 (transversalis capitis minor).

The cervical insertions of the levator scapulae muscle may extend from C1 to C7. An isolated belly may reach C1 or even the occipital bone or the mastoid process. One belly may join the angulus medialis scapulae instead of the margo superior (levator anguli scapulae muscle). A levator claviculae muscle may originate from the lateral part of the clavicle to join the levator scapulae, the lateral process of C1 or C2 or the nuchal ligament (6) (Fig. 1.11A). In a retrospective study of 300 CT scans, this muscle was found in 2% of cases (86). A short type has been described as the cleidotransversarius, which joins the transverse process of C6. Other aberrant muscles originating from the transverse process of C1 join the rhomboid muscles (rhomboatloideus muscle) (5).

Between the anterior and middle scalene muscles an accessory scalene muscle sometimes passes between the trunks of the brachial plexus, whereas a transversalis cervicis anterior muscle sometimes runs between the middle and posterior scalenes. In some cases a distinction between the middle and posterior scalenes cannot be made.

In the posterior region neck the trapezius muscle does not always reach the occipital bone. In that case the clavicular part of the muscle may exist as a separate cleidooccipital muscle (83). Another form of the cleidooccipital muscle is the separation of a belly from the lateral side of the sternocleidomastoid muscle that inserts next to the trapezius muscle (Fig. 1.11A). The splenius muscles may be completely fused, the splenius cervicis may be missing, and the splenius capitis may be separated into two parts—one that

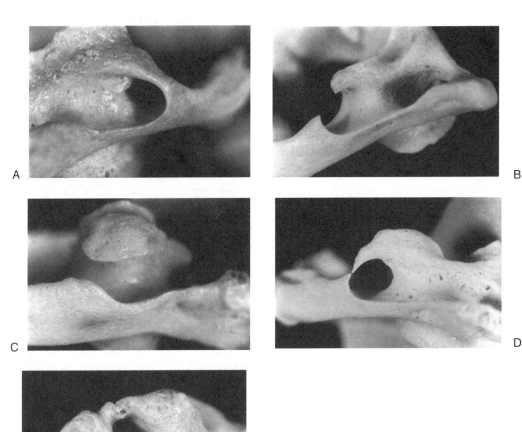

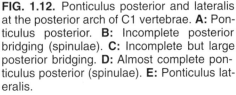

FIG. 1.12. Ponticulus posterior and lateralis at the posterior arch of C1 vertebrae. **A:** Ponticulus posterior. **B:** Incomplete posterior bridging (spinulae). **C:** Incomplete but large posterior bridging. **D:** Almost complete ponticulus posterior (spinulae). **E:** Ponticulus lateralis.

inserts on the occipital bone and a lower part that inserts on the mastoid process. A digit of the serratus posterior superior may be fused with splenius capitis or may even extend to the occipital bone. A small belly of semispinalis capitis may run beneath the normal semispinalis muscle between T2 and the occipital bone (complexus profundus muscle). A digastricus nuchae muscle may originate from three or four successive transverse processes between C2 and T1 on both sides of the spine and converge toward the midline, where the two parts join on an intermediate tendon. This muscle is more frequent in the lower part of the neck, but we have found it with its tendon at the level of the spinous process of C2 (Fig. 1.11B).

DISCUSSION

The anatomic configuration of the cervical spine may have a large number of interindividual and left-right differences. The findings that several aspects of articular tropism may occur in combination, at different cervical levels, and in combination with asymmetric muscular lever arms or asymmetric musculature is strong evidence against the basic assumption of a symmetric structure and function of the cervical spine, especially the degenerative cervical spine. It would be wise not to jump to conclusions when slightly deviating patterns of coupled motion are found in young and healthy volunteers. Nevertheless, advanced degeneration of the joints may substantially affect the coupling patterns. Because of the great variability of the cervical vertebrae, determination of the true diameter of the spinal canal with ratios from measurements of bony dimensions on radiographs or CT scans is unreliable (9).

Uncinate processes and intervertebral discs undergo substantial changes during the early decades of life that may be considered functional adaptations. Degenerative changes can alter the morphologic features of cervical motion segments and may not automatically cause symptoms. Because of the compact architecture of the cervical spine, marked degeneration of the intervertebral discs, uncinate processes, and zygapophyseal joints may endanger the neural structures and blood vessels of the central spinal canal and the lateral neurovascular foramina. They may progressively alter functional capabilities. The alteration is reflected in typical changes in ROM and posture.

The course of the vertebral artery can have interindividual variability in each of its four segments. The left vertebral artery often has a larger diameter than the right vertebral artery. Also the cervical bony canal for the vertebral artery, the surrounding veins, and the sympathetic nerves may have a variable appearance, eventually induced or accentuated by aging or degenerative processes.

ACKNOWLEDGMENTS

The authors wish to acknowledge Dr. D. Decraemer for placing dissected specimens of the aortic arch at their disposal, Mr. F. Van Roy for technical procedures in the dissection room, and Mr. R. Stien for preparing the photographs.

REFERENCES

1. Alleyne CHJr, Cawley CM, Barrow DL, et al. Microsurgical anatomy of the dorsal cervical nerve roots and the cervical dorsal root ganglion/ventral root complexes. *Surg Neurol* 1998;50:213–218.
2. Amevo B, Aprill C, Bogduk N. Abnormal instantaneous axes of rotation in patients with neck pain. *Spine* 1992;17:748–756.
3. Amevo B, Macintosh JE, Worth D, et al. Instantaneous axes of rotation of the typical cervical motion segments, I: an empirical study of technical errors. *Clin Biomech (Bristol, Avon)* 1991;6:31–37.

4. Amevo B, Worth D, Bogduk N. Instantaneous axes of rotation of the typical cervical motion segments: a study in normal volunteers. *Clin Biomech (Bristol, Avon)* 1991;6:111–117.

5. Barbaix E, Meeuwisse I, Janssens V, et al. Observation d'un muscle surnuméraire de la nuque: le muscle rhomboide de l'atlas (Macalister 1871). *Bull Assoc Anat (Nancy)* 1998;82:19–20.

6. Barbaix E, Van Roy P, Janssens V, et al. Observation de multiples variantes simultanées des muscles de la nuque et de la ceinture scapulaire, dont un m. levator claviculae. *Morphologie* 1999;83:13–14.

7. Barbosa Suero MB. Note sur la fréquence de quelques variations du rachis humain. *Bull Assoc Anat (Nancy)* 1926;1:51–59.

8. Bergman RA, Thompson SA, Afifi AK, et al. *Compendium of human anatomic variation.* Baltimore: Urban & Schwarzenberg, 1988:63–75, 374–378.

9. Blackley HR, Plank LD, Robertson PA. Determining the sagittal dimensions of the canal of the cervical spine: the reliability of ratios of anatomical measurements. *J Bone Joint Surg Br* 1999;81:110–12.

10. Bogduk N. The clinical anatomy of the cervical dorsal rami. *Spine* 1982;7:319–330.

11. Chen IH, Vasavada A, Panjabi MM. Kinematics of the cervical spine canal: changes with sagittal plane loads. *J Spinal Disord* 1994;7:93–101.

12. Chen J, Solinger AB, Poncet JF, et al. Meta-analysis of normative cervical motion. *Spine* 1999;24:1571–1578.

13. Cimen M, Elden H. Numerical variations in human vertebral column: a case report. *Okajimas Folia Anat Jpn* 1999;75:297–303.

14. Crock HV. *An atlas of vascular anatomy of the skeleton and spinal cord.* London: Martin Dunitz, 1996.

15. Crock HV, Yoshizawa H. The vascular supply of the cervical spine and the cervical spinal cord. In: Gunzburg R, Szpalski M, eds. *Whiplash injuries.* Philadelphia: Lippincott–Raven, 1998.

16. Dai L. Disc degeneration and cervical instability: correlation of magnetic resonance imaging with radiography. *Spine* 1998;23:1734–1738.

17. Dvořák J, Panjabi MM. Functional anatomy of the alar ligaments. *Spine* 1987;12:183–189.

18. Dvořák J, Panjabi MM, Grob D, et al. Clinical validation of functional flexion/extension radiographs of the cervical spine. *Spine* 1993;18:120–127.

19. Ebraheim NA, An HS, Xu R, et al. The quantitative anatomy of the cervical nerve root groove and the intervertebral foramen. *Spine* 1996;21:1619–1623.

20. Ebraheim NA, Fow J, Xu R, et al. The vertebral body depths of the cervical spine and its relation to anterior plate-screw fixation. *Spine* 1998;23:2299–2302.

21. Ebraheim NA, Haman ST, Xu R, et al. The anatomic location of the dorsal ramus of the cervical nerve and its relation to the superior articular process of the lateral mass. *Spine* 1998;23:1968–1971.

22. Ebraheim NA, Lu J, Biyani A, et al. Anatomic considerations for uncovertebral involvement in cervical spondylosis. *Clin Orthop* 1997;334:200–206.

23. Ebraheim NA, Lu J, Haman SP, et al. Anatomic basis of the anterior surgery on the cervical spine: relationships between uncus-artery-root complex and vertebral artery injury. *Surg Radiol Anat* 1998;20:389–392.

24. Ebraheim NA, Lu J, Yang H. The effect of translation of the C1-2 on the spinal canal. *Clin Orthop* 1998;351: 222–229.

25. Ebraheim NA, Xu R, Ahmad M, et al. The quantitative anatomy of the vertebral artery groove of the atlas and its relation to the posterior atlantoaxial approach. *Spine* 1998;23:320–323.

26. Ebraheim NA, Xu R, Bhatti RA, et al. The projection of the cervical disc and uncinate process on the posterior aspect of the cervical spine. *Surg Neurol* 1999;52:363–367.

27. Ebraheim NA, Xu R, Challgren E, et al. Quantitative anatomy of the cervical facet and the posterior projection of its inferior facet. *J Spinal Disord* 1997;10:308–316.

28. Ebraheim NA, Xu R, Lin D, et al. Quantitative anatomy of the transverse foramen and pedicle of the axis. *J Spinal Disord* 1998;11:521–525.

29. Eisenberg RA, Vines FS, Taylor SB. Bifid origin of the left vertebral artery. *Radiology* 1986;159:429–430.

30. Feipel V, Rondelet B, Le Pallec JP, et al. Normal global motion of the cervical spine: an electrogoniometric study. *Clin Biomech (Bristol, Avon)* 1999;14:462–470.

31. Fielding JW, Hensinger RN, Hawkins RJ. Os odontoideum. *J Bone Joint Surg Am* 1980;623:376–383.

32. Frykholm R. Lower cervical vertebrae and intervertebral discs: surgical anatomy and pathology. *Acta Chir Scand* 1951;101:345–349.

33. Gottlieb MS. Absence of symmetry in superior articular facets on the first cervical vertebra in humans: implications for diagnosis an treatment. *J Manipulative Physiol Ther* 1994;17:314–320.

34. Grilliot JR, Wiles MJ. Elongation of the anterior tubercle of a cervical vertebral transverse process. *J Manipulative Physiol Ther* 1988;11:221–223.

35. Hack GD, Koritzer RT, Robinson WL, et al. Anatomic relation between the rectus capitis posterior minor muscle and the dura mater. *Spine* 1995;20:2484–2486.

36. Harsch GR, Sypert GW, Weinstein PR, et al. Cervical spine stenosis secondary to ossification of the posterior longitudinal ligament. *J Neurosurg* 1987;67:349–357.

37. Hayashi K, Yabuki T. Origin of the uncus and of Luschka's joint in the cervical spine. *J Bone Joint Surg Am* 1985;67:788–791.

38. Humphreys SG, Hodges SD, Patwardhan A, et al. The natural history of the cervical foramen in symptomatic and asymptomatic individuals aged 20–60 years as measured by magnetic resonance imaging: a descriptive approach. *Spine* 1998;23:2180–2184.

39. Jones MD, Pais MJ, Omiya B. Bony overgrowths and abnormal calcifications about the spine. *Radiol Clin North Am* 1988;26:1213–1233.

40. Jovanovic MS. A comparative study of the foramen transversarium of the sixth and seventh cervical vertebrae. *Surg Radiol Anat* 1990;12:167–172.
41. Kevelaers I. *Morphometric study of the foramina transversaria of C2* [licentiate thesis]. Brussels: Vrije Universiteit Brussel, 1999.
42. Klausberger EM, Samec P. Foramen retroarticulare atlantis and das Vertebralisangiogramm. *MMW Munch Med Wochenschr* 1975;117:483–486.
43. Klein P, Burnotte J. Contribution à l'étude biomécanique de la moelle épinière et de ses enveloppes. *Ann Med Ostéopath* 1985;1:99–105.
44. Kobukun S, Sakurai M, Tanaka Y. Cartilaginous endplate in cervical disc herniation. *Spine* 1996;21:190–195.
45. Kotani Y, McNulty PS, Abumi K, et al. The role of anteromedial foraminotomy and the uncovertebral joints in the stability of the cervical spine: a biomechanical study. *Spine* 1998;23:1559–1565.
46. Lestini WF, Wiesel SW. The pathogenesis of cervical spondylosis. *Clin Orthop* 1989;239:69–93.
47. Lu J, Ebraheim NA. Anatomic consideration of C2 nerve root ganglion. *Spine* 1998;23:649–652.
48. Lu J, Ebraheim NA, Huntoon M, et al. Cervical intervertebral disc space narrowing and size of the intervertebral foramina. *Clin Orthop* 2000;370:259–264.
49. Lu J, Ebraheim NA, Yang H, et al. Cervical uncinate process: an anatomic study for anterior decompression of the cervical spine. *Surg Radiol Anat* 1998;20:249–252.
50. Lu J, Ebraheim NA, Yang H, et al. Anatomic bases for anterior spinal surgery: surgical anatomy of the cervical vertebral body and disc space. *Surg Radiol Anat* 1999;21:235–239.
51. Luzsa G. *X ray anatomy of the vascular system.* Philadelphia: Akaémiai Kiadó, 1974:147–223.
52. Lysell E. Motion in the cervical spine: an experimental study on autopsy specimens. *Acta Orthop Scand [Suppl]* 1969;123:5–61.
53. Madawi AA, Solanki G, Casey AT, et al. Variation of the groove in the axis vertebra for the vertebral artery: implications for instrumentation. *J Bone Joint Surg Br* 1997;79:820–823.
54. Matula C, Trattnig S, Tschabitscher M, et al. The course of the prevertebral segment of the vertebral artery: anatomy and clinical significance. *Surg Neurol* 1997;48:125–131.
55. Mazzara JT, Fielding JW. Effect of C1-2 rotation on canal size. *Clin Orthop* 1988;237:115–119.
56. McAfee PC, Regan JJ, Bohlman HH. Cervical cord compression from ossification of the posterior longitudinal ligament in non-Orientals. *J Bone Joint Surg Br* 1987;69:569–575.
57. Mercer S, Bogduk N. The ligaments and annulus fibrosus of human adult cervical intervertebral discs. *Spine* 1999;24:619–628.
58. Milne N. The role of zygapophyseal joint orientation and uncinate processes in controlling motion in the cervical spine. *J Anat* 1991;178:189–201.
59. Mitchell BS, Humphreys BK, O'Sullivan E. Attachments of the ligamentum nuchae to cervical posterior dura and the lateral part of the occipital bone. *J Manipulative Physiol Ther* 1998;21:145–148.
60. Monteiro H. Fréquence de l'occipitalisation de l'atlas chez les Portugais. *Comptes Rendus de l'association des Anatomistes (Nancy).* 1933;465–470.
61. Muhle C, Wiskirchen J, Weinert D, et al. Biomechanical aspects of the subarachnoid space and cervical cord in healthy individuals examined with kinematic magnetic resonance imaging. *Spine* 1998;23:556–567.
62. Murone I. The importance of the sagittal diameters of the cervical spinal canal in relation to spondylosis and myelopathy. *J Bone Joint Surg Br* 1974;56:30–36.
63. Mysorekar VR, Nandedkar AN. Surface area of the atlanto-occipital articulations. *Acta Anat (Basel)* 1986;126:223–225.
64. Nakamura H. A radiographic study of the progression of ossification of the cervical posterior longitudinal ligament: the correlation between the ossification of the posterior longitudinal ligament and that of the anterior longitudinal ligament. *Nippon Seikeigeka Gakkai Zasshi* 1994;68:725–736(abst).
65. Nizankowski C, Noczynski L, Suder E. Variability of the origin of ramifications of the subclavian artery in humans. *Folia Morphol (Warsz)* 1982;41:284–294.
66. Nowitzke A, Westaway M, Bogduk N. Cervical zygapophyseal joints: geometrical parameters and relationship to cervical kinematics. *Clin Biomech (Bristol, Avon)* 1994;9:342–348.
67. Oda J, Tanaka H, Tsuzuki N. Intervertebral disc changes with aging of human cervical vertebra: from neonate to the eighties. *Spine* 1988;13: 1205–1211.
68. Ogden JA. Radiology of postnatal skeletal development. *Skeletal Radiol* 1984;12:169–177.
69. Onan OA, Heggeness MH, Hipp JA. A motion analysis of the cervical facet joint. *Spine* 1998;23:430–439.
70. Ordway NR, Seymour RJ, Donelson RG, et al. Cervical flexion, extension, protrusion and retraction: a radiographic segmental analysis. *Spine* 1999;24:240–247.
71. Pait TG, Killefer JA, Amautovic KI. Surgical anatomy of the anterior cervical spine: the disc space, vertebral artery and associated bony structures. *Neurosurgery* 1996;39:769–776.
72. Pal GP, Routal RV. The role of the vertebral laminae in the stability of the cervical spine. *J Anat* 1996;188:485–489.
73. Panjabi M, Dvorak J, Duranceau J, et al. Three-dimensional movements of the upper cervical spine. *Spine* 1988;13:726–730.
74. Panjabi MM, Oda T, Crisco JJ III, et al. Posture affects motion coupling patterns of the upper cervical spine. *J Orthop Res* 1993;11:525–53.
75. Panjabi MM, Oxland T, Takata K, et al. Articular facets of the human spine. *Spine* 1993;18:1298–1310.
76. Pech P, Daniels DL, Williams AL, et al. The cervical neural foramina: correlation of microtomy and CT anatomy. *Radiology* 1985;155:143–146.

77. Penning L. Normal movements of the cervical spine. *AJR Am J Roentgenol* 1978;130:317–326.
78. Penning L. *Normale bewegingen van de hals: en lendenwervelkolom.* Utrecht: Lemma, 1998.
79. Penning L, Wilmink JT. Rotation of the cervical spine: a CT study in normal subjects. *Spine* 1987;12:732–738.
80. Prescher A. The craniocervical junction in man, the osseous variations, their significance and differential diagnosis. *Anat Anz* 1997;179:1–19.
81. Przybylski GJ, Carlin GJ, Patel PR, et al. Human anterior and posterior cervical longitudinal possess similar tensile properties. *J Orthop Res* 1996;14:1005–1008.
82. Przybylski GJ, Patel PR, Carlin GJ, et al. Quantitative anthropometry of the subatlantal cervical longitudinal ligaments. *Spine* 1998;23:893–898.
83. Rahman HA, Tamadori T. An anomalous cleido-occipitalis muscle. *Acta Anat (Basel)* 1994;150:156–158.
84. Rauschning W. Detailed sectional anatomy of the spine. In: Rothman SLG, Glenn WV, eds. *Multiplanar CT of the spine.* Baltimore: University Park Press, 1985;33–35.
85. Rauschning W. Anatomy and pathology of the cervical spine. In: Frymoyer JW. *The adult spine: principles and practice.* New York: Raven Press, 1991;907–928.
86. Rubinstein D, Escott EJ, Hendrick LL. The prevalence and CT appearance of the levator claviculae muscle: a normal variant not to be mistaken for an abnormality. *AJNR Am J Neuroradiol* 1999;20:583–586.
87. Rydevik BL. The effects of compression on the physiology of nerve roots. *J Manipulative Physiol Ther* 1992;15:62–66.
88. Sato K, Watanabe T, Yoshimoto T, et al. Magnetic resonance imaging of C2 segmental type of vertebral artery. *Surg Neurol* 1994;41:45–51.
89. Schwartz AM, Wechsler RJ, Landy MD, et al. Posterior arch defects of the cervical spine. *Skeletal Radiol* 1982; 8:135–139.
90. Singh S. Variations of the superior articular facets of atlas vertebrae. *J Anat* 1965;99:565–571.
91. Skopakoff C. Ober die Variabilität der Abzweigung der A subclavia und ihrer Hauptäste. *Anat Anz* 1964;115: 393–402.
92. Smoker WRK. Craniovertebral junction: normal anatomy, craniometry, and congenital anomalies. *Radiographics* 1994;14:255–277.
93. Smoker WRK. Congenital anomalies of the cervical spine. *Neuroimaging Clin N Am* 1995;5:427–449.
94. Taitz C, Arensburg B. Erosion of the foramen transversarium of the axis. *Acta Anat (Basel)* 1989;134:12–17.
95. Taitz C, Arensburg B. Vertebral artery tortuosity with concomitant erosion on the foramen of the transverse process of the axis. *Acta Anat (Basel)* 1991;141:104–108.
96. Taitz C, Nathan H, Arensburg B. Anatomical observations of the foramina transversaria. *J Neurol Neurosurg Psychiatry* 1978;41:170–176.
97. Takasato Y, Hayashi H, Kobayashi T, et al. Duplicated origin of right vertebral artery with rudimentary and accessory left vertebral arteries. *Neuroradiology* 1992;34:287–289.
98. ten Have HAMJ, Eulderink F. Mobility and degenerative changes of the ageing cervical spine: a macroscopic and statistical study. *Gerontology* 1981;27:42–50.
99. Testut L. *Les anomalies musculaires chez l'homme expliquées par l'anatomie comparée.* Paris: Masson, 1884.
100. Thiel HW. Gross morphology and pathoanatomy of the vertebral arteries *J Manipulative Physiol Ther* 1991;14: 133–141.
101. Töndury G, Theiler K. *Entwicklungsgeschichte und Fehlbildungen der Wirbelsäule.* Stuttgart: Hippokrates Verlag, 1990.
102. Trattnig S, Matula C, Karnel E, et al. Difficulties in examination of the origin of the vertebral artery by duplex and colour-coded Doppler sonography: anatomical considerations. *Neuroradiology* 1993;35:296–299.
103. Trott PH, Pearcy MJ, Ruston SA, et al. Three-dimensional analysis of active cervical motion: the effect of age and gender. *Clin Biomech (Bristol, Avon)* 1996;11:201–206.
104. Tulsi RS. Some specific anatomical features of the atlas and axis: dens, epitransverse process and articular facets. *Aust N Z J Surg* 1978;48:570–574.
105. Uflacker R. *Atlas of vascular anatomy, an angiographic approach.* Baltimore: Williams & Wilkins, 1997.
106. van Mameren H, Drukker J, Sanches H, et al. Cervical spine motion in the sagittal plane, II: position of segmental averaged instantaneous centers of rotation, a cineradiographic study. *Spine* 1992;17:467–474.
107. Van Roy P, Caboor D, De Boelpaep S, et al. Left-right asymmetries and other common anatomical variants of the first cervical vertebra. *Manual Ther* 1997;2:24–36.
108. Van Roy P, Lanssiers R, Vermoesen A, et al. Implementation of software adaptation for 3-D cervical kinematics by means of a magnetic tracking device. In: Arsenault A, McKinley P, McFadyen B, eds. Proceedings of the 12th Congress of the International Society of Electromyography and Kinesiology (ISEK), Montreal, June 27–30, 1998:10–11 (abst).
109. Walmsley RP, Kimber P, Culham E. The effect of initial position on active cervical axial rotation range of motion in two age populations. *Spine* 1996;21,2455–2442.
110. White AA III, Panjabi MM. *Clinical biomechanics of the spine,* 2nd ed. Philadelphia: Lippincott-Raven, 1990.
111. Woltring HJ, Huiskes R, De Lange A, et al. Finite centroid and helical axis estimation from noisy landmark measurements in the study of human joint kinematics. *J Biomech* 1985;18:379–389.
112. Xiuqing C, Bo S, Shizhen Z. Nerves accompanying the vertebral artery and their clinical relevance. *Spine* 1988; 13:1360–1364.

113. Yoo JU, Zou D, Edwards WT, et al. Effect of cervical spine motion on the neuroforaminal dimensions of human cervical spine. *Spine* 1992;17:1131–1136.
114. Yuan I, Dougherty L, Margulies S. In vivo human cervical spinal cord deformation and displacement in flexion. *Spine* 1998;23:1677–1683.
115. Zeidman SM, Ducker TB. Rheumatoid arthritis: neuroanatomy, compression and grading of deficits. *Spine* 1994;19:2259–2266.
116. Zimmerman HB, Farell WJ. Cervical vertebral erosion caused by vertebral artery tortuosity. *AJR Am J Roentgenol* 1970;108:767–770.

The Degenerative Cervical Spine,
edited by Marek Szpalski and Robert Gunzburg
Lippincott Williams & Wilkins, Philadelphia © 2001.

2

Cervical Spine Biomechanics

Malcolm H. Pope

Liberty Safework Research Center, Aberdeen AB9 2ZD, Scotland, United Kingdom

---

AGING
KINEMATICS
KINETICS
SUPPORT OF THE ACTIVE TISSUES
INJURY
BIOMECHANICS OF NECK PAIN
CONCLUSION

The cervical spine is a complex structure. It supports the mass of the head, moves the head, protects neurologic structures, and controls motion. Mobility is needed for the many physical tasks of daily living and work, which tend to compromise the structure of the spine. The basic functional unit of the spine is called the *functional spinal unit* (FSU). The FSU is defined as the superior vertebra, the inferior vertebra, the intervertebral disc, and the associated ligaments. The motions of the individual FSUs are important because they contribute to the total motion of the cervical spine and determine the stress distribution therein.

AGING

He who is of a calm and happy nature will hardly feel the pressure of age, but to him who is of an opposite disposition youth and age are equally a burden. Plato 427–347 BC

Physiologic conditions, aging, and degeneration affect both the static and dynamic viscoelastic behavior of the intervertebral discs. Degeneration of an intervertebral disc includes nuclear desiccation, formation of anular tears, disc fragmentation, and loss of height (2,7,12). The viscoelastic properties of the disc determine the creep rate and the degree of deformation of the disc. A degenerated disc creeps faster than a nondegenerated disc, and rheologic conditions strongly influence the creep response. Repetitive loading deforms the disc more than does static loading. It seems probable that the changes in the viscoelastic properties that accompany degeneration also influence the stability of the FSU. In central spinal stenosis and in degenerative retrolisthesis or spondylolisthesis, disc abnormalities probably affect spinal dynamics and initiate pathophysiologic changes that cause pain. Aging or degenerative processes can be found in the intervertebral discs during the third decade of life. The discs are particularly vulnerable because of their lack of direct blood supply, at least in adults. The lack of a vascular supply limits the capability of the disc to regenerate and repair itself.

Aging decreases the range of motion of the cervical spine, largely in the middle and lower portions (2). This effect is caused by degeneration of the intervertebral disc, osteoarthritis of the zygapophyseal joints or facets, and the development of uncovertebral joints (7). The uncovertebral spaces of the lower cervical spine transform into the uncovertebral joints as a reaction to the load moment caused by the weight of the head (12). This process is preceded by degeneration and transverse tearing of the disc anulus. This reduces the load-absorbing function of the disc, and the uncovertebral joints remodel. The transformation of the structure and shape of the uncovertebral processes is mainly responsible for the decreased range of motion with aging.

KINEMATICS

There is a great deal of clinical interest in accurate measurement of intervertebral motion. Abnormal kinematics of the cervical vertebrae are widely considered to play an important role in neck pain. Most studies have used radiographic techniques and most have measured coupled motions at the end points of normal clinical motions. Evaluation of spinal instability depends on the correct application of biomechanical principles. This involves understanding kinematic patterns, anatomic relations and functions, and stability criteria. Clinical instability is conveniently defined as the loss of ability of the spine under physiologic loads to maintain its pattern of displacement so that there is no initial or additional neurologic deficit, no major deformity, and no incapacitating pain.

The FSU exhibits coupled motion, which means that a force in one direction may induce motion in another (3). This phenomenon may be important in unstable motion segments. These studies allow one to assess the effects of all the loads and torques experienced by the FSU in vivo. The coupled motion is normally presented in the form of a flexibility or stiffness matrix, which gives the motion in three dimensions (6 degrees of freedom) with respect to imposed forces and moments (8). The facet (zygapophyseal) joints are essential to the control of normal motion, and they serve as a constraint because of their orientation. Thus the motion of each segment is controlled actively by muscles and passively by ligaments and the orientation of the facets.

The atlantooccipital joint is a spheroid joint connected with a tight joint capsule that limits motion to flexion and extension with a small amount of lateral bending and axial rotation. The summary of motion in the cervical joints is shown in Table 2.1. The medial joint capsule is loose and allows considerable axial rotation (Table 2.1). The motion

TABLE 2.1. *Possible movements in the cervical joints*

Joint	Flexion/extension	Lateral bending (one side)	Axial rotation (one side)
Occipital-C1	13.0–50.0	5.5–40.0	0.0–7.2
C1-2	0.0–30.0	0.0–10.0	14.5–80.0
C2-3	8.0–12.0	4.7–10.0	3.0–9.0
C3-4	13.0–17.0	4.7–11.0	6.5–11.0
C4-5	12.0–21.0	4.7–11.0	6.7–12.0
C5-6	17.0–23.0	4.7–8.0	6.9–10.0
C6-7	16.0–19.0	4.7–7.0	5.4–9.0

All values are degrees.
Data from references 22–28.

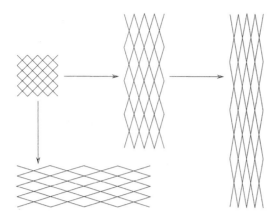

FIG. 2.1. Orientation of the collagen fibers of the transverse ligament resembles a folding lattice and allows extensive stretching of the ligament during flexion and axial rotation without damage to the fibers.

within the upper cervical spine is mainly limited by the ligaments. The alar ligaments are particularly active in restricting axial rotation. The cruciate ligament restricts anterior gliding of the atlas during flexion of the head while it allows the atlas to turn freely around the dens during axial rotation. The transverse ligament is a unique biomechanical structure. The collagen fibers are in a lattice structure that allows extensive stretching of the ligament during axial rotation (Fig. 2.1).

The kinematics of the lower cervical spine are different than those of the rest of the cervical spine, partly because the uncovertebral joints and the articular processes of the cervical spine are inclined approximately 45 degrees from the horizontal plane with steeper inclinations in the lower segments. The laminae are connected by the stiff ligamentum flavum, which limits flexion, the dominant motion in the lower cervical spine. Lateral bending of the cervical spine is normally coupled with axial rotation.

KINETICS

Kinematics and kinetics usually are measured at the level of the FSU. Like other materials and structures, the FSU and its components can be injured through cyclic loading, which can cause failure or an adaptive response. The tissues of the FSU are viscoelastic, which means that the rate of loading is important and that in normal functioning they absorb energy. The FSU is susceptible to creep caused by the viscoelasticity and particularly the composition of the disc. Degenerated discs have increased creep rates and thus less ability to absorb energy. The energy absorbed in the FSU is produced by both fluid migration from the disc and cyclic plastic strain of the viscoelastic materials that compose the FSU. The response of the FSU to sustained loading shows not only a creep response but also increased compliance in one or more of the six degrees of freedom of motion.

SUPPORT OF THE ACTIVE TISSUES

The neck muscles are important and necessary components of normal spinal function. The mechanical role of the muscles includes providing stability, controlling movement, and generating the force necessary to perform essential activities of daily living and work. With pain, the muscles no longer work in harmony; the result is a loss of coordination and loss of strength and endurance. The spine is unstable without the support of the muscles (20). Without muscles, movements could not be initiated and controlled; thus proper muscle function is a prerequisite for normal spinal function. Important attributes of muscle function are strength, speed of response, coordination, and endurance. Strength is needed in many activities, particularly sports, to prevent injury. Endurance is exceeded when a contraction cannot be sustained at a certain level (isometric fatigue), or when repetitive work can no longer be maintained at a certain output (dynamic fatigue). The mechanical events are preceded by biochemical and physiologic changes within the muscle.

Tests of muscle fatigue generally include maintaining a posture or repeatedly performing an activity. Electromyography (EMG) is an objective method of measuring muscle fatigue through measurement of a shift in the median frequency in the power density spectrum. Another important attribute is the ability of the muscles to contract quickly to minimize injury. Examination of the muscles is part of a standard physical examination of a patient with cervical spinal pain, dysfunction, or deformity. The cervical muscles are routinely examined for tenderness, spasm, and asymmetry. However, the mechanical function of the neck muscles usually is not specifically evaluated. Although an active motion examination can be considered a test of muscle function, tests of strength and endurance are infrequently performed, and tests of muscle coordination are almost nonexistent. Poor muscle function can cause painful conditions in the neck. Conditions such as myelopathy, radiculopathy, and other degenerative diseases can cause abnormal muscle function due to biomechanical interaction between the FSU and the neural elements.

INJURY

Injury can be thought of as a continuum of failure at the tissue level. An injury to the cervical spine may be triggered by direct trauma, a single overexertion, or frequent or sustained loading. The strengths of the tissues are influenced by age, fatigue, medications, and concomitant diseases. Therefore the loading level at which an injury occurs may vary greatly. In cases of direct trauma, several structures may be damaged at the same time. Repetitive loading may fatigue a ligament to the point at which there may be partial tissue rupture. However, the partial tear may not propagate to failure if rest periods allow healing to occur. Therefore, temporal factors and healing properties are critical.

Traumatic spinal injuries can be produced by a predominantly compressive or tensile load, shear forces, excessive rotation about any of the three principal axes, and in varying combinations. Acute, high speed injuries to the vertebrae and associated soft tissue can be conveniently classified as follows: (a) anterior wedge fractures, (b) burst fractures, (c) dislocations and fracture dislocations, (d) rotational injuries, (e) hyperextension injuries, and (f) soft-tissue injuries. The first three modes injury are caused by combined axial compression and forward flexion, sometimes accompanied by moments and forces outside the sagittal plane. Vertical compression and flexion-extension mechanisms tend to predominate. Flexion-extension injuries include the relatively more common whiplash, facet dislocation, and hangman's fractures. Because of its shape and flexibility, the ligamentous vertebral column is frequently subjected to bending loads that are superimposed on the axial load from support of the head and torso. Impact accelerations in the horizontal plane exert bending loads on the spine. Muscle contraction is a factor in the injury. The articular facets have been found to play an important role in the mechanism of spinal support and in the mechanisms of injury to the spine. The three column concept often is used to describe the biomechanics of acute spinal trauma. The three columns are the anterior vertebral column and the two sides of the neural arch. The degree of stability after injury depends on the integrity of the three columns. Many classifications of spinal injuries rely on an estimate of forces producing the injury (8). For example, White and Panjabi (20) introduced the idea of the major injury vector to classify the cause of injuries. Figure 2.2 shows how the effects of biomechanical and anatomic factors act produce a fracture of the ring of C1.

Whiplash injuries (19) have increased in recent years, possibly because of increased traffic density. In Japan, 50% of car-to-car traffic accidents cause neck injury (16). In

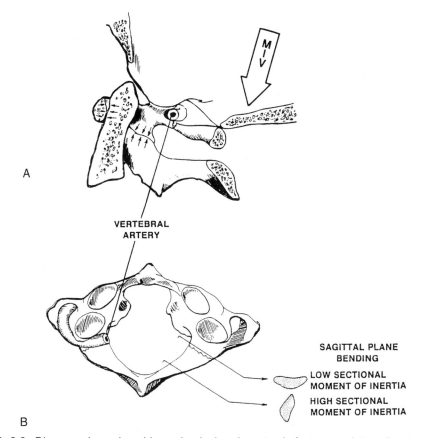

FIG. 2.2. Diagram shows how biomechanical and anatomic factors work together to produce a typical fracture of the posterior arch of C1. **A:** Midsagittal section of the occipitoatlantoaxial complex shows a possible mechanism of injury, one that causes fracture of the ring of C1. A force causing extension (x-axis rotation) results in fixation of the anterior ring of C1 against the dens and bilateral fixation at the articular condyles between the ring of C1 and C2. With this fixation, it is possible for impingement of the occiput against the posterior ring of C1 to cause a bending moment about the ring of C1. The position of the vertebral artery at which the ring of C1 is grooved and weakened is evident. **B:** Top view of the ring of C1 shows the vertebral artery on the left in the region of the fracture. On the *right* side, the sectional moment of inertial counter bending in the sagittal plane is much smaller where the fracture occurs than it is in the more posterior area, where the resistance to bending in that plane is much greater. The areas are shown in cross section at these two points. In addition to the considerations of the effects of sectional moment of inertia on the location of the fracture site, there is another factor. Forces are applied at the tip of the ring of C1 by the occiput; thus the maximum bending moment is also at the site where the fracture occurs.

Canada, 68% of vehicle accident insurance claims were whiplash injuries (13). The most common scenario in whiplash is a rear-end low-velocity impact of one motor vehicle against another. The driver of the stationary vehicle often has no warning of the impending collision (1). As shown in Fig. 2.3, the torso undergoes a sequence of acceleration and deceleration, whereas the head and cervical spine undergo hyperextension followed by hyperflexion. Injuries to the cervical spine include tears of the anterior, posterior, and in-

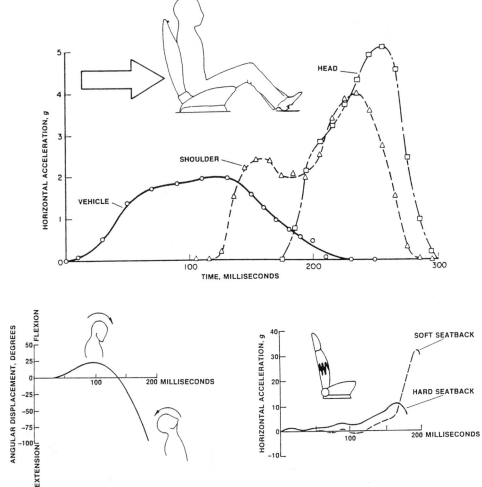

FIG. 2.3. A: The shoulder and the head lag behind as the vehicle accelerates when hit, but they catch up and within 0.3 s and reach accelerations 2 to 2.5 times the maximum vehicle acceleration. **B:** The head first goes into flexion and then into hyperextension within the first 0.2 s. **C:** The horizontal acceleration of the head for two different degrees of stiffness of the seat back. The harder seat back has a lower acceleration and therefore is associated with less injurious loading. (Data in **A** from Severy DM, Mathewson JH, Bechtol CO. Controlled automobile related engineering and mechanical phenomena: medical aspects of traffic accidents. In: Proceedings of the Montreal Conference, Montreal, Quebec, 1955:152. Data in **B** and **C** from McKenzie JA, Williams JF. The dynamic behavior of the head and cervical spine during "whiplash." *J Biomech* 1971;4:477.)

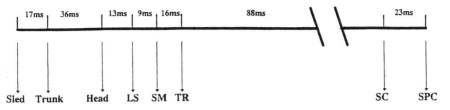

FIG. 2.4. Muscle activation patterns in whiplash.The reaction times of each muscle with respect to sled acceleration. The typical pattern of motion and muscular activity events. (LS, levator scapulae; SM, sternocleidomastoid; TR, trapezius; SC, semispinalis capitis; SPC, splenius capitis.)

terspinous ligaments, fractures of spinous processes, disc rupture, end-plate avulsion, dens fracture, strain of the cervicooccipital joint complex, rupture of ligamenta flava, fracture and disruption of facet joints, overstretching of the anterior muscles, and stretching of the vertebral artery and superficial branches of the cervical plexus (1,11,15,18).

In a survey of 10,000 cases, Dvorak et al. (4) found that 86% of the injuries were to the soft tissue and that only 14% were fractures. Soft-tissue injury usually is a subfailure injury to the ligament. Studies (14) have been conducted in which low-speed tests were performed in which the subjects wore both surface and wire electrodes to record the EMG features of the paraspinal musculature. The investigators found that muscle activation occurs 125 to 285 ms after the front or back collision (Fig. 2.4). The sternocleidomastoid muscle is a powerful flexor of the head and neck and may protect the spine during whiplash by dissipating kinetic energy with an eccentric contraction.

There is undoubtedly a positive relation between occupation and neck pain. It is self-evident that mechanical stressors such as flexion, twisting, and static postures or whole-body vibration have the potential of injuring the components of the spine if the magnitude or the duration of exposure is excessive. There is therefore a place for primary prevention of neck pain in the workplace and early return to work if emphasis is placed on physical work factors, specifically work posture (including sitting) and cyclic loading.

In a seated posture, the dorsal musculature must contract to support the load-moment caused by the mass of the head. A fixed posture also produces sustained static loading of tissues and interference with the circulation of blood in a muscle, and thereby with oxygen, and removal of breakdown products. This occurs at as little as 10% of maximum voluntary contraction. At higher percentages of maximum voluntary contraction, muscle naturally fatigues more rapidly, and secondary changes in the muscle may occur. The intervertebral disc can lose nutrition while in a fixed posture because of the avascular nature of the disc. An immobilized intervertebral disc does not receive nutrition through either of the two main routes—the end plate or the outer anulus. Thus there is an increased risk of neck pain among persons who work in a fixed posture and an increase in symptoms among persons with preexisting neck pain who are required to sit for prolonged periods. Persons with a sedentary occupation should be encouraged to stretch, stand up, or rotate their tasks as much as possible.

BIOMECHANICS OF NECK PAIN

A herniated or bulging disc may affect an adjacent spinal nerve root and dorsal root ganglion and excite nociceptors. Some bulging is inevitable under axial load, and an intervertebral disc abnormality seen on a magnetic resonance image may be symptom free.

Mechanical impingement of the intervertebral disc that causes inflammation lowers the threshold of nociceptors, which then can fire spontaneously. Pain fibers (nociceptors) normally have high mechanical thresholds. Under pathologic conditions such as inflammation, they may become activated and sensitized, firing at lower thresholds (17) with the dorsal root ganglion more sensitive than the roots. The types of loading that activate dorsal root ganglion neurons include sustained, high rate, and cyclic loading. There is no agreement about the extent to which the intervertebral disc itself is innervated. Yoshizawa et al. (21) reported profuse innervation in pathologic discs. The intervertebral disc may contain silent nociceptors (6) that respond to algesic chemicals produced with inflammation.

The facet joints undergo degenerative and inflammatory changes with rheumatoid or osteoarthritis and are a source of symptoms. High strain in innervated tissues such as the facet joint capsules can trigger a pulse of action potentials (5). The facet is highly innervated and contains free and encapsulated nerve endings (10,17) that are at a high threshold and thus likely to signal pain. They can be activated by both pressure and capsule stretch. However, nociceptors fire at much lower strain in the presence of certain chemicals and thus may be a mechanism of chronic pain (9).

CONCLUSION

The cervical spine is a complex structure. The functions are to support the mass of the head, to provide mobility of the head, to protect neurologic structures, and to control motion. The ligamentous human spine has intricately arranged joints that constitute a complex system that behaves much like a mechanical linkage. The role of various components in a normal or diseased spine can be investigated with well-established engineering principles. In addition to the experimental and clinical studies, engineering studies are an indispensable part of investigations into satisfactory delineation of the biomechanics of the human musculoskeletal system. The biomechanics of the cervical spine are determined by the shape of the vertebral bodies and the orientation of the zygapophyseal joints.

The upper cervical spine, consisting of the occiput, atlas, and axis, is responsible for most of the axial rotation and some of the flexion-extension and lateral bending of the head. In addition to allowing large rotation, it must be stable enough to support the weight of the head and protect the spinal cord. The alar ligaments limit axial rotation. Lateral bending of the cervical spine is normally coupled with axial rotation. Aging decreases the motion, largely in the middle and lower cervical spine owing to disc degeneration, facet osteoarthritis, and the development of uncovertebral joints. The neck muscles provide stability, control movement, and generate forces. The viscoelastic properties of the intervertebral disc determine the creep rate and the deformation of the disc. A degenerated intervertebral disc creeps faster than a nondegenerated disc. Repetitive loading deforms the intervertebral disc more than static loading.

Changes in the viscoelastic properties accompanying degeneration influence the stability of the FSU. Tolerance data on the FSU and its components in both acute and chronic trauma are not complete. There is a particular need to study the ability of the intervertebral disc, ligaments, facets, and capsule to tolerate both single and repetitive loading. A priority is simulation of high-risk injury when the facets are loaded to produce dislocation. These high-speed events must be simulated with high-strain-rate tests. The types and mechanisms of both low and high-speed trauma should be identified as a function of aging, sex, race, stature, and other characteristics.

REFERENCES

1. Cammack KV. Whiplash injuries to the neck. *Am J Surg* 1957;93:663–666.
2. Coventry M, Ghormley R, Kernohan IW. The intervertebral disc: its microscopic anatomy and pathology, 2: changes in the intervertebral disc concomitant with age. *J Bone Joint Surg Am* 1945; 27:233–247.
3. Dvorak J, Panjabi MM, Novotny JE, et al. In vivo flexion/extension of the normal cervical spine. *J Orthop Res* 1991;9:828–834.
4. Dvorak J, Valach L, Schmid ST. Cervical spine injuries in Switzerland. *J Manual Med* July 6-9, 1989;4:7–16.
5. El-Bohy AA, Goldberg SJ, King AL. Measurements of facet capsular stretch. In: 1987 Conference of the American Society of Mechanical Engineers, Cincinnati, March 4-7, 1987:161–164.
6. Grigg P, Schaible HG, Schmidt RF. Mechanical sensitivity of group III and IV afferents from posterior articular nerve in normal and inflamed cat knee. *J Neurophysiol* 1986;55:635–643.
7. Hansen HJ. A pathologic-anatomical study on disc degeneration in dog. *Acta Orthop Scand Suppl* 1952;11: 111–118.
8. Holdsworth F. Fractures, dislocations, and fracture dislocations of the spine. *J Bone Joint Surg Am* 1970;52: 1534–1551.
9. Howe JF, Loeser JD, Calvin WH. Mechanosensitivity of dorsal root ganglia and chronically injured axons: a physiological basis for the radicular pain of nerve root compression. *Pain* 1977;3:25–41.
10. Jackson HC, Winkelmarin RK, Bickel WH. Nerve endings in the human spinal column and related structures. *J Bone Joint Surg Am* 1966;48:1272–1281.
11. Jeffreys ET, McSweeney T. *Disorders of the cervical spine.* London: Butterworths, 1980.
12. Keyes DC, Compere EL. The normal and pathological physiology of the nucleus pulposus of the intervertebral disc: an anatomical, clinical and experimental study. *J Bone Joint Surg Am* 1932;14:897–938.
13. Lubin S, Sehmer J. Are automobile head restraints used effectively? *Can Fam Physician* 1993;39:1584–1588.
14. Magnusson ML, Pope MH, Hasselquist L, et al. Cervical electromyography during low-speed rear impact. *Eur Spine J* 1999;8:118–125.
15. McNab I. *Acceleration extension injuries of the cervical spine.* Philadelphia: WB Saunders, 1982.
16. Ono K, Kanno M. Influences of the physical parameters on the risk to neck injuries in low impact speed rear-end collisions. *Accid Anal Prev* 1996;28:493–499.
17. Ozaktay AC, Cavanaugh JM, Blagoev DC, et al. Effects of a carrageenan-induced inflammation in rabbit lumbar facet joint capsule and adjacent tissues. *Neurosci Res* 1994;20:355–364.
18. Ozaktay AC, Yamashita T, Cavanaugh JM, et al. Fine nerve fibers of the fibrous capsule of the lumbar facet joint. In: Proceedings of the 37th Annual Meeting of the Orthopaedic Research Society, Anaheim, California, August 3-5, 1991:353.
19. Svensson MY. *Neck injuries in rear-end collisions: sites and biomechanical causes of the injuries, test methods and preventive measures.* Gothenburg, Sweden: Chalmers University of Technology, 1993.
20. White AA, Panjabi MM. *Clinical biomechanics of the spine,* 2nd ed. Philadelphia: JB Lippincott, 1990.
21. Yoshizawa H, O'Brien JP, Smith WT, et al. The neuropathology of intervertebral discs removed for low back pain. *J Pathol* 1980;132:95–104.

The Degenerative Cervical Spine,
edited by Marek Szpalski and Robert Gunzburg
Lippincott Williams & Wilkins, Philadelphia © 2001.

3

Where Does the Pain Come From?

Björn Rydevik, Helena Brisby, Kjell Olmarker

Department of Orthopaedics, Göteborg University, Sahlgrenska University Hospital,
SE-413 45 Göteborg, Sweden

TISSUE ORIGIN OF CERVICAL SPINE PAIN AND RADICULAR PAIN
ETIOLOGY OF CERVICAL SPINE PAIN SYNDROMES
Tumors • Infection • Inflammatory Conditions • Severe Disc Degeneration • Disc Herniation • Other Causes of Neck Pain

Pain is defined by the International Association for the Study of Pain (8) as "an unpleasant sensory and emotional experience associated with actual or potential tissue damage or described in terms of such damage." Pain not only is a peripheral phenomenon but also is a product of interpretation by the brain of complex afferent impulses. The experience of pain often is influenced by physical and psychological factors. In this context, the duration of pain seems to be of utmost importance when considering the prognosis of neck pain syndromes. It is clinically important to differentiate acute from chronic neck pain. A duration of pain exceeding approximately 6 months is considered the critical time limit in this regard (6,18).

TISSUE ORIGIN OF CERVICAL SPINAL PAIN AND RADICULAR PAIN

A limited amount of scientific data is presented in the literature regarding the exact underlying causes of cervical spinal pain syndromes, including radicular pain (2). Some of the clinical and experimental knowledge in this field has been derived from studies of the lumbar spine. In this respect, there are some interesting observations by MacNab (11) and Smyth and Wright (17). These investigators found that if a nerve root is the site of chronic irritation, even minor mechanical deformation might induce radiating pain. This was demonstrated by placing sutures or inflatable catheters around nerve roots at the time of surgery for disc herniation and postoperatively inducing stretching or compression of the nerve root. These phenomena have been investigated experimentally by, for example, Howe et al. (7).

Clinical data have been obtained by Kuslich et al. (10) regarding the response of various tissues in the lumbar spine to mechanical stimulation. The subjects were patients undergoing spinal surgery under local anesthesia (Fig. 3.1). These investigators found that back pain could be produced by means of stimulation of several tissues, but by far the most common tissue of origin of pain was the outer layer of the anulus fibrosus and to certain extent the posterior longitudinal ligament. Buttock pain could be produced by si-

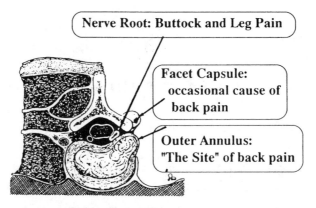

FIG. 3.1. Schematic shows tissue origin of low back pain and leg pain based on intraoperative observations of patients undergoing lumbar spinal surgery under local anesthesia. (From Kuslich SD, Ulstrom CL, Michael CJ. The tissue origin of low back pain and sciatic: a report of pain response to tissue stimulation during operations on the lumbar spine using local anesthesia. *Orthop Clin North Am* 1991;22:181–187, with permission.)

multaneous stimulation of the anulus fibrosus and the nerve root. The facet joint capsule rarely generated back pain. The facet capsule synovial layer and the cartilage surfaces of the facet joint were never found to generate pain. Kuslich et al. (10) also found that sciatic leg pain could be produced only by means of stimulation of a swollen, stretched, or compressed nerve root. The basic biologic principles of pain generation are likely to be applicable to the entire spinal column. Therefore the findings on pain mechanisms in the lumbar spine reported in the literature should be relevant to understanding of pain production in the cervical spine.

Cervical spinal pain and other types of pain require action potentials to ascend in the pain pathways. Such action potentials generated in the free nerve endings of the pain receptors (nociceptors) continue up the axons of small C delta and A delta fibers and enter the dorsal horn of the spinal cord at the first synapse. Various systems of neurons transfer the neurophysiologic message through the spinal cord and thalamus to the somatosensory cortex of the brain (3).

Nociceptive nerve fibers can be divided into two main groups—C polymodal nociceptors and A mechanoheat fibers, also known as A delta fibers. The C polymodal nociceptors are nonmyelinated sensory fibers, which constitute most of the nerve fibers in many sensory peripheral nerves. These polymodal nociceptors respond to all three types of noxious stimuli—thermal, mechanical, and chemical. These sensory neurons also contain neuropeptides. The A delta fibers respond mainly to mechanical and thermal stimulation of noxious magnitude but also respond to a certain chemical stimuli (17).

Pain generation may under certain conditions occur at sites on the pain pathway other than peripherally at the free nerve endings in tissues. Such a phenomenon is called *ectopic impulse generation.* This may occur in damaged or regenerating nerve fibers (neuroma), dorsal root ganglia, or inflamed nerve roots (7).

Long-standing tissue injury or inflammation can initiate a pronounced input of nociceptive impulses into the spinal cord. This may lead to sensitization of neurons in the dorsal horn of the spinal cord, which has been called *central sensitization* (3,4). If a patient has established such central sensitization, nerve impulses in A beta touch afferents can evoke pain whether they arise normally or ectopically (5). Furthermore, mechanical thresholds are reduced, so stimulation of low-threshold mechanoreceptors may cause firing in pain transmitting neurons in the dorsal horn of the spinal cord. Such pain mechanisms may explain certain chronic conditions, including long-standing neck pain, in which no obvious peripheral cause of the condition can be found.

ETIOLOGY OF CERVICAL SPINAL PAIN SYNDROMES

When examining a patient with neck pain, one must attempt to verify or exclude certain conditions of the cervical spine. Specific diagnoses lead to different therapeutic interventions. This chapter discusses conditions likely related to the production of neck pain with or without radiating nerve root pain in the arm (16) (Fig. 3.2).

Tumors

Metastatic tumors in the spine are much more common than primary bone tumors. Primary tumors such as myeloma, chondrosarcoma, and chordomas are found in the cervical spine. Vertebral metastases may originate from primary tumors of, for example, the breast, prostate, thyroid, or kidney. A typical symptom of vertebral tumors is unremitting pain, including pain at night (19). Neurologic symptoms may occur at fairly early stages because of mechanical deformation of the spinal cord or nerve roots.

Infection

Discitis and spondylitis, sometimes in combination, are frequently associated with pronounced neck pain. As with tumors, the pain may be of a constant nature and occur

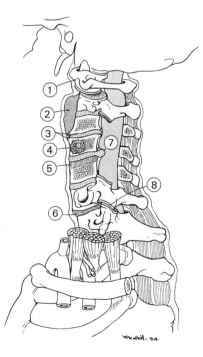

FIG. 3.2. Schematic shows specific underlying causes of pain in the cervical spine. *1,* Instability of C1-2, which often is related to rheumatoid arthritis; *2,* prevertebral tumor or infection; *3,* severe disc degeneration; *4,* vertebral tumor (primary or secondary); *5,* spondylitis or discitis; *6,* instability, posttraumatic or degenerative; *7,* disc herniation; *8,* severe degenerative changes in intervertebral joints. The clinical relevance of these possible underlying causes, which can be seen radiologically, vary with the specific diagnosis. (From Rydevik B. Spine adult. In: Lindgren U, Svensson O, eds. *Ortopedi.* Stockholm: Almqvist Wiksell Medicin/Liber, 1996:421–460, with permission.)

at night. Common pathogens are *Staphylococcus aureus* and *Mycobacterium tuberculosis.*

Inflammatory Conditions

Rheumatoid arthritis may affect the cervical spine. Changes at C1-2 can cause pain in the occipital, retroauricular, and temporal regions. Involvement of the middle part of the cervical spine may give rise to pain in the neck, sometimes radiating down to the collar bones. Rheumatoid arthritis affects the lower cervical spine and can cause pain that radiates to the shoulders. Pronounced inflammatory changes at any level can cause instability and compression of the spinal cord. Ankylosing spondylitis, which occurs among approximately 2% of the population, also may affect the cervical spine and cause neck pain (9).

Severe Disc Degeneration

With disc degeneration, the relation between radiologic findings and the existence of neck pain is not well established. However, pronounced disc degeneration, especially if present at multiple levels, seems to be related to increased risk of neck pain (12).

Disc Herniation

In the cervical spine, disc herniation may cause involvement of nerve roots, the spinal cord, or both, depending on the location of the disc herniation. Sometimes disc herniation is combined with osteophyte formation from the vertebral bone structures. For lumbar disc herniation, there is a considerable amount of evidence from experiments that autologous nucleus pulposus tissue in the intervertebral disc may biochemically sensitize the nerve root when disc herniation occurs so that mechanical nerve root compression causes radiating sciatic pain (13–15). The biologic and pathophysiologic mechanisms of various pain conditions in different regions of the spine are likely to be analogous. Therefore the biologic principles established for the lumbar spine apply to the generation of radiating nerve root pain in the arm caused by cervical disc herniation. Centrally located disc herniation in the cervical spine may compress the spinal cord and cause symptoms in the legs. It is important to recognize that cervical disc herniation can occur without clinical symptoms (1). Thus the sensitivity and specificity of diagnostic tests, including magnetic resonance imaging and computed tomography, must be considered in the diagnosis and treatment of patients with cervical spinal disorders (5).

Other Causes of Neck Pain

One should always consider the possibility of nonspinal causes of neck pain, such as prevertebral tumor or infection and various neurologic diseases, such as multiple sclerosis and inflammatory conditions or tumors of the nervous system. For a large number of patients with neck pain, no specific cause of the pain can be identified. Through careful review of the history and a thorough physical examination, including radiologic investigations when appropriate, one can exclude or verify specific diagnoses with a very high accuracy. These considerations are important in the care of patients with neck pain.

REFERENCES

1. Boden S, McCowin P, Davis D, et al. Abnormal magnetic-resonance scans of the cervical spine in asymptomatic subjects. *J Bone Joint Surg Am* 1990;72:1178–1184.
2. Brower RS. Cervical disc disease: clinical syndromes and differential diagnosis of cervical disc disease. In: Herkowitz HN, ed. *Rothman-Simeone: the spine.* Philadelphia: WB Saunders, 1999:455–461.
3. Cavanaugh JM. Neural mechanisms of lumbar pain. *Spine* 1995;20:1804–1809.
4. Coderre TJ, Katz J, Vaccarino AL, et al. Contribution of central neuroplasticity to pathological pain: review of clinical and experimental evidence. *Pain* 1991;52:259–285.
5. Devor M, Basbaum AI, Bennet GJ, et al. Mechanisms of neuropathic pain following peripheral injury. In: Basbaum A, Besson J-M (eds). *Towards a New Pharmacology of Pain.* Dalheim Konferenzen. Chichester: Wiley, 1991:417–440.
6. Deyo RA. Understanding the accuracy of diagnostic tests. In: Weinstein JN, Rydevik BL, Sonntag V, eds. *Essentials of the spine.* New York: Raven Press, 1995:55–70.
7. Fordyce WE. *Behavioral methods for chronic pain and illness.* St. Louis: Mosby, 1976.
8. Howe JF, Loeser JD, Calvin WH. Mechanosensitivity of dorsal root ganglia and chronically injured axons: a physiological basis for the radicular pain of nerve root compression. *Pain* 1977;3:25–41.
9. International Association for the Study of Pain (Subcommittee on Taxonomy). Pain terms: a list with definitions and notes on usage. *Pain* 1979;6:249–252.
10. Jayson MIV. *Back pain: the facts.* New York: Oxford University Press, 1981.
11. Kuslich SD, Ulstrom CL, Michael CJ. The tissue origin of low back pain and sciatic: a report of pain response to tissue stimulation during operations on the lumbar spine using local anesthesia. *Orthop Clin North Am* 1991;22:181–187.
12. MacNab I. The mechanism of spondylogenic pain. In: Hirsch C, Zotterman Y, eds. *Cervical pain.* New York: Pergamon Press, 1972:89–95.
13. Nachemson A, Bigos S. The low back. In: Cruess RL, Rennie WRJ, eds. *Adult orthopaedics.* Vol II. New York: Churchill Livingstone, 1984:843–935.
14. Olmarker K, Myers RR. Pathogenesis of sciatic pain: role of herniated nucleus pulposus and deformation of spinal nerve root and DRG. *Pain* 1998;78:9–105.
15. Olmarker K, Rydevik B. Pathophysiology of spinal nerve roots as related to sciatica and disc herniation. Herkowitz HN, ed. In: *Rothman-Simeone: the Spine,* 4th ed. Philadelphia: WB Saunders, 1999:175–182.
16. Olmarker K, Rydevik B, Nordborg C. Autologous nucleus pulposus induces neurophysiologic and histologic changes in porcine cauda equina nerve roots. *Spine* 1993;18:1425–1432.
17. Rang HP, Bevan S, Dray A. Chemical activation of nociceptive peripheral neurons. *Br Med Bull* 1991;47:534–548.
18. Rydevik B. Spine adult. In: Lindgren U, Svensson O, eds. *Ortopedi.* Stockholm: Almqvist Wiksell Medicin/Liber, 1996:421–460.
19. Smyth MJ, Wright V. Sciatica and the intervertebral disc: an experimental study. *J Bone Joint Surg Am* 1958;40:1401–1418.
20. Sternbach RA. *Pain patients: traits and treatment.* New York: Academic Press, 1974.
21. Weinstein JW. Differential diagnosis and surgical treatment of primary benign and malignant spine neoplasm. In: Frymoyer J, et al., eds. *Adult spine: principles and practice.* New York: Raven Press, 1991:829–860.

SECTION 2

Clinical Presentation

The Degenerative Cervical Spine,
edited by Marek Szpalski and Robert Gunzburg
Lippincott Williams & Wilkins, Philadelphia © 2001.

4

Clinical Presentation

Federico Balagué, *Jean Dudler

*Department of Rheumatology, Physical Medicine and Rehabilitation, Hospital Cantonal,
1708 Fribourg and *Department of Rheumatology, CHUV, 1011 Lausanne, Switzerland*

DEGENERATIVE DISORDERS OF THE CERVICAL SPINE
  Common clinical syndromes • Uncommon clinical syndromes
INFLAMMATORY DISORDERS OF THE CERVICAL SPINE
  Case Report • Rheumatoid Arthritis • Spondylarthropathies • Tumors and Infiltrative
  Lesions • Spondylodiscitis and Other Infectious Diseases • Microcrystalline and Mis-
  cellaneous Diseases
CONCLUSIONS

This chapter focuses on the symptoms of patients suffering from degenerative or inflammatory diseases of the spine. Most nontraumatic disorders of the neck are degenerative, inflammatory, or idiopathic in origin. As is often the case, various rare and often exotic diagnostic origins have been described in the literature. It is the general expectation in medical practice that with detection of a spectrum of clinical signs and symptoms, an accurate diagnosis can be made, other sources of neck pain excluded, and appropriate therapy prescribed. This is considered the task of physicians (11,15). The flaw in this expectation is that in the case of the cervical spine, a clinical-pathologic correlation has never been made and different medical authorities view similar symptoms in greatly different ways (11).

According to Spangfort (72), there are three main ways to classify patients' clinical presentations: by etiology, by morbid anatomic features, or by the topography of symptoms. Topography is the best criterion for application at the bedside. This means that the diagnosis relies mainly on the information obtained from the patient. Although many authors believe that "a highly probable diagnosis can be made prior to physical examination" on the basis of historical data alone (6), others contend that historical elicitation and physical examination are the "least likely to be done well" (19). Moreover, despite these common beliefs, the usefulness of many clinical variables still has to be proved (16,35).

Cervical pain can be caused by lesions of various anatomic structures (13,16,36). However, not all abnormalities are painful. It is well known that many persons without symptoms have radiologic images that show degeneration of the cervical spine. The incidence of degeneration increases with age. Degeneration is nearly ubiquitous in the later decades of life without a concomitant increase in the prevalence of symptoms (14,30,36, 43,76,77). Physical signs of cord involvement have been found among patients free of any spinal or neurologic symptoms (12). This high prevalence of asymptomatic abnormalities increases the difficulty of the diagnosis.

Epidemiologic studies have shown that the point prevalence of pain in the neck, shoulder, or arm is approximately 10% among the general population 15 years and older (43). The annual prevalence has been found to be higher than 33% (18). More recent surveys have shown an unexpectedly high prevalence of neck pain among otherwise healthy schoolchildren. These figures are much higher than the overall prevalence of inflammatory and degenerative disorders of the cervical spine among these age groups. For example, Mikkelson et al. (51) reported on two groups totaling 1,756 children with mean ages of 9.8 and 11.8 years. They found a prevalence of neck pain at least once a week of 15%. One year later, 48.3% of these children still reported neck pain with the same frequency. According to these figures and many others, symptoms arising from the cervical spine represent a major public health issue (30).

A review of the literature has shown us that clinicians are faced with four main situations when evaluating pathologic conditions of the cervical spine:

1. Cervical disorders caused by local pathologic changes in the cervical spine or by a systemic disorder that affects the cervical spine
2. Cervical symptoms due to a nonmusculoskeletal disorder, such as a visceral, vascular, or neurologic disorder (10)
3. A known diagnosis that necessitates systematic evaluation of the cervical spinal despite the absence of specific symptoms, because there is a definite risk of silent lesions that can cause severe complications
4. Cervical spinal involvement recognized as the source of atypical or noncervical symptoms, such as angor (12,75), rare cases of sciatica due to cervical cord compression (39), or infections of the spine that mimic disease of the internal organs (48).

This chapter does not discuss acute traumatic lesions or symptoms due to whiplash, which are clearly different from spontaneous pain (16). Accidents are common, so it is not surprising that a patient with a pathologic conditions of the cervical spine also has been involved in a recent or remote accident; however, no clear causal relation between the two has been established (4,21,55,63,77,84). It is not the purpose of this chapter to examine other clinical approaches to cervical pain, such as the manual medicine approach (25) or trigger and tender points (71,90). According to Bogduk (16), trigger points are "neither reliable nor valid in neck pain." This chapter also does not discuss congenital problems or disorders of infancy and childhood (5,7).

DEGENERATIVE DISORDERS OF THE CERVICAL SPINE

The various degenerative lesions recognized, such as spondylosis, disc space narrowing, or zygapophyseal joint osteoarthritis, do not seem to give rise to different clinical manifestations (16). As such, degenerative disorders are discussed as a single entity and divided into common and uncommon clinical syndromes.

Common Clinical Syndromes

Pathologic processes in the cervical spine can manifest as a wide diversity of symptoms ranging from asymptomatic lesions to potentially lethal ones (62). It is customary to approach any patient by trying to classify the clinical presentation according to four different clinical syndromes—cervical vertebral syndrome, radicular syndrome, myelopathy, and vertebrobasilar insufficiency (37,78). A patient can have one or any combination of these syndromes. This classification is flawed because these syndromes have only been defined empirically (11). Despite this limitation, this system is used herein for the purpose of clarity.

Vertebral Syndrome

Vertebral syndrome is characterized by pain and impaired range of motion (78). The pain usually has mechanical characteristics, although nocturnal pain also is frequent (78). Patients usually report a long history of relapsing pain with a reduction or absence of pain between crises (78). Localization of the pain can vary from pure cervical pain to pain radiating to the occipital area or to the shoulder or scapula (78). Headaches are reported by one third of patients and unilateral or bilateral shoulder pain by 71% (37). Using the criteria of the International Headache Society, Nilsson (54) found the prevalence of cervicogenic headache to be 2.5% (95% confidence interval, 1.1–4.8) in the general population. On the basis of his clinical experience, Maigne (47) differentiated three typical localizations of pain in cervicogenic headaches—isolated occipital pain, pain in the mastoid-maxillary area, and pain in the supraorbital area with or without occipital pain. Nevertheless, it is always the C2-3 facet joints, which were reported to be painful on palpation (47). This topic was reviewed by Bontoux (17), who concluded that if the arguments to define the causation of a headache as cervicogenic deserve consideration they also require confirmation. Cervical problems also can manifest as pain limited to the interscapular thoracic area (47).

Dwyer et al. (26) investigated whether pain arising from the cervical zygapophyseal joints has characteristic topographic radiating patterns. Injections into the C2-3 to C6-7 joints were performed on healthy volunteers, and the distribution of pain was recorded (26). The composite map published by these authors suggests the presence of considerable overlap, particularly between adjacent levels (26). The same group reported later on 318 patients with intractable neck pain evaluated by means of discography and zygapophyseal joint block (2). The investigators concluded that symptomatic zygapophyseal joints "were encountered in 25% of the sample with a possibility that a further 38% suffered zygapophyseal pain but were not appropriately investigated" (2).

A current trend is toward use of questionnaires specifically designed and validated (in English) for the study of cervical pain (44,87). These tools are used to assess the intensity of pain, its interference with different aspects of living (vocational, recreational, social, and functional), and the presence and extent of associated emotional factors (87). These questionnaires allow physicians to calculate a numerical score, which should be a better way to evaluate outcomes than a simple clinical impression.

After an extensive review of the literature, Bogduk (16) stated that "factors found to be positively associated with neck pain are educational level, occupation, physical stress at work, mental stress at work and working with machines." In the same article it is clearly stated that personal psychological factors are not associated with neck pain (16).

Neck pain reported in questionnaires has been found to be associated with limited and painful spinal mobility (31). Range of motion can be more or less impaired, but most often a moderate reduction in mobility is found (78). The reduction in range of motion has been reported to be typically predominant in some directions and sectors, whereas others are more or less normal (78). Among patients with acute torticollis, the neck is fixed in side flexion toward or away from the painful side. There is a typical limitation of one lateral and one rotational movement, and the sternocleidomastoid and trapezius muscles are very tender (8).

The clinical evaluation of patients is influenced by the lack of a gold standard for the measurement of cervical motion (20). Some clinical tests commonly used are either unreliable (80) or insensitive (70). Bogduk (16) stated that "with respect to neck pain with no associated neurological features, physical examination has proven neither reliable nor valid." The limits of the clinical examination have been highlighted by Hawk et al. (35). In a similar approach, these authors looked at the intraexaminer and interexaminer reliability of chiropractic evaluation of the lumbar spine and concluded that interexaminer reliability is poor to slight (35).

Muscle spasm usually is considered to be part of the vertebral syndrome. However, loss of lordosis on a lateral radiograph of the cervical spine does not allow one to conclude that this finding is caused by a muscle spasm (38). Muscle strain, muscle imbalance, and postural faults can cause cervical clinical problems. Bland (8) differentiated syndromes characterized by soreness, fatigue, and burning pain depending on the posture associated with the typical signs, such as the presence of focal points of tenderness and shortening of some muscles.

Radicular Syndrome and Myelopathy

Radicular syndrome and myelopathy are discussed in Chapter 6. Other excellent review and epidemiologic articles have been published (27,28,58,66,67,73,74). Although symptomatic cervical disk herniation usually manifests as a radicular syndrome, compression of the spinal trigeminal tract by C3-4 disk herniation has been reported (4). Juxtafacet cysts of the cervical spine are rare lesions that can cause myelopathy, radiculopathy, or both (41). Another rare pathologic condition is cervical intradural disc herniation; only six cases had been reported as of 1994 (55). Five of the six patients had signs of cord compression, and one patient had root compression (55). To cite Boden et al. (15), the "first major decision" of a physician facing a patient with a cervical problem is "to rule in or out the presence of a cervical myelopathy."

Compression of the Vertebral Arteries

Degenerative disorders of the cervical spine can cause compression on the vertebral arteries and vertebrobasilar insufficiency. Minor and major types of compressions have been described (78). The former can cause Barré-Lieou syndrome (12,17,47), perhaps through irritation of the perivascular sympathetic nervous system (78). From an anatomic point of view, autonomic symptoms can be explained at the levels of the stellate ganglion or the rami communicantes (37). Many different symptoms have been described under this label, including headaches, dizziness, vertigo, tinnitus, visual symptoms (blurring, diplopia, hallucination, photophobia, photopsia, scotomata, visual anosognosia), facial pain or numbness, pharyngeal and laryngeal symptoms, sweating, lacrimation, rhinorrhea, flushing, and hiccups (12,37,47,78). According to Bontoux (17), a cervical origin for vertigo is considered possible, but in an individual case this etiology can be accepted only after all other possibilities have been ruled out. Autonomic pathways could also be an explanation to cervical angina or pseudoangina (6,37). Variations of blood pressure between the right and left arms resulting from cervical spinal disorders have been described and attributed to irritation of the sympathetic nerve supply and to arterial vasoconstriction (6).

Major compression of the vertebral arteries can cause transient ischemic attacks or permanent lesions such as Wallenberg syndrome. Cervical degenerative lesions usually are one factor associated with atherosclerotic lesions of the vessels (78). Vascular lesions are a major concern during any manipulation of the spine. A test has been described that helps practitioners avoid performing manipulation on patients with symptoms of verte-brobasilar insufficiency (64,65).

Uncommon Clinical Syndromes

Hundreds of reports have highlighted uncommon clinical presentations of local pathologic conditions of the cervical spine, nonmusculoskeletal disorders manifesting with cervical symptoms, and noncervical symptoms caused by cervical spinal diseases. The following discussion is far from exhaustive. The following choices are based on personal interest or clinical relevance.

Degenerative disorders localized at C1-2 have been reported to induce a few specific symptoms and signs. The prevalence of symptomatic forms of such lesions was reported to be 4% among a population with peripheral osteoarthritis or degenerative joint disease of the spine without cervical symptoms (33). Most patients were older women (33,57) with a history of occipital or postauricular neck pain often interpreted by the subjects as a headache (33). Clinical examination showed a rotational head tilt deformity in about 50% of cases that was nonreducible in two thirds of these. All patients had reduced active and passive head rotation (33). Prost et al. (57) found rotation and lateral flexion movements to be extremely painful. Other distinctive signs are tender or trigger points confined to the occipital area and palpable cervical crepitus (33).

In the presence of spinal pain and neurologic signs, mainly myelopathy or radiculopathy, experienced by a patient who has undergone an operation on the cervical spine, one should entertain the diagnosis of a rarely reported lesion—transdural herniation of the spinal cord (84). A review of the topic identified 25 cases in the literature and described 5 more (84), but only 6 cases were localized in the cervical spine. More important, all were considered iatrogenic (84). The delay before the onset of clinical manifestations was 3 to 18 years (84).

The term "neck-tongue syndrome" has been used to describe patients reporting unilateral tongue dysesthesia accompanying ipsilateral neck and occipital pain induced by sudden neck movements (8,85). These symptoms have been found among patients with ankylosing spondylitis as well as among patients with cervical spondylosis or a radiologically "normal" cervical spine (85).

Dysphagia can be caused by very large anterior osteophytes, particularly among patients with diffuse idiopathic skeletal hyperostosis (DISH) (8,37,74). In his review, Bontoux (17) reported a prevalence of dysphagia of 2/1,000 among patients with radiologic signs of degeneration. This figure increased to 17% to 28% among persons with DISH. Dysphagia occurs mainly after ingestion of solid food with or without pharyngeal pain and sometimes is relieved by anterior flexion of the neck (17). In a case reported by Warnick et al. (83), DISH interfered with the swallowing mechanism to the point that the patient had aspiration pneumonia. DISH can mimic inflammatory diseases, patients reporting morning and evening stiffness increased by immobilization and activated by cold (8).

Neck pain induced by temporomandibular joint disorder has been clinically differentiated from neck pain of cervical origin on the basis of six variables—jaw symptoms, symptoms of the ears, symptoms of the eyes, joint sounds, symptoms of the shoulders, and pain in the joints. Use of these criteria led to correct classification in 91% of cases (23).

Neck pain and torticollis due to neurologic disease have been reported (21). In a retrospective review of 21 cases divided into acute, chronic, relapsing, and progressive, Croisile et al. (21) found that all the acute cases were caused by vascular diseases. The chronic cases were caused by benign tumors. The one patient with relapsing torticollis had Chiari malformation (21). In the progressive cases, characterized by a lack of response to the usual analgesic treatment, intracranial brain tumor, myeloma of a cervical vertebra, and epidural hematoma were found (21). A neurologic origin of acute torticollis should be suspected in the presence of certain clinical characteristics—extremely acute onset, unusual pain without the characteristics of mechanical pain, lack of pain on palpation, and flexion of the neck much more limited than rotation (21).

Muscle contractures of unknown origin with an extremely rigid cervical spine ("rigid spine syndrome") have been described. The condition usually begins during childhood and has typical clinical musculoskeletal and cardiac signs (53). Niamane et al. (53), however, described a 39-year-old man with a 5-year history of progressive stiffness of the neck without pain or other symptoms. A clinical examination showed limitation of all movement except cervical extension (53). This uncommon disorder can mimic a number of other muscle or joint diseases (53).

In complete contrast are the syndromes of flaccid neck paralysis that occur in a variety of diseases (8) and are characterized by extreme weakness of the muscles with the head falling about and restricting the person to immobility. These symptoms are caused by compression and collapse of pharyngeal and esophageal structures (8).

Athletes involved in collision sports sometimes report piercing, burning pain radiating from the neck to the finger tips after a blow to the head, the shoulder, or both (46). These symptoms have been called a "burner" or a "stinger" (46). According to a literature review by Levitz et al. (46), the career incidence of such symptoms can be as high as 65% among players of American football, and the recurrence rate can reach 87%. Many cases are acute and not always reported to the team physician. Levitz et al. (46) evaluated 55 chronic and recurrent cases in a prospective study. Although the subjects were young (mean age 23 years), 93% had either disc disease or degenerative narrowing of the foramina on magnetic resonance (MR) images (46). The Spurling test had a positive result in 71% of cases, and persistent weakness of the deltoid and spinatus muscle groups was present (46). Burner has been defined as neurapraxia or axonotmesis of a nerve root due to stretch or blow injury to the brachial plexus or due to compression in the foramina caused by disc disease or degenerative changes (46).

Symptoms remote from the cervical spine can be caused by cervical disorders. Ito et al. (39) reviewed 13 cases of sciatica due to cervical or thoracic spinal cord compression, mainly from tumors. A clue to this rare diagnosis was the absence of a history of low back pain and a negative straight leg raising test (39).

According to Maigne (47), as many as two-thirds of cases of lateral epicondylar pain are caused at least in part by problems at C5-6 or C6-7. Maigne also has stated that many cases of shoulder pain labeled tendinitis are frequently related to C4-5 or C5-6 mechanical dysfunction. The embryologic origin of the dermatomes, myotomes, and sclerotomes gives credence to this hypothesis (8,9).

A food and drug combination may be the cause of head and cervical pain without any abnormalities of the spine. As many as 25 syndromes have been identified that range from pure local pain to more complex features such as gastrointestinal, neurologic, renal, or other symptoms (8).

INFLAMMATORY DISORDERS OF THE CERVICAL SPINE

Case Report

A 41-year-old man arrives in the emergency department with acute posterior neck pain and impaired motion, which had appeared approximately 3 weeks earlier. The patient attributed his symptoms to unusual physical activity (helping someone move to a new house) and ruled out any injury, contusion, or sprain. The pain did not radiate to the upper limbs. Cervical rotation and lateral bending to the left increased the intensity of pain. Pain had increased despite treatment with naproxen and tolperisone and wearing a cervical collar. The clinical examination showed lowering of the right shoulder and antalgic left-sided cervical scoliosis. The cervical rotations were limited to 10–0–10 degrees, and the lateral bending range of motion was 30 degrees to the right side and 20 degrees to the left. For flexion-extension, the chin on chest distance varied from 2.5 to 15 cm. Palpation of the cervical spinous processes was painless, and palpation of the zygapophyseal joints was painful in the upper cervical spine.

A neurologic examination showed no relevant findings. The findings on conventional radiographs were considered normal (Fig. 4.1). Physiotherapy with analgesic techniques

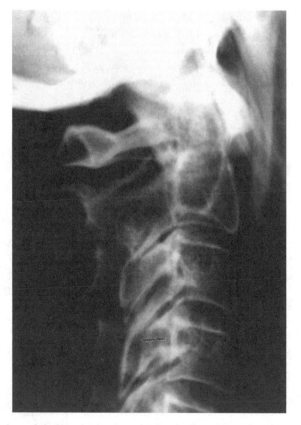

FIG. 4.1. Lateral view of the cervical spine obtained a few days after the pain began was described as normal by the radiologist and the treating physicians.

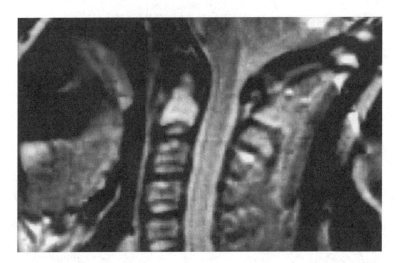

FIG. 4.2. Magnetic resonance image obtained 2 weeks after the pain began shows high signal intensity at C2.

and mobilization had not improved the patient's symptoms. MR images obtained 2 weeks later (Fig. 4.2) showed increased signal intensity at C2. The erythrocyte sedimentation rate increased to 56 mm/h, and the patient was admitted to the hospital for a complete evaluation. Multiple myeloma IgG-κ was diagnosed because of the presence of a monoclonal peak of γ-globulins (IgG-κ) and increased plasmocytosis in a bone marrow biopsy

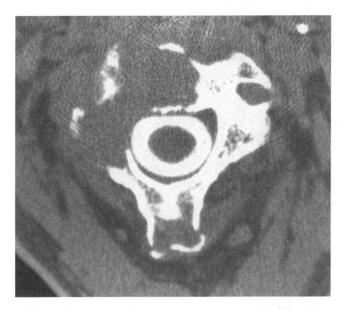

FIG. 4.3. Computed tomographic scan obtained a few weeks after the magnetic resonance image in Fig. 4.2 shows extensive destructive lesions of C2 that necessitated surgical stabilization.

specimen. Computed tomography performed a few weeks later showed extensive destructive vertebral lesions (Fig. 4.3) that necessitated surgical stabilization (C1-4 spondylodesis with a plate and bone cement). Despite aggressive chemotherapy and radiation therapy, the patient died 3 years after the emergency department visit.

Rheumatoid Arthritis

Involvement of the cervical spine that produces clinical and radiographic findings is common in rheumatoid arthritis. Any segment of the spine can be affected, but lesions of the occipitoatlantoaxial junction are most common. They cause atlantoaxial subluxation, basilar invagination, subaxial subluxation, or any combination of these conditions. Depending on the series and the criteria used, cervical involvement has been reported among 17% to 86% of all patients with rheumatoid arthritis (24,61,62). Recognition of such involvement is critical because even patients without symptoms are at risk of severe neurologic complications or sudden death from cord compression (61). As many as 10% of patients with rheumatoid arthritis die of unrecognized spinal cord or brainstem compression (52).

Pain is the most common and earliest clinical manifestation. It is nonspecific among 40% to 80% of patients, who describe it as a deep ache. The pain classically occurs in the neck and the occipital, retroorbital, or temporal area (24,61,62). The pain may not have the typical inflammatory quality of peripheral disease, probably because it is caused by not only synovitis of the zygapophyseal joints but also by instability and disc degeneration.

Apart from the nonspecific cervical pain syndrome, patients with rheumatoid arthritis can have a host of vague neurologic signs and symptoms, which often are difficult to evaluate because of coexisting severe peripheral arthritis, wasting, neuropathy, and loss of joint motion (24,61,62). Patients may report root compression symptoms or myelopathic symptoms, such as weakness, gait disturbance, loss of endurance, paresthesia in the extremities with loss of dexterity, or even urinary retention and incontinence, while physical examination shows increased deep tendon reflexes, spasticity, and sometimes a Babinski sign. Flexion of the neck can cause a Lhermitte sign. Vertebrobasilar insufficiency and brainstem compression can induce symptoms such as tinnitus, vertigo, diplopia, and dysphagia. It is estimated that true objective neurologic signs are observed among only 7% to 34% of patients (61). Numerous clinical tests for subluxation have been described (6); however, their prevalence, sensitivity, and specificity have not been reported. As many as 15% of patients with rheumatoid arthritis and atlantoaxial subluxation may have no cervical signs at all (6).

Risk factors for severe involvement of the cervical spine in rheumatoid arthritis have been classically regarded as similar to those of severe rheumatoid arthritis: disease duration, male sex, severe peripheral joint involvement, use of glucocorticoids, high-titer rheumatoid factor, or the presence of vasculitis (24,61,62). Some studies have challenged these views. Cervical spinal involvement occurs early in rheumatoid arthritis, and as many as 30% of patients have radiographic evidence of involvement after a mean follow-up period of 6.5 years (56). A study conducted in England (89) showed that conventional clinical and laboratory values did not have a statistically significant association with cervical spinal changes, unlike the case for peripheral joint disease. On the other hand, an age at onset of 45 years or older and the presence of HLA-B27 or Dw2 were powerful discriminant factors for the presence of severe atlantoaxial subluxation. These data were not reproduced in a study conducted in Finland (56). In the Finnish cohort, the presence of rheumatoid factor, a high initial level of C-reactive protein, and radiologic progression of peripheral joint disease correlated with cervical involvement. The presence of the HLA-DR4 or B27 did not influence early cervical involvement.

Because of the large number of patients without symptoms and the low specificity of history and physical examination, clinical presentation is of limited value in assessing cervical involvement in rheumatoid arthritis. It does not allow the exclusion of severe and impending complications. Clinical presentation can be useful for the planning of surgical treatment, as is shown by use of the Ranawat classification (60). This emphasizes the importance of regular clinical and radiologic evaluations of the cervical spine for patients with rheumatoid arthritis. Again, lack of specific symptoms is not synonymous with absence of a lesion.

Spondylarthropathies

Cervical involvement in ankylosing spondylitis usually occurs among patients with classic thoracolumbopelvic symptoms and signs of the disease (8). It results in limitation of neck motion and progressive kyphosis (62). Radiographic evidence of squaring of the vertebral bodies and of eventually complete bony ankylosis is accompanied by osteoporosis. Ankylosis of the zygapophyseal joint is probably essential to this process. It has been observed in relation to syndesmophytes in 22% of cervical zygapophyseal joints affected by ankylosing spondylitis (22).

Neck pain in spondylarthropathies is much more typical than in rheumatoid arthritis. It has the classic features of inflammation: pain is worse in the morning and is mitigated by activity or a hot shower (62). Atlantoaxial instability also occurs among more than 20% of patients with spondylarthropathies (59) and has even been described as a presenting feature (34). Because of the combination of ankylosis and osteoporosis, fractures are not uncommon, even after minor trauma. Any patient with new neck pain or modification in head position, even in the absence of clear trauma, should be assumed to have a fracture until proved otherwise (62). An overlooked fracture can cause epidural hematoma, which also should be recognized.

Reiter syndrome and psoriatic arthritis also affect the cervical spine. If rare in Reiter syndrome (3.4%), cervical involvement is very common, at least radiologically, in psoriatic arthritis, with incidence as high as 70% (68). Psoriatic arthritis also can cause lesions similar to those of rheumatoid arthritis—bony erosions and subluxation—which should be managed in a similar manner (62).

Tumors and Infiltrative Lesions

Although severe night pain is considered the hallmark of neoplasia, as it is with any inflammatory disease of the cervical spine, the initial clinical manifestations of tumor involvement of the cervical spine vary widely. Tumors may appear as incidental findings on radiographs. Physical examination and symptoms may range from very mild pain to stiffness, scoliosis, or even a mass (1). Neurologic deficit also can be the presenting symptom. Constitutional symptoms such as weight loss and anorexia or a history of malignant disease should raise the suspicion of metastatic disease (1).

Primary tumors are rare, less than 0.5% of all tumors, and cervical tumors are much less common than the thoracic and lumbar counterparts (1). Primary tumors can be distributed throughout the cervical spine, except for C1, and occur typically in the first two decades of life. Neck pain and stiffness with or without torticollis or scoliosis are the classic presentation (1). Pain is typically worst at night and is not relieved with analgesics and rest (1). Pain induced by osteoid osteoma typically is relieved with salicylates, at least initially (82). Neurologic symptoms are uncommon at presentation, and the course of the disease can be extended, although certain tumors such as aneurysmal bone cyst and eosinophilic granuloma tend to have a more rapid evolution (1). Most cases are diagnosed only after an initial observation period. This emphasizes the importance of a complete history and examination to detect red flags that suggest a specific process as the origin of the symptoms (1).

Manifestations of malignant tumors do not differ from those of benign tumors. Pain, often nocturnal and associated with spasm, is the primary symptom in both cases (1). Nevertheless, malignant tumors tend to occur more often among persons older than 50 years with a male predominance, and neurologic deficits are much more common in this population (1,21,40). At the time of diagnosis, the tumor often involves not only the vertebral body but also the surrounding tissues (1). Again, all levels are represented equally except C1. Multiple myeloma, as in the case presented earlier, is the most common form of primary malignant tumor, followed by chordoma, osteosarcoma, and Ewing sarcoma (1).

Metastatic disease of the spine is common. Metastatic disease occurs among 30% to 70% of patients with known neoplastic disease, and it is the first sign of metastasis among 20% of patients (1). Nevertheless, cervical involvement is less frequent than that of the other spinal sites, occurring among 8% to 20% of patients with known metastatic disease (1). It also is frequently less worrisome than other localizations, given the lower frequency of neurologic complications and the less pronounced tendency toward instability (1). The incidence of neurologic compromise is low, approximately 5%, because of the relatively wide area of the cervical spinal canal. If present, neurologic compromise is more likely to be caused by direct extension of a tumor inside the canal than by kyphotic deformity (1). It is important to recognize that neck pain and torticollis can be symptomatic of not only local neoplastic involvement but also of an intracranial tumor (21).

Spondylodiscitis and Other Infectious Diseases

The most common sites of hematogenous osteomyelitis among adults are the vertebrae, usually of the thoracic and lumbar spine (81). In one study, cervical involvement represented only 58 of 997 locations, mainly between C3 to C6 (48). The classic manifestations are acute pain, high fever, high erythrocyte sedimentation rate, intense muscle spasms, and eventually a palpable mass or neurologic symptoms from radicular or meningeal involvement. As for the other cervical diseases, the clinical presentation is not as standardized as one would think. Diagnosis often is delayed because symptoms can range in severity and intensity. The onset can be acute with high fever, violent pain, and malaise, but it also can be subacute with moderate fever and pain or chronic with a subfebrile temperature and local pain that does not disturb general well-being (48). Again, if the classic case with high fever, neck pain, and muscle spasms is easy to diagnose, a high degree of alertness is necessary to diagnose cases with chronic or less typical presentations, such as involvement limited to the posterior elements (3). Fever, even low grade, a high erythrocyte sedimentation rate, and any special context, such as a case reported after removal of a fishbone (79), are crucial clinical elements. Radiographic evaluation usually provides enough information for a diagnosis, but cervical epidural abscesses can have the same clinical presentation without radiographic anomalies (69). A patient with neck pain, fever, and neurologic symptoms without abnormalities on conventional radiographs should undergo MR evaluation.

In addition to classic osteomyelitis, tuberculosis can affect the cervical spine, although rarely. The presentation follows a chronic course. Patients report fever, night sweats, weight loss, and neck and upper back pain of several weeks' to months' duration (88). Signs and symptoms related to spread of the tuberculous process outside the cervical spine can also be the first clue to diagnosis.

If a patient with a systemic illness has neck stiffness and pain and a high fever, the diagnosis of Grisel syndrome has to be entertained. Grisel syndrome is the presence of atlantoaxial instability in association with pharyngeal infection or other inflammation of the adjacent peripharyngeal tissues (50,86). The pathogenesis is still unclear, and the syndrome usually affects children younger than 13 years. Neck stiffness and pain with attempts at motion are the most common symptoms, and dysphagia is frequent (50,86). Patients appear to have a systemic illness, have a high fever, and experience occipital pain that radiates to the head or ears. The head is held immobile in a pathologic position. Neurologic symptoms are rare, but quadriplegia has been reported (86). True septic arthritis of the C1-2 lateral zygapophyseal joint has been reported to mimic Grisel syndrome, and a high degree of alertness is needed to reach a diagnosis (32).

Microcrystalline and Miscellaneous Diseases

Both calcium pyrophosphate dihydrate and apatite crystal deposition in soft spinal or neck tissue may manifest as an acute, febrile, neck pain syndrome evoking meningitis (29,45,63). Pain is severe. The onset is extremely rapid and often is associated with a high fever and a marked decrease in cervical range of motion in all three planes. Apatite crystal disease usually manifests in the third through sixth decades of life, and calcium pyrophosphate dihydrate deposition disease manifests in the eighth decade (29,45,63). The erythrocyte sedimentation rate often is high. The findings at radiographic evaluation confirm the diagnosis.

Destructive spondylarthropathy among patients undergoing long-term hemodialysis was initially reported by Kuntz et al. (42). The pathophysiologic mechanism is not clear and may involve crystal deposition, amyloidosis, or hyperparathyroidism. Nonspecific local pain was the reported clinical presentation in initial studies, but it is now recognized that most cases are asymptomatic. Systematic radiologic study of the cervical spine is mandatory for these patients (49).

CONCLUSIONS

Evaluation of the contribution of the clinical presentation to the diagnosis and management of cervical disorders is difficult. Important differences exist between various experts' statements in books or review articles and what has been definitely proved in scientific studies. Although most patients with neck pain have nonspecific pain, "the obvious diagnosis is not always the correct one" (6). Most authors believe that the physician should perform a complete medical evaluation of each patient with cervical symptoms to establish a differential diagnosis. In the care of each patient, the physician should not focus on an initial assumption but should give attention and thought to all possible diagnoses (6). We agree with Bogduk's opinion about possible red flags (16). Patients with inflammatory diseases should undergo systematic evaluation of the cervical spine even if there is a lack of specific symptoms. Clinicians should always keep in mind the four possible combinations of anatomopathologic lesions and clinical features: asymptomatic abnormality of the cervical spine, cervical spine abnormality with cervical symptoms, abnormality of the cervical spine with noncervical symptoms, and systemic or nonspinal disorder of the neck with cervical symptoms.

REFERENCES

1. Abdu WA, Provencher M. Primary bone and metastatic tumors of the cervical spine. *Spine* 1998;23:2767–2777.
2. Aprill C, Bogduk N. The prevalence of cervical zygapophyseal joint pain: a first approximation. *Spine* 1992;17: 744–747.
3. Babinchak TJ, Riley DK, Rotheram EB Jr. Pyogenic vertebral osteomyelitis of the posterior elements. *Clin Infect Dis* 1997;25:221–224.
4. Barakos J, D'Amour P, Dillon W, et al. Trigeminal sensory neuropathy caused by cervical disk herniation. *AJNR Am J Neuroradiol* 1990;11:609.
5. Bland J. Cervical spine in infancy and childhood. In: Bland JH, ed. *Disorders of the cervical spine: diagnosis and medical management.* Philadelphia: WB Saunders, 1994:405–416.
6. Bland J. Clinical methods. In: Bland JH, ed. *Disorders of the cervical spine: diagnosis and medical management.* Philadelphia: WB Saunders, 1994:113–146.
7. Bland J. Congenital anomalies. In: Bland JH, ed. *Disorders of the cervical spine: diagnosis and medical management.* Philadelphia: WB Saunders, 1994:417–431.
8. Bland J. Differential diagnosis and specific treatment. In: Bland JH, ed. *Disorders of the cervical spine: diagnosis and medical management.* Philadelphia: WB Saunders, 1994:223–270.
9. Bland J. Embryology: practical clinical implications and interpretation. In: Bland JH, ed. *Disorders of the cervical spine: diagnosis and medical management.* Philadelphia: WB Saunders, 1994:11–39.
10. Bland J. Epidemiology and demographics: phylogenesis and clinical implications. In: Bland JH, ed. *Disorders of the cervical spine: diagnosis and medical management.* Philadelphia: WB Saunders, 1994:3–10.
11. Bland J. New anatomy and physiology with clinical and historical implications. In: Bland JH, ed. *Disorders of the cervical spine: diagnosis and medical management.* Philadelphia: WB Saunders, 1994:71–91.
12. Bland J. Problem-oriented approach. In: Bland JH, ed. *Disorders of the cervical spine: diagnosis and medical management.* Philadelphia: WB Saunders, 1994:211–221.
13. Bland J, Boushey D. Anatomy and physiology of the cervical spine. *Semin Arthritis Rheum* 1990;20:1–20.
14. Boden S, McCowin P, Davis D, et al. Abnormal magnetic-resonance scans of the cervical spine in asymptomatic subjects. *J Bone Joint Surg Am* 1990;72:1178–1184.
15. Boden S, Wiesel S, Laws E, et al. The aging spine. Philadelphia: WB Saunders, 1991.
16. Bogduk N. The neck. *Baillieres Clin Rheumatol* 1999;13:261–285.
17. Bontoux D. Dysphagie, céphalée, vertige et rachis cervical. *Rev Rhum Ed Fr* 1998;65:374–379.
18. Bovim G, Schrader H, Sand T. Neck pain in the general population. *Spine* 1994;19:1307–1309.
19. Brain W. Some unsolved problems in cervical spondylosis. *Br Med J* 1963;5333:771–777.
20. Chen J, Solinger A, Poncet J, et al. Meta-analysis of normative cervical motion. *Spine* 1999;24:1571–1578.
21. Croisile B, Aimard G, Vighetto A, et al. Cervicalgies et torticolis isolés révélateurs de lésions neurologiques. *Presse Med* 1989;18:1513–1515.
22. De Vlam K, Mielants H, Veys EM. Involvement of the zygopophyseal joint in ankylosing spondylitis: relation to the bridging syndesmophyte. *J Rheumatol* 1999;26:1738–1745.
23. De Wijer A, de Leeuw J, Steenks M, et al. Temporomandibular and cervical spine disorders. *Spine* 1996;21: 1638–1646.
24. Dreyer SJ, Boden SD. Natural history of rheumatoid arthritis of the cervical spine. *Clin Orthop* 1999;366: 98–106.
25. Dvorák J, Dvorák V, Schneider W, et al. *Manuelle medizin: diagnostik.* Stuttgart: Georg Thieme Verlag, 1997: 448.
26. Dwyer A, Aprill C, Bogduk N. Cervical zygapophyseal joint pain patterns, I: a study in normal volunteers. *Spine* 1990;15:453–457.
27. Ellenberg M, Honet J. Clinical pearls in cervical radiculopathy. *Phys Med Rehabil Clin N Am* 1996;7:487–508.
28. Ellenberg M, Honet J, Treanor W. Cervical radiculopathy. *Arch Phys Med Rehabil* 1994;75:342–352.
29. Fahlgren H. Retropharyngeal tendinitis. *Cephalalgia* 1986;6:169–174.
30. Hadler NM. Osteoarthritis as a public health problem. *Clin Rheum Dis* 1985;11:175–185.
31. Hagen K, Harms-Ringdahl K, Enger N, et al. Relationship between subjective neck disorders and cervical spine mobility and motion-related pain in male machine operators. *Spine* 1997;22:1501–1507.
32. Halla JT, Bliznak J, Hardin JG, et al. Septic arthritis of the C1-C2 lateral facet joint and torticollis: pseudo–Grisel's syndrome. *Arthritis Rheum* 1991;34:84–88.
33. Halla J, Hardin J. Atlantoaxial (C1-C2) facet joint osteoarthritis: a distinctive clinical syndrome. *Arthritis Rheum* 1987;30:577–582.
34. Hamilton MG, MacRae ME. Atlantoaxial dislocation as the presenting symptom of ankylosing spondylitis. *Spine* 1993;18:2344–2346.

35. Hawk C, Phongphua C, Bleecker J, et al. Preliminary study of the reliability of assessment procedures for chiropractic adjustments of the lumbar spine. *J Manipulative Physiol Ther* 1999;22:382–389.
36. Heller C, Stanley P, Lewis-Jones B, et al. Value of x ray examinations of the cervical spine. *Br Med J* 1983;287: 1276–1278.
37. Heller J. The syndromes of degenerative cervical disease. *Orthop Clin North Am* 1992;23:381–394.
38. Helliwell P, Evans P, Wright V. The straight cervical spine: does it indicate muscle spasm? *J Bone Joint Surg Br* 1994;76:103–106.
39. Ito T, Homma T, Uchiyama S. Sciatica caused by cervical and thoracic spinal cord compression. *Spine* 1999;24: 1265–1267.
40. Khosla A, Martin DS, Awwad EE. The solitary intraspinal vertebral osteochondroma: an unusual cause of compressive myelopathy–features and literature review. *Spine* 1999;24:77–81.
41. Krauss W, Atkinson J, Miller G. Juxtafacet cysts of the cervical spine. *Neurosurgery* 1998;43:1363–1368.
42. Kuntz D, Naveau B, Bardin T, et al. Destructive spondylarthropathy in hemodialyzed patients: a new syndrome. *Arthritis Rheum* 1984;27:369–375.
43. Lawrence J. *Rheumatism in populations.* London: William Heinemann, 1977.
44. Leak A, Cooper J, Dyer S, et al. The Northwick Park Neck Pain Questionnaire: devised to measure neck pain and disability. *Br J Rheumatol* 1994;33:469–474.
45. Le Goff P, Pennec Y, Schwarzberg C. Cervicalgies aiguës fébriles simulant un syndrome méningé révélatrices de la chondrocalcinose articulaire. *Rev Rhum Ed Fr* 1980;47:507–509.
46. Levitz C, Reilly P, Torg J. The pathomechanics of chronic, recurrent cervical nerve root neurapraxia: the chronic burner syndrome. *Am J Sports Med* 1997;25:73–76.
47. Maigne R. Algies rachidiennes et radiculaires. In: Grossiord A, Held JP, eds. *Médecine de rééducation.* Paris: Flammarion Médecine-Sciences, 1981:446–467.
48. Malawski S, Lukawski S. Pyogenic infection of the spine. *Clin Orthop* 1991;272:58–66.
49. Maruyama H, Gejyo F, Arakawa M. Clinical studies of destructive spondyloarthropathy in long-term hemodialysis patients. *Nephron* 1992;61:37–44.
50. Mathern GW, Batzdorf U. Grisel's syndrome: cervical spine clinical, pathologic, and neurologic manifestations. *Clin Orthop* 1989;244:131–146.
51. Mikkelsson M, Salminen J, Kautiainen H. Non-specific musculoskeletal pain in preadolescents: prevalence and 1-year persistence. *Pain* 1997;73:29–35.
52. Mikulowski P, Wollheim FA, Rotmil P, et al. Sudden death in rheumatoid arthritis with atlanto-axial dislocation. *Acta Med Scand* 1975;198:445–451.
53. Niamane R, Birouk N, Benomar A, et al. Rigid spine syndrome: two case reports. *Rev Rhum Engl Ed* 1999;66: 347–350.
54. Nilsson N. The prevalence of cervicogenic headache in a random population sample of 20–59 year olds. *Spine* 1995;20:1884–1888.
55. Özer A, Özek M, Pamir M, et al. Intradural rupture of cervical vertebral disc. *Spine* 1994;19:843–845.
56. Paimela L, Laasonen L, Kankaanpaa E, et al. Progression of cervical spine changes in patients with early rheumatoid arthritis. *J Rheumatol* 1997;24:1280–1284.
57. Prost A, Tanguy G, Audran M, et al. Arthroses erosives atloïdo-axoïdiennes: a propos de trois observations. *Rev Rhum Ed Fr* 1982;49:365–369.
58. Radhakrishnan K, Litchy W, O'Fallon M, et al. Epidemiology of cervical radiculopathy: a population-based study from Rochester, Minnesota, 1976 through 1990. *Brain* 1994;117:325–335.
59. Ramos-Remus C, Gomez-Vargas A, Guzman-Guzman JL, et al. Frequency of atlantoaxial subluxation and neurologic involvement in patients with ankylosing spondylitis. *J Rheumatol* 1995;22:2120–2125.
60. Ranawat CS, O'Leary P, Pellicci P, et al. Cervical spine fusion in rheumatoid arthritis. *J Bone Joint Surg Am* 1979;61:1003–1010.
61. Rawlins BA, Girardi FP, Boachie-Adjei O. Rheumatoid arthritis of the cervical spine. *Rheum Dis Clin North Am* 1998;24:55–65.
62. Reiter MF, Boden SD. Inflammatory disorders of the cervical spine. *Spine* 1998;23:2755–2766.
63. Ring D, Vaccaro AR, Scuderi G, et al. Acute calcific retropharyngeal tendinitis: clinical presentation and pathological characterization. *J Bone Joint Surg Am* 1994;76:1636–1642.
64. Rivett D. The premanipulative vertebral artery testing protocol. *N Z J Physiother* 1995;April:9–12.
65. Rivett D, Sharples K, Milburn P. Effect of premanipulative tests on vertebral artery and internal carotid artery blood flow: a pilot study. *J Manipulative Physiol Ther* 1999;22:368–375.
66. Ross J. Myelopathy. *Neuroimaging Clin N Am* 1995;5:367–384.
67. Ruggieri P. Cervical radiculopathy. *Neuroimaging Clin N Am* 1995;5:349–365.
68. Salvarani C, Macchioni P, Cremonesi T, et al. The cervical spine in patients with psoriatic arthritis: a clinical, radiological and immunogenetic study. *Ann Rheum Dis* 1992;51:73–77.
69. Sanchez J, Jimenez-Escrig A, Saldana C, et al. Cervical epidural abscess: approaches to diagnosis. *J Neurosurg Sci* 1992;36:121–125.
70. Sandmark H, Nisell R. Validity of five common manual neck pain provoking tests. *Scand J Rehabil Med* 1995; 27:131–136.
71. Sheon R. Soft tissue cervical spine syndromes. In: Bland JH, ed. *Disorders of the cervical spine: diagnosis and medical management.* Philadelphia: WB Saunders, 1994:365–372.

72. Spangfort E. Clinical aspects of neck and shoulder pain. *Scand J Rehabil Med* 1995;[Suppl 32]:43–46.
73. Sweeney P. Clinical evaluation of cervical radiculopathy and myelopathy. *Neuroimaging Clin N Am* 1995;5: 321–327.
74. Swezey R. Chronic neck pain. *Rheum Dis Clin North Am* 1996;22:411–437.
75. Tandan R. Rheumatologic neurology. In: Bland JH, ed. *Disorders of the cervical spine: diagnosis and medical management.* Philadelphia: WB Saunders, 1994:17–73.
76. Teresi L, Lufkin R, Reicher M, et al. Asymptomatic degenerative disk disease and spondylosis of the cervical spine: MR imaging. *Radiology* 1987;164:83–88.
77. Trojan D, Pouchot J, Pokrupa R, et al. Diagnosis and treatment of ossificatio of the posterior longitudinal ligament of the spine: report of eight cases and literature review. *Am J Med* 1992;92:296–306.
78. Valat JP, Lioret E. Arthroses cervicales. *Rev Prat* 1996;46:2206–2211.
79. Van Ooij A, Manni JJ, Beuls EA, et al. Cervical spondylodiscitis after removal of a fishbone: a case report. *Spine* 1999;24:574–577.
80. Viikari-Juntura E. Interexaminer reliability of observations in physical examinations of the neck. *Phys Ther* 1987;67:1526–1532.
81. Waldvogel FA, Papageorgiou PS. Osteomyelitis: the past decade. *N Engl J Med* 1980;303:360–370.
82. Walker AP. The presentation, diagnosis and treatment of cervical osteoid osteoma. *Postgrad Med J* 1980;56: 724–729.
83. Warnick C, Sherman M, Lesser R. Aspiration pneumonia due to diffuse cervical hyperostosis. *Chest* 1990;98: 763–764.
84. Watters M, Stears J, Osborn A, et al. Transdural spinal cord herniation: imaging and clinical spectra. *AJNR Am J Neuroradiol* 1998;19:1337–1344.
85. Webb J, March L, Tyndall A. The neck-tongue syndrome: occurrence with cervical arthritis as well as normals. *J Rheumatol* 1984;11:530–533.
86. Wetzel FT, La Rocca H. Grisel's syndrome. *Clin Orthop* 1989:141–152.
87. Wheeler A, Goolkasian P, Baird A, et al. Development of the neck pain and disability scale. *Spine* 1999;24:1290–1294.
88. Wurtz R, Quader Z, Simon D, et al. Cervical tuberculous vertebral osteomyelitis: case report and discussion of the literature. *Clin Infect Dis* 1993;16:806–808.
89. Young A, Corbett M, Winfield J, et al. A prognostic index for erosive changes in the hands, feet, and cervical spines in early rheumatoid arthritis. *Br J Rheumatol* 1988;27:94–101.
90. Zohn D. Relationship of joint dysfunction and soft-tissue problems. *Phys Med Rehabil Clin N Am* 1997;8:69–86.

The Degenerative Cervical Spine,
edited by Marek Szpalski and Robert Gunzburg
Lippincott Williams & Wilkins, Philadelphia © 2001.

5

Natural Evolution

Michel Benoist, *Pierre Guigui

*Department of Orthopedic Surgery and Section of Rheumatology,
University of Paris VII, 75116 Paris, France; *Department of Orthopedic Surgury, Hôpital Beaujon,
92110 Clichy, France*

NATURAL EVOLUTION AND PROGNOSIS OF CERVICAL SPONDYLOSIS
Anatomic Changes • Clinical Complications • Axial Neck Pain • Cervical Radiculopathy • Myelopathy
INFLAMMATORY ARTHROPATHY
Rheumatoid Arthritis • Seronegative Spondylarthropathy

This chapter focuses on the evolution of the anatomic lesions and clinical symptoms and complications of the various forms of cervical arthropathy. A wide range of degenerative and inflammatory conditions can affect the cervical spine. The most common are listed in Table 5.1. Knowledge of the course of degenerative arthropathy is limited (11). There is more precise information about the epidemiology and evolution of inflammatory disorders.

EVOLUTION AND PROGNOSIS OF CERVICAL SPONDYLOSIS

Cervical spondylosis (osteoarthritis) can be defined as degenerative changes in the disc, facets, and uncovertebral joints caused by failure of the cells to produce, maintain, and repair the matrix. The biomechanical changes induce structural modifications, including uncovertebral and facet enlargement and osteophytosis, protrusion of the disc, and thickening of the ligaments. These modifications cause progressive narrowing of the spinal canal and of the foramina. Because of the proximity of the neural structures, these hypertrophic changes can cause radicular or spinal cord compression.

Anatomic Changes

There have been few studies concerning the evolution of the anatomic changes of cervical spondylosis. However, good correlation between radiologic findings and anatomic modifications has been demonstrated (10,31). Gore et al. (13) studied the incidence of degeneration seen on the lateral radiographs of 200 persons without symptoms in five age groups from 20 to 65 years. Tables 5.2 and 5.3 show the number of men and women with degenerative changes in the various age groups. Radiologic findings included disc-space narrowing, end-plate sclerosis, and the presence of anterior and posterior osteophytes. The results of this study showed the progressive evolution of spondylosis with aging. Per-

TABLE 5.1. *Degenerative and inflammatory cervical arthropathies*

Degenerative
　Osteoarthritis (spondylosis)
　Crystal-induced arthropathy
　Diffuse idiopathic skeletal hyperostosis
Inflammatory
　Rheumatoid arthritis
　Ankylosing spondylitis
　Juvenile rheumatoid arthritis
　Psoriatic arthritis
　Reiter syndrome
　Inflammatory bowel disease

TABLE 5.2. *Degenerative changes with aging: Women*

Degenerative change	20–25 yr	30–35 yr	40–45 yr	50–55 yr	60–65 yr
Narrowing	0	2	6	9	13
Sclerosis	0	0	5	7	6
Anterior osteophytes	0	3	6	13	11
Posterior ostoephytes	0	1	5	8	12
Any of the above	0	4	7	14	14

Values are numbers of women.
From Gore DR, Sepic SB, Gardner GM. Roentgenographic findings of the cervical spine in asymptomatic people. *Spine* 1986;11521–525, with permission.

TABLE 5.3. *Degenerative changes with aging: Men*

Degenerative change	20–25 yr	30–35 yr	40–45 yr	50–55 yr	60–65 yr
Narrowing	0	1	4	13	15
Sclerosis	0	1	1	10	13
Anterior osteophytes	1	5	7	16	19
Posterior ostoephytes	0	1	4	10	14
Any of the above	1	5	7	16	19

Values are numbers of men.
From Gore DR, Sepic SB, Gardner GM. Roentgenographic findings of the cervical spine in asymptomatic people. *Spine* 1986;11521–525, with permission.

sons 20 to 25 years of age had normal cervical spines. By 60 to 65 years of age, 95% of the men and 70% of the women had spondylotic changes on the radiographs. More information on anatomic evolution was provided by the same study (12). Cervical lordosis decreases considerably with age in association with disc-space narrowing. Loss or reversal of cervical lordosis was found among 9% of subjects without any relation to age or to degenerative changes. This finding indicates that kyphotic deformities are not necessarily abnormal. This information should be kept in mind in clinical practice. Sagittal diameters of the spinal canal tended to be smaller among older persons. A decrease in sagittal diameter correlated strongly with the size of posterior osteophytes. It appears clearly that the slow, progressive evolution of spondylosis with subsequent narrowing of the spinal canal and foramina is not necessarily correlated with symptoms. Additional factors such as a constitutionally narrow canal or foramen probably are necessary for compression of the cord or the nerve roots.

TABLE 5.4. *Major abnormalities among subjects without symptoms*

Abnormality	Younger than 40 yr (n = 40)	Older than 40 yr (n = 23)	Total (N = 63)
Herniated disc	10	5	8
Bulging disc	0	3	2
Foraminal stenosis	4	20	9

Values are percentages.
From Boden SD, McCown PR, Davis DO, et al. Abnormal magnetic-resonance scans of the cervical spine in asymptomatic subjects. *J Bone Joint Surg Am* 1990;72:1178–1184, with permission.

Magnetic resonance imaging (MRI) shows anatomic modifications more accurately than does plain radiography. Abnormal MR images of the cervical spine among 63 volunteers without symptoms were studied by Boden et al. (3). Table 5.4 presents the abnormalities found in two age groups—persons younger than 40 years and persons older than 40 years. Major abnormalities were found among 19% of the entire group, among 14% of those younger than 40 years, and among 28% of those older than 40 years. The older group had a high prevalence of degenerative changes such as foraminal stenosis, disc bulging, and narrowing at one or several intervertebral spaces. The results of the study (3) confirmed the slow progression of the degenerative lesions that are part of the aging process. A similar MRI study was performed by Teresi et al. (45). Among a group of persons without symptoms, at 65 years of age 23% of the subjects had major structural spondylotic changes causing cord compression. Matsumoto et al. (27) confirmed a high prevalence of degenerative changes with increasing age. Almost 90% of 497 subjects without symptoms had MRI signs of disc degeneration. Moreover, 7.6% of those older than 40 years had disc protrusion, usually median or paramedian, impinging on the cord. How often do osteoarthritic changes cause symptoms? Why and how do they do so? Answers to these questions are controversial.

Clinical Complications

The clinical complications of cervical spondylosis can be divided into four main syndromes—neck pain with or without referred pain, radiculopathy, myelopathy, and vertebral artery compromise. The last complication is discussed in Chapter 7.

In the case of pure neck pain, the local receptors are located in the anulus, ligaments, and facets. In the case of radiculopathy, the nociceptive message starts at the inflamed nerve root and ganglion. Studies of the degenerative lumbar spine have shown that the mechanical stimulus, such as compression or instability, is associated with inflammatory, chemical, and neurogenic factors that sensitize the local receptors perpetuating the nociceptive message at a low level of stimulation. The nociceptive message is transmitted through the dorsal horn of the spinal cord to the ascending pathways and high centers for ultimate cortical processing. In discussion of the evolution of the painful syndromes, neck pain, or radiculopathy, it is important to consider not only peripheral nociception but also the role of the central nervous system. In chronic conditions the central nervous system can become sensitized through a complex cascade of chemical, cellular, and molecular events (7).

Axial Neck Pain

Chronic neck pain without a radicular component is a common symptom. Few studies have evaluated the epidemiologic aspects and evolution of neck pain. Prevalence, deter-

TABLE 5.5. *Changes in severity of pain
between initial and final evaluation*

Change in pain	Percentage
Completely gone	43
Mild but still present	36
Same or worse	21

From Gore DR, Sepic SB, Gardner GM, et al.
Neck pain: a long term follow-up of 205 patients.
Spine 1987:12;1–5, with permission.

minants and consequences of chronic neck pain were investigated in Finland by Makela et al. (24). Using a population-based questionnaire distributed to 8,000 adults, the investigators diagnosed chronic neck syndrome for 9.5% of the men and 13.5% of the women. The most important determinants were age, presence of mental and physical stress at work, having sustained an injury, and being overweight. Frequency and duration of neck pain were assessed by Bovim et al. (4) with a questionnaire sent to a random sample of 10,000 adult Norwegians. Overall 34.4% of the responders had experienced neck pain within the previous year. A total of 13.8% reported neck pain that had lasted more than 6 months. Prevalence increased with age and was higher among women.

The evolution of neck pain and of the various syndromes related to pathologic changes in the neck is poorly known. Moreover, criteria of prognosis have not been established. Gore et al. (13) reviewed the symptoms and radiologic findings of 205 patients with neck pain observed for a minimum of 10 years. The population studied included 106 women and 99 men with a mean age of 43 ± 13 years at the initial evaluation and 58 ± 13 years at the last follow-up evaluation. One hundred twenty-one patients were evaluated after an injury; 76 of them had a whiplash injury. Most of these patients underwent the usual medical treatment that included drugs, collars, and physiotherapy. All patients had neck pain. Approximately 25% of them had a radiating pain in the upper limb. The authors did not indicate whether the arm pain was radicular or referred. Table 5.5 shows the changes in pain after 10 years. Approximately 21% had residual moderate or severe pain. These figures are consistent with those from studies of patients with late whiplash syndrome (1). Unsatisfactory outcome was related to severity of pain at onset, the presence of injury, and the presence of arm pain, especially if bilateral. There was no statistically significant relation between the presence of radiologic findings of degeneration and level of pain, between changes in pain and changes in radiologic abnormalities, or between pain and changes in cervical lordosis or measurements of the sagittal diameter of the cervical canal. There also was no difference in the radiologic evidence of degenerative changes between patients with neck pain and a matched group of subjects without neck pain.

Cervical Radiculopathy

Cervical radiculopathy can be caused by herniation of the nucleus pulposus (lateral soft disc) in the intervertebral foramen or by bony proliferation at the posterolateral margins of the intervertebral space that encroaches the nerve root in the foramen (hard disc). There is little information on the epidemiologic aspects of cervical radiculopathy. According to Hult (16) half of the adult population will have neck and arm pain in its lifetime. No randomized trial has compared nonoperative treatment with observation and the evolution of cervical radiculopathy of nonoperative treatment with operative treatment.

Lees and Turner (22) analyzed the evolution of cervical spondylosis among 51 patients and had complete follow-up data on 85%. Of the 41 patients observed for 10 years or less (range 2 to 11 years), 10 still had moderate disability at final evaluation. In this series no patient's condition progressed to a myelopathic state. Other open-ended studies (5,39) have provided strong indications that cervical radiculopathy usually improves without surgery. However, in a study by Radhakrishnan et al. (34), the frequency of surgery was 26% among 561 patients. The evolution of cervical radiculopathy caused by bony osteophytic spurs has not been investigated. The foramina are larger in persons without symptoms than among those with symptoms, and the foraminal measurements decrease with age (17). There is no clear explanation for the switch from the asymptomatic to the symptomatic state or vice versa after nonoperative treatment.

Information has been acquired about the evolution of cervical soft-disc herniation. Maigne and Deligne (23) conducted a study with 21 patients who underwent repeated computed tomographic examinations after healing of the radiculopathy. In 20 of 21 patients, cervical soft-disc herniation decreased in size or disappeared progressively over 1 year. The largest herniations had the greatest tendency to resolve. Mochida et al. (29) found regression of cervical disc herniation at MRI. Thirty-three patients underwent repeated MRI during conservative therapy for cervical radiculopathy. In 15 patients the herniation decreased progressively in size; in 18 there was no change. Migrating herniation on the sagittal view and lateral herniation on the axial view showed the greatest tendency to regression. All of the patients healed with nonoperative treatment, which shows that soft-disc herniation can be asymptomatic. Regression of disc herniation has been shown to be related to phagocytosis by macrophages with neovascularization, especially in sequestrated lesions (21).

Myelopathy

Understanding the course of cervical spondylosis is especially important in relation to myelopathy. A clinical follow-up study involving 44 patients with radiologic and myelographic evidence of cervical osteoarthritis and signs of cord damage was performed by Lees and Turner (22). The follow-up periods lasted 1 year to 32 years, and 26 patients were observed for 5 years or more. As shown in Table 5.6, the duration of symptoms to follow-up evaluation or death was more than 5 years for 34 patients and more than 10 years for 20 patients. The pattern of evolution was as follows: a few patients' conditions did not deteriorate, but the conditions of most of the patients worsened over the years.

TABLE 5.6. *Myelopathy: Duration of symptoms to follow-up or death*

Duration (yr)	No. of patients
3–5	10
6–10	12
11–15	11
16–20	5
21–30	4
32–40	2

Adapted from Lees F, Turner J. Natural history and prognosis of cervical spondylosis. *Med J* 1963;2:1607–1610, with permission.

Deterioration was slow and progressive among about 20% of the patients, but the common clinical pattern involved periods of worsening followed by static periods. The episodes were prolonged for weeks or months with long intervals of relative stability. At the final follow-up evaluation most of the patients had moderate or severe disability. Ten patients died, but only two deaths were related to myelopathy. A similar pattern of evolution has been found in other studies (6). An acute onset of cord damage after development of soft-disc herniation in a spondylotic small canal and severe hyperextension injury have been documented.

The prognostic value of changes in signal intensity at MRI of the spinal cord is unclear (see Chapter 9). Changes on early T2-weighted images probably are related to edema of the cord, usually are reversible, and have no prognostic value. Severe changes in signal intensity on T1-weighted images usually are irreversible and carry a poorer prognosis. Further prospective studies are needed to clarify the exact significance of cord signal abnormalities. Better understanding of the evolution of myelopathy related to cervical spondylosis is a prerequisite for treatment. For example, is surgery indicated for patients with imaging evidence of compression with abnormal results of electrophysiologic studies but without clinical cord compression symptoms and signs? Such a situation may be encountered in the care of patients with isolated cervical radiculopathy. The evolution of the condition must be borne in mind in discussions of surgery in older patients who have early clinical symptoms, such as those of stage 1 of the Nurik classification.

Cervical spondylosis has a high prevalence among older persons. It is frequently asymptomatic. Axial neck pain is not always self-limiting and becomes chronic among about one third of patients. The epidemiologic characteristics and course of cervical radiculopathy are largely unknown, but few cases necessitate surgery. Patients with myelopathy may have long periods without development of new or worsening symptoms and signs.

INFLAMMATORY ARTHROPATHIES

Rheumatoid Arthritis

Involvement of the cervical spine is a well-known complication of rheumatoid arthritis. All synovial joints of the cervical spine can be affected. Synovitis, however, occurs primarily in the upper segment. Loss of cartilage, bone erosion, and destruction of the transverse ligament are considered the cause of atlantoaxial instability and subluxation, and of superior migration of the odontoid process. The mechanical implications of involvement of the cervical spine in rheumatoid arthritis and indications for surgery are discussed in Chapter 3. The incidence of subluxation at the upper level varies between 40% and 88% according to the radiologic criteria applied (37). Subaxial subluxation occurs among 10% to 20% of patients (38). Severity and duration of the disease, seropositivity, and glucocorticoid therapy are associated with slow evolution of the cervical spinal arthropathy (37,38). Most authors have concentrated on the deformities at C1-2 (20,36,42).

Atlantoaxial instability and subluxation typically are the first anatomic events. Various rates of radiologic progression have been reported. In a 10-year prospective study of 41 cases of atlantoaxial subluxation, 27% of patients had radiologic progression (36). In the same study, 10% of patients had upward translocation of the odontoid process with a resulting decrease in the atlantoaxial interval. Similar rates of radiologic progression have been reported (26,42). The course of subaxial subluxation is less well documented. However, the incidence of subaxial subluxations is lower than that of subluxation at the higher level (8). Patients who have had rheumatoid arthritis for a long time may have subluxation at one or several levels, C3-4 being the most common site (40). Subaxial canal diameter must be carefully studied and followed with MRI to determine operative management before symptoms and signs of cord compression occur. Subaxial subluxation can occur with atlantoaxial instability. Thirty-six percent of patients with multiple-level subluxations described by Pellici et al. (32) had progressive neurologic signs.

Cervical subluxation often is asymptomatic, but it can cause intractable neck pain. Possible neural complications have been well described and do not necessarily correspond with the severity of subluxation (26,36,42). The frequency of complications varies from study to study. Boden et al. (2) have conducted a follow-up study of 73 patients with cervical involvement in rheumatoid arthritis. Fifty-seven percent had a neural complication. Most of the patients underwent surgery. Seven patients were not operated on, and their neurologic status deteriorated (2). Sudden deaths of patients with cervical subluxations have been attributed to fatal medullary compression. Two of the 12 deaths among 41 patients observed by Rana (36) were attributed to neurologic problems. In another study, 10% of the deaths were related to medullary compression (28). The cervical spinal lesions associated with rheumatoid arthritis have been well documented, and indications for surgery have been determined. As indicated by Reiter and Boden (38), however, predicting progression of the anatomic changes and of neural complications is impossible. Careful clinical and imaging surveillance is mandatory at the individual level. Patients with several subluxations and basilar invagination are at high risk of neural complications. Understanding the course of disease is a prerequisite for management and surgical decision making.

Juvenile rheumatoid arthritis is a chronic synovitis of childhood associated with a number of extraarticular manifestations. The cervical spine frequently is affected among patients with systemic and polyarticular disease (9). Cervical subluxation can occur at one or several levels, as can rheumatoid arthritis among adults, but neural complications are rare.

Seronegative Spondylarthropathy

Ankylosing spondylitis is the most frequent of the seronegative forms of spondyloarthropathy, which include psoriasis, Reiter syndrome, and inflammatory bowel disease. Alteration of the cervical spine in ankylosing spondylitis usually is noticed late in the course of disease, after the thoracolumbar and lumbosacral segments and junctions have become involved. Cervical involvement predominantly affects women. Anterior syndesmophyte formation and bony ankylosis of the facets can cause fusion of anterior and posterior elements of the cervical spine and resultant restriction of motion. Vigorous drug treatment, physiotherapy, and patient education should prevent progressive ankylosis and a kyphotic posture.

Cervical kyphosis occurs in severe cases of ankylosing spondylitis. The patients have a spinal flexion deformity that restricts the ability to look forward. Osteotomy at the cervicothoracic junction can correct the line of sight. Corrective osteotomy was performed on 7 of 19 patients who underwent cervical spinal surgery in a retrospective cross-sectional study. Patients' perception of outcome was success in 5 cases, failure in 1 case, and unknown in 1 case. There were no complications of surgery in 4 cases; the 3 other patients had paresthesia in the limbs, which resolved (15).

Inflammation of the synovial tissue of the atlantoaxial joint and of the bursa behind the odontoid process and in front of the transverse ligament can cause rupture of the transverse ligament and deterioration of the odontoid process. These lesions allow anterior atlantoaxial subluxation, which is the most common spinal complication at the cervical level. The prevalence of this complication varies according to the radiologic measurements used to diagnose anterior subluxation. In early reports (25,41) anterior atlantoaxial subluxation was considered a rare complication of ankylosing spondylitis. A more recent study (35) disclosed a higher prevalence than previously reported. One hundred three consecutively registered patients were evaluated within a period of 6 months. The mean duration of disease was 10 years. Anterior atlantoaxial subluxation was found among 22 patients (21%). Atlantoaxial subluxation usually is a late complication, but it can occur early in the course of disease (43). Ramos-Remus et al. (35) found that anterior atlantoaxial subluxation was associated with a prevalence of grade IV radiologic sacroiliitis but not with peripheral arthritis or uveitis.

Anterior atlantoaxial subluxation can be asymptomatic or produce pain in the upper cervicooccipital region. Progressive myelopathy can cause quadriplegia and death (41). The frequency of neural complications has not been systematically assessed. Ramos-Remus et al. (35) found a statistical association between the presence of neural complications and symptoms and signs of vertebrobasilar insufficiency and between the presence of neural complications and abnormal somatosensory-evoked potentials. Two patients in the series needed surgical fusion because of severe cervical cord compression. To avoid neural complications during surgery, any patient with ankylosing spondylitis should be screened with dynamic lateral views before surgery. Upward subluxation of the axis was detected in 2 patients described by Ramos-Remus. This is an uncommon complication of ankylosing spondylitis but is important to recognize because, as in rheumatoid arthritis, it can cause cord and brainstem compression.

Ossification of the posterior longitudinal ligament has been detected in a few cases of ankylosing spondylitis (18,30). A high prevalence of this disorder (16%) has been reported. Association with anterior atlantoaxial subluxation increases the risk of cord compression. Fracture of the ossified ligament after minor trauma can cause sudden neurologic complications (14,33).

Spinal fractures in the ankylosed and often osteoporotic spine can occur after minor trauma. The lower cervical spine is a frequent site. Five of the 13 cases reported by Weinstein et al. (46) were located at the cervical level. Two of the patients eventually had quadriplegia. Radiologic diagnosis of the fracture often is difficult, especially at the cervicothoracic junction. It is therefore essential to use bone scans, computed tomography, or MRI if such lesions are suspected after trauma. Risk of neurologic complications increases with development of epidural hematoma. Nine of 54 patients with ankylosing spondylitis and spinal fractures had a severe epidural hematoma (19). Treatment of patients with cervical fractures complicating ankylosing spondylitis can be conservative by means of reduction with traction and application of a halo vest for cervical immobilization. Spinal decompression and fusion are recommended when reduction cannot be achieved or the structures fail to unite. Early recognition of fractures and appropriate therapy are crucial to reduce the high risk of mortality and permanent neurologic deficit (46).

Involvement of the cervical spine can be detected in other forms of spondyloarthropathy, such as psoriasis, Reiter syndrome, and inflammatory bowel disease. In psoriatic spondylitis, the cervical spine often is the only segment involved. Ankylosis and loss of function are less severe and frequent than in idiopathic ankylosing spondylitis. Abnormalities of the cervical spine, including paravertebral ossification, can occur in Reiter syndrome but are milder and less often encountered than in psoriatic spondylitis. Spondylitis of inflammatory bowel disease is similar to that of classic idiopathic ankylosing spondylitis and has the same pattern of spinal involvement.

The prevalence of anterior atlantoaxial subluxation is high among patients with spondylitis associated with peripheral arthritis. For example, Suarez-Almazor and Russell (44) conducted a study with a group of 17 patients with axial and peripheral arthritis. Three had psoriasis, 4 had Reiter syndrome, and 1 had inflammatory bowel disease, and all 8 eventually had anterior atlantoaxial subluxation. Two other patients with anterior atlantoaxial subluxation had a family history of psoriasis or Reiter syndrome. None of the 21 patients with a pure axial spondylitis had subluxation (44).

Inflammatory arthropathy can involve the cervical spine and generate various structural disorders, which can cause severe neurologic complications. Subluxation appears to be more frequent and severe in association with rheumatoid arthritis than with seronegative arthropathy. Subluxation can be asymptomatic or induce pain, which must not be confused with the pain and stiffness of inflammation of ligaments and facets. The cervical spine should be regularly assessed radiologically, especially before an operation, to detect subluxation and to determine appropriate treatment before cord compression. An ankylosed osteoporotic spine is fragile and prone to fractures. Recurrence of pain after minor trauma may signal the presence of a fracture. Precautions must be taken to avoid severe complications and death.

REFERENCES

1. Benoist M. Natural evolution and resolution of the cervical whiplash syndrome. In: Gunzburg R, Szpalski M, eds. *Whiplash injuries.* Philadelphia: Lippincott-Raven, 1998:117–126.
2. Boden SD, Dodge LD, Bohlman HH, et al. Rheumatoid arthritis of the cervical spine: a long term analysis with predictors of paralysis and recovery. *J Bone Joint Surg Am* 1993;75:1282–1227.
3. Boden SD, McCown PR, Davis DO, et al. Abnormal magnetic-resonance scans of the cervical spine in asymptomatic subjects. *J Bone Joint Surg Am* 1990;72:1178–1184.
4. Bovim G, Schrader H, Sand T. Neck pain in the general population. *Spine* 1994;19:1307–1309.
5. Bush K, Hillier S. Outcome of cervical radiculopathy treated with periradicular, epidural corticosteroid injections: a prospective study with independent clinical review. *Eur Spine J* 1996;5:319–325.
6. Clark CR. *Degenerative conditions of the spine.* In: Frymoyer JW, ed. New York: Raven Press, 1991:1145–1165.
7. Codere TJ, Katz Y, Vaccharino AI, et al. Contributions of central neuroplasticity to pathological pain. *Pain* 1993; 52:259–285.
8. Conaty JP, Mongan ED. Cervical fusion in rheumatoid arthritis. *J Bone Joint Surg* 1981;63:1218–1227.
9. Fried JA, Arthreya B, Gregg JR, et al. The cervical spine in juvenile rheumatoid arthritis. *Clin Orthop* 1983;179:102–108.
10. Friedenberg ZB, Edeiken J, Spencer N, et al. Degenerative changes of the cervical spine. *J Bone Joint Surg Am* 1959;41:61–102.
11. Garfin SR. Spine focus: cervical spine [Editorial]. *Spine* 1998;23:2661–2662.
12. Gore DR, Sepic SB, Gardner GM. Roentgenographic findings of the cervical spine in asymptomatic people. *Spine* 1986;11:521–525.
13. Gore DR, Sepic SB, Gardner GM, et al. Neck pain: a long term follow-up of 205 patients. Spine 1987;12:1–5.
14. Ho EKW, Xeong JY. Traumatic tetraplegia: a rare neurologic complication in ankylosing spondylitis with ossification of the posterior longitudinal ligament of the cervical spine. *Spine* 1987;12:403–405.
15. Howe Koh W, Garrett SL, Calin A. Cervical spine surgery in ankylosing spondylitis: is the outcome good? *Clin Rheumatol* 1997;16:466–470.
16. Hult L. The Munkfors investigation. *Acta Orthop Scand Suppl* 1959;16:1–10.
17. Humphrey SC, Hodges SD, Patwardhan A, et al. The natural history of the cervical foramen in symptomatic and asymptomatic individuals aged 20–60 years as measured by magnetic resonance imaging: a descriptive approach. *Spine* 1998;20:2180–2184.
18. Hunter T. The spinal complications of ankylosing spondylitis. *Semin Arthritis Rheum* 1989;19:172–182.
19. Hunter T, Dubo H. Spinal fractures complicating ankylosing spondylitis. *Ann Intern Med* 1978;88:546–549.
20. Isdale JC, Conlon PW. Atlanto-axial subluxation: a six year follow-up report. *Ann Rheum Dis* 1971;30:387–389.
21. Ito T, Yamada M, Ikuta F, et al. Histologic evidence of absorption of sequestration: type herniated disc. *Spine* 1996;21:230–234.

22. Lees F, Turner J. Natural history and prognosis of cervical spondylosis. *Med J* 1963;2:1607–1610.
23. Maigne JY, Deligne L. Computed tomography follow-up study of 21 cases of nonoperatively treated cervical soft disc herniations. *Spine* 1994;19:189–191.
24. Makela M, Heliovaara M, Sievers K, et al. Prevalence, determinants and consequences of chronic neck pain in Finland. *Am J Epidemiol* 1991;134:1356–1367.
25. Martel W. The occipito-atlanto-axial joints in rheumatoid arthritis and ankylosing spondylitis. *AJR Am J Roentgenol* 1961;86:223–240.
26. Mathews JA. Atlanto-axial subluxation in rheumatoid arthritis: a five year follow-up study. *Ann Rheum Dis* 1974;33:526–531.
27. Matsumoto M, Fujimura Y, Suzuk N, et al. Magnetic resonance imaging of cervical intervertebral disc in asymptomatic subjects. *J Bone Joint Surg Br* 1998;80:19–24.
28. Mikulowski P, Wolheim FA, Rotmil D, et al. Sudden death in rheumatoid arthritis with atlanto-axial dislocation. *Acta Med Scand* 1975;198:445–451.
29. Mochida K, Komori H, Okawa A, et al. Regression of cervical disc herniation observed on magnetic resonance images. *Spine* 1998;23:990–997.
30. Olivieri I, Trippi D, Gemignani G, et al. Ossification of the posterior longitudinal ligament in ankylosing spondylitis. *Arthritis Rheum* 1988;31:452–457.
31. Payne EE, Spillane JD. An anatomopathological study of 70 specimens with particular reference to the problem of cervical spondylosis. *Brain* 1957;80:571–596.
32. Pellici PM, Ranawat CS, Tsairis P, et al. A prospective study of the progression of rheumatoid arthritis of the cervical spine. *J Bone Joint Surg Am* 1981;63:342–350.
33. Pouchot J, Watts CS, Esdaile JM, et al. Sudden quadriplegia complicating ossification of the posterior longitudinal ligament and diffuse idiopathic skeletal hyperostosis. *Arthritis Rheum* 1987;30:1069–1072.
34. Radhakrishnan K, Litchy WJ, Fallon NM, et al. Epidemiology of cervical radiculopathy: a population based study from Rochester Minnesota, 1976 through 1994. *Brain* 1994;117:125–130.
35. Ramos-Remus C, Gomez-Vaigus A, Guzman-Guzman JL, et al. Frequency of atlantoaxial subluxation and neurologic involvement in patients with ankylosing spondylitis. *J Rheumatol* 1995;22:2120–2125.
36. Rana NA. Natural history of atalanto-axial subluxation in rheumatoid arthritis. *Spine* 1989;14:1054–1056.
37. Rasker J, Cosh JA. Radiological study of cervical spine and hand in patients with rheumatoid arthritis of 15 years duration: an assessment of the effects of corticosteroid treatment. *Ann Rheum Dis* 1978;37:529–535.
38. Reiter MF, Boden SD. Inflammatory disorders of the cervical spine. *Spine* 1998;23:2755–2766.
39. Saal JS, Saal JA, Yurth EF. Nonoperative management of herniated cervical intervertebral disc with radiculopathy. *Spine* 1996;21:1877–1883.
40. Santavirta S, Konhinen YT, Sandelin J, et al. Operations for unstable cervical spine in rheumatoid arthritis: sixteen cases of subaxial subluxation. *Acta Orthop Scand* 1990;61:106–110.
41. Sharp J, Purser DW. Spontaneous atlanto-axial dislocation in ankylosing spondylitis and rheumatoid arthritis. *Ann Rheum Dis* 1961;20:47–89.
42. Smith PH, Benn RT, Sharp J. Natural history of rheumatoid cervical luxations. *Ann Rheum Dis* 1972;31:431–439.
43. Sorin S, Askari A, Moskowitz RW. Atlantoaxial subluxation as a complication of early ankylosing spondylitis: two case reports and a review of the literature. *Arthritis Rheum* 1979;22:273–276.
44. Suarez-Almazor ME, Russell AS. Anterior atlanto-axial subluxation in patients with spondyloarthropathies: association with peripheral disease. *J Rheumatol* 1988;15:973–975.
45. Teresi LM, Lufkin RB, Reicher MA. Asymptomatic degenerative disc disease and spondylosis of the cervical spine: MR imaging. *Radiology* 1987;164:83–88.
46. Weinstein PR, Karmpan RR, Gall EP, et al. Spinal cord injury, spinal fracture and spinal stenosis in ankylosing spondylitis. *J Neurosurg* 1982;39:609–616.

The Degenerative Cervical Spine,
edited by Marek Szpalski and Robert Gunzburg
Lippincott Williams & Wilkins, Philadelphia © 2001.

6

Neurologic Symptoms

A. Müller, Jiri Dvorak

Spine Unit, Department of Neurology, Schulthess Clinic, Zurich, Switzerland

---

SYMPTOMS AND SIGNS
History and Examination • Pain • Motor and Muscular Weakness • Sensory Loss • Changes In or Loss of Muscle Jerk Reflexes
GAIT
Normal Gait • Abnormal Gait
DIAGNOSIS AND DIFFERENTIAL DIAGNOSIS
Segmental Root Patterns • Cervical Myelopathy • Multiple Sclerosis • Motor-Neuron Disease, Amyotrophic Lateral Sclerosis, Charcot Disease • Polyradiculitis, Guillain-Barré Syndrome • Neuralgic Shoulder Amyotrophy • Lyme Disease, Borreliosis • Double Crush Combination of Nerve Root and Peripheral Nerve Compression • Psychogenic Disorders
CONCLUSION

Syndromes involving the cervical spine are caused by a lesion affecting the spinal cord, the nerve roots, or the vertebrae. Many arthritic disorders produce changes in the cervical spine that eventually affect the cervical cord and roots. Many of these conditions are degenerative or inflammatory and cause problems mostly by directly compressing neural tissue.

Radiologic evidence of degenerative changes in the cervical spine is common with aging. Within the fourth decade of life, 30% of persons without symptoms have degenerative changes in the intervertebral discs. In the seventh decade, as many as 90% have degenerative alterations (9). It is always important to interpret radiologic findings within the framework of the clinical signs and symptoms. If symptoms and radiologic findings cannot be logically correlated, the presence of a different pathologic condition should be suspected and appropriate investigations performed.

SYMPTOMS AND SIGNS

The spinal cord and its associated roots are susceptible to many types of injury, infection, congenital disturbances, and other destructive processes. *Cervical spondylosis* denotes progressive degenerative changes in the spine that begin in the cervical intervertebral discs and extend to the surrounding bones and soft tissues. The fundamental elements of a correct diagnosis of cervical spinal syndromes are the history and precise

TABLE 6.1. *Cervical disorders: Main points for first differential diagnosis*

Central
   Cervical myelopathy
   Brain or brain stem disorder
Peripheral
   Root
   Peripheral nerves of upper limb
Upper extremity
   Shoulder
   Upper limb
   Elbow
   Hand
Other

neurologic and musculoskeletal examinations. It is important to differentiate whether the patterns stem from a central or peripheral cervical disorder (Table 6.1), both, or another condition. If physical, the syndrome patterns may stem from nerve root compression (Table 6.2), a disorder of a peripheral nerve of the upper limb, or a disorder of the shoulder, elbow, or hand.

TABLE 6.2. *Segmental root patterns of neck and the upper extremity*

Nerve root	Pain	Motor weakness	Sensory loss	Reflex	Comments
C1	—	—	—	—	Vestigeal nerves
C2	Neck—suboccipital, occipital	Paraspinal	Suboccipital	—	Sensory loss may not be present
C3-4	Neck—suboccipital Auricular—mandibular Paravertebral interscapular	Neck muscle	Lateral neck, acromioclavicular joint area	Scapulohumoralis	Phrenic nerve paralysis if severely involved
C5	Neck—shoulder anterior arm	Deltoid, biceps	Deltoid area Lateral arm	Biceps	—
C6	Neck, shoulder, medial scapula, lateral arm, dorsum, forearm	Biceps selectively Wrist extension	Lateral forearm Thumb and index finger	Biceps, Brachioradialis	Wrist extension is not pure C6 Pronation may be selectively involved
C7	Neck, shoulder, medial scapula, lateral arm, dorsum forearm	Triceps	Index, middle, and forefinger	Triceps	May also test strength of wrist flexors and finger extensors
C8-T1	Neck, medial scapula, medial arm and forearm	Intrinsic hand muscles	Ring and little finger medial upper arm	—	Painless weakness and atrophy may be only signs T1 check for Horner syndrome

History and Examination

We generally ask patients to give us an unstructured account of problems involving the neck or upper limb and of headaches. We then systematically explore the various features.

Pain

Pain arising from the cervical spine and felt in the neck and back of the head, even though projected into the shoulder, arm, and hand, is evoked or enhanced by certain movements and positions of the neck. The pain is accompanied by limitation of motion of the neck and by tenderness to palpation over the cervical spine. Details of the onset, severity, and quality of pain are important for diagnosis. Also important is localization of the pain. For patients with chronic pain, important details are the beginning of increases, the pattern and quality of spread, frequency, and duration.

Motor and Muscular Weakness

Muscle weakness, paralysis, and reduced strength of muscle contraction are manifested by diminished power of single contractions, resistance to opposition (peak power), and by endurance during sustained performance of demanded movements. In such testing, patients may be reluctant to contract muscles fully in a painful limb, and pain itself may cause reflex diminution in the power of contraction (algesic paresis). Weakness of muscle contraction is important when it is associated with other abnormalities, such as tenderness or atrophy of muscles and changes in or loss of jerk reflexes. Atrophy of muscle is the main trophic disturbance caused by interruption of the motor nerves. With trophic changes, a number of chronic forms of polyneuropathy occur, and the feet, hands, and spine can become deformed. This is most likely to occur when the disease begins during childhood.

Sensory Loss

Accurate testing of sensory modalities can be difficult. It depends a great deal on the cooperation of the patient. During testing differential diagnostic patterns, such as central, root, peripheral nerve, diffuse, and glovelike, must be considered. Sensory modalities—touch, pressure, pain, temperature, and vibration, and joint position—must be evaluated thoroughly. Sensory abnormalities—tickling, prickling, electric stimulation, bandlike sensations, paresthesia, pins and needle, dysesthesia, and numbness—also must be evaluated. It needs to be determined whether the pattern is segmental or peripheral nerve distribution or polyneuropathy.

Changes In or Loss of Muscle Jerk Reflexes

Muscle jerk reflexes or tendon stretch reflexes are an important and often not easy investigation in addition to muscle testing to evaluate abnormalities in muscle pattern if there is a peripheral or central pattern of pathologic reflexes. Diminution or loss of jerk reflexes is an invariable sign of peripheral nerve disease. Pathologically increased tendon reflexes, hyperreflexia, is a typical sign of a central nerve system disorder. It also is possible that both central and peripheral nervous disorders are present.

GAIT

Normal Gait

The normal gait seldom attracts attention, but it should be observed with care if slight deviations from normal are to be appreciated. The body is erect, the head is straight, and the arms hang loosely and gracefully at the sides, each moving rhythmically forward with the opposite leg. When analyzed in detail, the requirements for locomotion in an upright position can be reduced to the following elements: antigravity support of the body, stepping, maintenance of equilibrium, and a decrease of propulsion.

Abnormal Gait

Because normal body posture and locomotion require intact labyrinthine function, proprioception, and vision (we see where we are going and pick our steps), the effect of deficits in these senses on normal function is worth documenting in an examinations of a patient with an abnormal gait. When confronted with a disorder of gait, the examiner must observe the patient's stance and the attitude and dominant positions of the legs, trunk, and arms. It is good practice to watch patients as they walk into the examination room, when they are apt to walk more naturally than during special tests. For example, cerebellar gait is characterized by a wide base (separation of legs), unsteadiness, irregularity of steps, and lateral veering. Steps are uncertain, some are shorter and others longer than intended, and the patient may compensate for these abnormalities by shortening the steps and shuffling, that is, keeping both feet on the ground simultaneously. In the differential diagnosis of gait disorders, it is important to perform differentiate cerebellar ataxia, sensory ataxia, and hemiplegic and paraplegic (spastic) gait with its typical lesions from spastic-ataxic gait disorders due to cervical myelopathy.

DIAGNOSIS AND DIFFERENTIAL DIAGNOSIS

On the basis of the history and physical signs and symptoms, a neurologic evaluation should be designed to confirm the diagnosis and determine treatment. The steps are as follows:

1. Electromyography (EMG)
2. Electroneurography
3. Sensory-evoked potentials
4. Motor-evoked potentials
5. Computed tomography
6. Magnetic resonance imaging (MRI)
7. Analysis of cerebrospinal fluid (CSF)

The following patterns of disorders are important in the differential diagnosis of degenerative cervical disorders (Table 6.3):

TABLE 6.3. *Differential diagnosis of degenerative cervical disorders*

Neurologic disorders
    Multiple sclerosis
    Amyotrophic lateral sclerosis
    Cerebrovascular disease
    Syringomyelia
    Peripheral nerve entrapment neuropathy, double crush
    Brachial plexus injury or neuritis, thoracic outlet syndrome
Inflammatory disorders
    Polyradiculitis, Guillain-Barré syndrome
    Neuralgic shoulder amyotrophy (Turner, Parsonage)
    Osteoarthritis (upper and lower cervical spine)
    Rheumatoid arthritis, ankylosing spondylitis
    Fibrositis (trigger point syndrome)
    Polymyalgia rheumatica
Neoplasia
    Metastatic disease, primary bone tumors, intradural tumors
    Extraspinal tumors (Pancoast tumor, intracerebral tumors, shoulder girdle tumors)
Infection
    Lyme disease, borreliosis
    Vertebral osteomyelitis, discitis
Primary shoulder and upper extremity problems
    Subacromial bursitis, tendinitis
    Impingement syndrome or rotator cuff tear
    Shoulder instabilities, glenohumeral arthritis, adhesive capsulitis
    Tennis elbow
    Reflex sympathetic dystrophy
Psychogenic disorders
Visceral and miscellaneous disorders
    Cardiac ischemia
    Gastrointestinal disorders, gallbladder disorders
    Vertebral artery compression
    Temporomandibular joint disease
    Thyroid and lymph node masses

Segmental Root Patterns

Segmental root patterns are important in the overall understanding of the various disorders of the cervical spine (Table 6.3). The C2 sensory ramus also is important. It serves as a pain pathway from an arthritic atlantoaxial articulation or subluxation. Compression or irritation of this root produces unilateral pain or paresthesia in the upper neck, suboccipital area, or retromastoid region. This pain usually is aggravated by neck motion and is associated with localized tenderness in this region. The C3 and C4 roots are rarely involved in cervical disc herniation but may be impinged upon with arthrosis of the posterior articulations. In compression of these roots, there usually is no motor deficit. Pain, however, is characteristic in that it spreads from the side of the neck to the region of the acromioclavicular joint, stopping just short of the deltoid muscle.

Cervical Myelopathy

Cervical spondylotic myelopathy (Table 6.4) is a syndrome that includes spastic lower extremity weakness, lack of coordination, paresthesia, proprioceptive abnormalities, and sphincter dysfunction. Specific myelopathic syndromes depend on the etiologic process. Myelopathy can occur alone or with radiculopathy. Neck pain may or may not be associ-

TABLE 6.4. *Differential diagnosis of cervical myelopathy*

Cervical spondylotic myelopathy
   Syringomyelia, Chiari malformation, Klippel-Feil abnormality, congenital osteopetrosis,
Congenital dystonic cerebral palsy
Ossification of the posterior longitudinal ligament
Vascular, vasculopathy
   Malformation, vasculitis, anterior cord syndrome (anterior spinal artery), spinal cord infection
Rheumatoid arthritis
   Atlantoaxial dislocation
Arthropathy
Neoplasia
   Neurofibroma, meningioma
   Metastasis, carcinomatosis, lipoma
Motor neuron disease
Amyotrophic lateral sclerosis, multiple sclerosis, degeneration

ated with myelopathy. Cervical cord compression often does not produce neck or limb pain, but neck flexion, extension, or axial loading induces an electrical shock sensation that shoots down the cord and into the extremities. This sign is called the *Lhermitte sign.*

Neurologic Signs of Cervical Myelopathy

Motor

- Increased tone or spasticity in the lower extremities
- Weakness of the lower extremities
- Ataxia or difficulty controlling lower extremities while walking

Sensory

- Impaired sensation to pin prick, light touch, or temperature that may correspond to a level
- Impaired position or vibration in the lower extremities with dorsal column involvement

Reflexes

- Hyperactive deep tendon reflexes in the lower extremities
- Hypoactive deep tendon reflexes in the upper extremities in nerve roots C5, C6, or C7 in association with cervical radiculopathy
- Hyperactive reflexes in the upper extremities if the cervical spinal cord above C4 is involved
- Positive Babinski sign

Multiple Sclerosis

It is not always easy to differentiate cervical spondylosis with myelopathy from the predominantly spinal form of multiple sclerosis. Progressive paraparesis or tetraparesis can occur in both conditions. However, patients with cervical myelopathy are usually older, oligoclonal bands in the CSF are absent, and visual evoked potentials are normal. It is well recognized that both conditions can occur simultaneously. In an excellent monograph, Kesselring (10) describes the role of MRI in evaluations for multiple sclerosis.

MRI is the most sensitive means of detecting CNS lesions in demyelinating disease. However, the MRI findings must be interpreted in light of the clinical findings and results of other studies, such as abnormal evoked potentials, including motor evoked potentials, and the presence of oligoclonal bands in the CSF. Caution must be exercised in evaluations of elderly patients, among whom white-matter abnormalities, probably vascular in origin, appear with increasing frequency.

It is also possible that both diseases can cause progressive symptoms, especially weakness and gait disturbances. The indications for decompressive surgery must be determined in light of the radiologic and clinical findings. Surgery should be considered only if considerable narrowing of the spinal canal and compression of the spinal cord are verified.

Motor Neuron Disease, Amyotrophic Lateral Sclerosis, Charcot Disease

Motor neuron disease usually begins in the fourth to sixth decade of life. The disease is characterized by a combination of muscle atrophy due to degeneration of the anterior horn cells in the spinal cord and spasticity with other pyramidal signs due to involvement of the lateral corticospinal tract. Early in the course of disease, the patient reports painful muscle cramps, often nocturnal, and observes muscle fasciculations. Muscle atrophy, increased muscle tone, and hyperreflexia usually occur later, and sensation remains normal. The clinical diagnosis is supported by typical findings during quantitative and qualitative EMG. These findings include markedly increased duration of motor unit potentials, signs of denervation, such as fibrillations, sharp positive waves, and fasciculations in the upper and lower extremity muscles. The prognosis is unfavorable, and the disease progresses rapidly. Motor neuron disease must be differentiated from involvement of the anterior horn cells at the level of the cervical spine due to spinal cord compression, called *myelopathic hand.* In this condition the EMG tracing for the lower limb muscles is normal, but for the muscles of upper extremities, typical signs of motor neuron degeneration are present.

Polyradiculitis, Guillain-Barré Syndrome

Polyradiculitis is an acute, most probably viral inflammatory disease characterized by ascending paralysis of the muscles of the extremities, commonly paraesthesia, and not infrequently diffuse pain in the limbs. Areflexia, hypotonia, and sensory disturbance are characteristic. Pyramidal tract signs are absent. CSF analysis typically reveals an increased amount of protein in the presence of a normal cell count. Electroneurography shows diminished peripheral conduction velocity, and signs of denervation are common on EMG tracings of affected muscles. Central motor conduction time measured with motor evoked potentials usually is normal. Spontaneous recovery occurs within months in most cases. Use of steroids usually is not indicated. In selected cases, especially those of younger patients or patients with recurrent symptoms, plasmapheresis or use of immunoglobulins may be useful.

Neuralgic Shoulder Amyotrophy

Acutely occurring shoulder and neck pain followed by weakness and atrophy of the shoulder girdle and upper limb muscles was first described as acute brachial radiculitis and later by the same authors as neuralgic amyotrophy. Bilateral neuralgic amyotrophy occurs in approximately one-fourth of cases. An inflammatory allergic cause is postulated. Clinical examination reveals weakness and atrophy of the shoulder girdle and arm muscles, hyporeflexia, and hyperesthesia in about one fourth of cases. EMG of the affected muscles shows typical signs of denervation with fibrillation and sharp positive waves. Most patients recover within 9 to 12 months, although longer periods of recovery have been observed. Shoulder amyotrophy, which has an acute onset and commonly is associated with neck pain, should be differentiated from acute radicular syndromes due to disc herniation or narrowing of the intervertebral foramina.

Lyme Disease, Borreliosis

Lyme disease is a spirochetal infection characterized by exacerbations and remissions in different stages. It has dermatologic, neurologic, rheumatic, and cardiac manifestations. Meningoradiculitis with sensory and motor dysfunction can mimic vertebral disc herniation or radicular compression due to foraminal stenosis. If the central nervous system is involved, inflammatory changes—increases in lymphocyte count and the amount of total protein—are found in the CSF. These changes are caused by intrathecal production of immunoglobulins. Oligoclonal bands also may be detected. A *Borrelia* titer in the IgA fraction of the serum of 1:124 suggests the presence of Lyme disease. A titer greater than 1:1,062 is almost certain proof of infection. Therapy for the neurologic complications of Lyme disease is high doses of penicillin.

Double Crush Combination of Nerve Root and Peripheral Nerve Compression

Not infrequently, a combination of nerve root and peripheral nerve compression can occur coincidentally. The primary pathologic process usually can be elucidated by means of neurophysiologic assessment, including electroneurography with measurement of sensory and motor conduction velocities, F-wave latency, and sensory and motor evoked potentials. Somatosensory evoked potentials following nerve and segmental stimulation do not reliably confirm a diagnosis of unilateral radiculopathy with sensory and motor deficits (23). Schmid et al. (23) concluded that sensory evoked potentials are not helpful in the electrophysiologic investigation of neck-arm pain of unknown origin. It appears that the sensitivity of motor evoked potentials is high for nerve root or spinal cord compression, although the specificity is not yet known. It is also not known whether the sensitivity can be increased with a combination of motor evoked and sensory evoked potentials.

The most common peripheral nerve compression is the presence of cervical radiculopathy of the median nerve at the level of the carpal tunnel (19). If marked slowing of conduction velocity is present over the carpal tunnel, carpal tunnel syndrome should be managed first, either conservatively or surgically, even if additional nerve root compression is suspected. A similar approach should be taken in the management of suspected compression of the ulnar and radial nerves.

Psychogenic Disorders

A psychogenic disorder is understood to be a neurotic disorder with somatic or psychosomatic symptoms. The most common of these are sensory symptoms such as hypesthesia or hyperesthesia. The localization of the sensory disturbance depends on what the patient perceives as being an anatomic distribution, for example the forearm or one side of the body, with a strict boundary in the midline. Other than the nonanatomic distribution of the sensory signs, findings such as intact skin reflexes, such as the cremasteric reflex, should alert the physician to the possibility of a psychosomatic disorder. The motor symptoms usually affect one extremity or part of an extremity. Persons with hysteria may enjoy the role of having an illness and sometimes go as far as readily accepting surgery if it is suggested (furor operatorius passivus). Malingerers want to appear sick; persons with hysteria want to be sick.

In the clinical assessment, it is not always easy to differentiate psychogenic disorders from those of somatic origin, especially if marked degenerative changes can be radiologically documented. Besides a careful clinical examination, EMG electroneurography, and especially the motor evoked potentials may be useful to verify or disprove motor palsy.

CONCLUSION

Care must be exercised in interpreting clinical and radiologic findings when evaluating cervical spondylosis and involvement of neural structures, especially if surgery is discussed as a therapeutic procedure. If the historical, neurologic, and musculoskeletal findings do not explain the radiologic findings, further investigation is indicated to exclude systemic disease. Investigations include electrophysiologic tests, transcranial magnetic stimulation, CSF analysis, and MRI.

REFERENCES

1. Bleuler E. *Lehrbuch der Psychiatrie,* 11th ed. Berlin: Springer Verlag, 1969.
2. Brain W, Wilkinson M. The association of cervical spondylosis and multiple sclerosis. *Brain* 1957;80:456–478.
3. Burgdorfer W, Barbour A, Hayes S. Lyme disease: a tick-born spirochaetosis? *Science* 1982;216:1317.
4. Dvorak J. The neurologist's view of differential diagnosis in patients with cervical spine disorders. In: *Cervical spondylosis and similar disorders.* Ono K, Dvorak J, Dunn E, eds. London: World Scientific, 1998:287–295.
5. Dvorak J, Herdmann J, Theiler R. Magnetic transcranial brain stimulation: painless evaluation of central motor pathways: normal values and clinical application in spinal cord diagnostics—upper extremities. *Spine* 1990;15: 155–160.
6. Ebara S, Yonenobu K, Fujiwara K, et al. Myelopathy hand characterized by muscle wasting: a different type of myelopathic hand in patients with cervical spondylosis. *Spine* 1988;13:785–791.
7. Guillain G. Sur un syndrome de radiculo-névrite avec hyperalbuminose du liquide céphalo-radidien sans réaction cellulaire. *Bull Soc Med Hop Paris* 1916;40:1462–1470.
8. Janssen BA, Theiler R, Grob D, et al. The role of motor evoked potentials in psychogenic paralysis. *Spine* 1995; 20:608–611.
9. Kellgren J, Lawrence J. Osteo-arthrosis and disc degeneration in an urban population. *Ann Rheum Dis* 1958;17: 288–397.
10. Kesselring J. *Multiple sklerose,* 2nd ed. Berlin: Kohlhammer 1993.
11. Kesselring J, Miller D, McManus D, et al. Quantitative magnetic resonance imaging in multiple sclerosis: the effect of high dose intravenous methylprednisone. *J Neurol Neurosurg Psychiatry* 1989;1989a:14–17.
12. Kesselring J, Miller D, Robb S, et al. Acute disseminated encephalomyelitis: MRI findings and the distinction from multiple sclerosis. *Brain* 1990;113:291–302.
13. Kesselring J, Ormerod I, Miller DE, et al. *Magnetic resonance imaging in multiple sclerosis.* New York: Georg Thieme, 1989.
14. Lambert E. *Electromyography in amyotrophic lateral sclerosis in motor neuron diseases.* New York: Grune & Stratton, 1969.
15. Lane RJM, Dewar JA. Bilateral neuralgic amyotrophy. *Br Med J* 1978;I:895.
16. Lawrence J. Disc degeneration: its frequency and relationship to symptoms. *Ann Rheum Dis* 1969;28:121–136.
17. Löffel NB, Rossi LN, Mumenthaler M, et al. The Landry-Guillain-Barré syndrome: complications, prognosis and natural history in 123 cases. *J Neurol Sci* 1977;33:71–79.
18. Ludin HP. *Praktische elektromyographie,* 4th ed. Stuttgart: F Enke Verlag, 1993.
19. Marie P, Roix C. Atrophie isolée de l'eminence thénar d'origine névritique: rôle du ligament annulaire antérieur du carpe dans la pathogénie de la lésion. *Rev Neurol (Paris)* 1913;26:647–649.
20. Meier C, Grahmann F, Englehardt A, et al. Peripheral nerve disorders in Lyme-borreliosis: nerve biopsy study from eight cases. *Acta Neuropathol (Berl)* 1989;79:271–278.

21. Meier C, Reulen H, Huber P, et al. Meningoradiculoneuritis mimicking vertebral disc herniation: a "neurosurgical" complication of Lyme-borreliosis. *Acta Neurochir (Wien)* 1989;89:42–46.
22. Mumenthaler M. Charakteristische Krankheitsbilder nicht rheumatischer peripherer Nervenschäden: Ursachen und Diagnose. *Nervenarzt* 1974;45:61–66.
23. Schmid UD, Hess CW, Ludin HP. Somatosensory evoked potentials following nerve and segmental stimulation do not confirm cervical radiculopathy with sensory deficit. *J Neurol Neurosurg Psychiatry* 1988;51:182–187.
24. Tepe HJ. Die Häufigkeit osteochondrotischer Röntgenbefunde der Halswirbelsäule bei 400 symptomfreien Erwachsenen. *Rofo Fortschr Geb Rontgenstr Neuen Bildgeb Verfahr* 1985;6:659–663.
25. Tsairis P, Jordan B. Neurological evaluation of cervical spinal disorders. In: Camins MB, O'Leary PF, eds. *Disorders of the cervical spine.* Baltimore: Williams & Wilkins, 1992:11–22.
26. Turner JWA, Parsonage M. Acute brachial radiculitis. *Br Med J* 1944;2:592–594.
27. Turner JWA, Parsonage M. Neuralgic amyotrophy (paralytic brachial neuritis): with special reference to prognosis. *Lancet* 1957;2:209–212.

The Degenerative Cervical Spine,
edited by Marek Szpalski and Robert Gunzburg
Lippincott Williams & Wilkins, Philadelphia © 2001.

7

The Vertebral Arteries in Degenerative and Inflammatory Spine Disease

Philippe Gutwirth

Department of Vascular Surgery, Centenary Clinic, B-2018 Antwerp, Belgium

THE VERTEBRAL ARTERIES
    Anatomy • Physiology
EXTRINSIC COMPRESSION
    Mechanism and Occurrence • Clinical Presentation • Diagnostic Techniques • Medical
    Therapy • Surgical Therapy
IATROGENIC INJURY TO THE VERTEBRAL ARTERY
CONCLUSION

Degenerative and inflammatory disease of the cervical spine may produce osteophytic spurs, hernial protrusions, or structural instability. Squeezing of neighboring structures may ensue and cause pain or functional loss. The same structures are indirectly at risk when surgical or physical therapy is used to manage the spinal problem. The vertebral arteries are discussed in this context.

THE VERTEBRAL ARTERIES

Anatomy

Normally both vertebral arteries arise as side branches of the subclavian arteries. Their origin and initial course are directed upward and slightly inward and rearward. They reach and enter the transverse canal at C6. After a vertical and straight to slightly winding ascent, they run somewhat laterally through the transverse foramen of C2 and then take a remarkably warped bend through the C1 foramen, around the lateral bodies. At the upper edge of C1 they run posteromedially in a bony gutter and take another remarkable bend to perforate from behind the atlantooccipital membrane in the anterior direction. Both arteries then run along the medulla and converge on the clivus, finally merging into the one basilar artery. Figure 7.1 shows the effect of the anatomic bends in the frontal or sagittal plane and illustrates the traditional segmental numbering. Many anatomic variations exist in branching, sideways uniqueness, point of entry in the transverse canal, size and possible unilateral dominance (even possible one-sided aplasia), possible duplication, and tortuosity (8). The tortuosity can be anything from mere exaggeration of the natural bends to curious buckling or looping (Fig. 7.1A). Disease may increase the tortuosity (1,16). Sympathetic fibers and veins run along the arteries. Small muscular, vertebral,

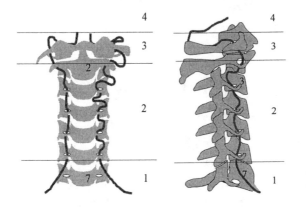

FIG. 7.1. Effect of the anatomic bends of the vertebral arteries in the frontal and sagittal planes. Traditional segmental numbering.

and spinal branches originate at the cervical level. The cranial branches include spinal, meningeal, medullary, and cerebellar arteries (7).

Physiology

The role and function of the vertebral arteries is to help perfuse the brain and medulla. This is achieved through connection to the encephalic common arterial manifold—the circle of Willis (Fig. 7.2). Despite the numerous bony and ligamentous cliffs along the course, blood flow through the vertebral arteries must not be hindered by normal movement of the head and cervical spine. Some of the bends help accommodate these movements. Extreme rotation can obstruct the contralateral suboccipital vertebral artery (1,12).

In the ideal case, hemodynamic resistance within the circle of Willis would be negligible, and a set well-developed carotid and vertebral arteries would exist. Mean arterial pressure would then be the same at all four injection points of the circle. Should one or more of the four injective vessels fail, there would be immediate and sufficient compensation of the arterial supply to any part of the brain. In other words, the crude territorial partition indicated in Fig. 7.2 would not matter. In persons with healthy and fully developed cervical arteries, however, the arteries of the circle of Willis are rather thin, pre-

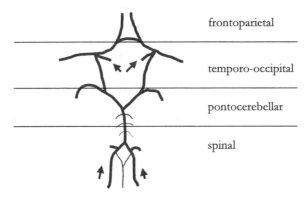

FIG. 7.2. The circle of Willis. The cranial branches include the spinal, meningeal, medullary, and cerebellar arteries. Their role and function is to perfuse the brain and medulla.

cisely because of equal pressures at all corners; flow and function in the circle are therefore modest. Then the circle of Willis does not function as a distributor or equalizer of flow (7). Moreover the circle may lack completeness and symmetry either by constitution or by disease. The same is true of the vertebral and carotid arteries. For these reasons, territorial partition is absolutely meaningful only in the general case. To assess the possible effect of a particular arterial shut-off on a particular person, one needs to know the exact situation of the entire network. Vertebrobasilar insufficiency is a typical example of territorial ischemia. It can be visualized on radionuclide scans (19).

EXTRINSIC COMPRESSION

With knowledge of the essential anatomy and physiology, it is possible to understand the mechanical problems sometimes suffered by the vertebral arteries in the course of degenerative and inflammatory spinal disease.

Mechanism and Occurrence

In the course of degenerative and inflammatory disease, the vertebral arteries may be compressed by osteophytes or unstable vertebral elements (1,7,8,11,17). Levels C4 to C7 seem to be affected most (15). Fig. 7.3 is a cross-sectional schematic of the cervical spine. This figure and Fig. 7.1 show that typical hernial protrusions do not directly affect the vertebral arteries, which are situated a safe distance away from the lesion and are protected by the uncinate rim.

External compression of the vertebral arteries by osteophytes is a rare disorder (2). In a series of 51 cases of external compression, George and Laurian (7) found only 4 cases due to osteophytes, the other causes being tumor (34 cases), constitutional elements such as fibrous bands and nerve strings (7 cases), trauma (4 cases), and infection (2 cases). Only 13 patients had vertebrobasilar symptoms. The total number of such problems is perhaps underestimated because of compensating collateral arterial flow, as through side branches or the circle of Willis.

Osteophytic compression develops gradually and is most likely to produce extreme or complete occlusion on bending and rotating the head and cervical spine. Figures 7.4 and 7.5 illustrate the problem related to articular and uncinate spurs, respectively. Figure 7.6 clarifies the role of rotation in compression of the vertebral artery when an osteophyte is present. Rotation of the head moves the ipsilateral vertebral artery (to which the chin points) backward, possibly squeezing the vessel against an articular spur. Squeezing of

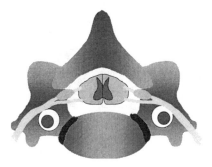

FIG. 7.3. Cross-sectional schematic of the cervical spine.

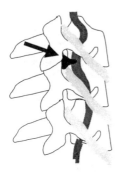

FIG. 7.4. Problem related to articular spur.

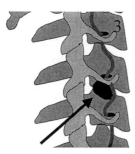

FIG. 7.5. Problem related to uncinate spur.

the contralateral artery may occur if an uncinate spur is present. This simple mechanism must be understood for correct interpretation and correlation of clinical and imaging findings.

Instability of cervical elements due to extreme and destructive disease, such as occipitoatlantoaxial subluxation in rheumatoid arthritis, can threaten the vertebral arteries.

Compression follows one of several courses. Either the condition remains intermittent with impaired flow with specific movements of the head and neck, or arterial disease

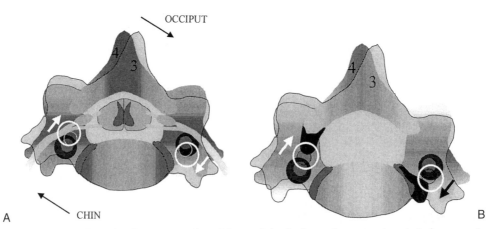

FIG. 7.6 Role of rotation in compression of the vertebral artery when an osteophyte is present. **A**, normal situation: vertebral arteries follow the movement. **B**, with ostophytes: possible squeezing of the arteries.

gradually is induced (secondary arterial lesion). The latter situation can evolve into embolism or complete thrombotic occlusion.

Clinical Presentation

Typical Situations

Intermittent compression or embolism from a secondary lesion may cause transient ischemia in the posterior territories (Fig. 7.2). So-called vertebrobasilar signs and symptoms occur in varying degrees and combinations. The patient has acute episodes of vertigo, nausea, diplopia, cranial nerve palsy, ataxia, falling (drop attacks), or any combination of these. Much depends on the size of the ischemic territory, according to the individual characteristics of the arterial network. The causative event (e.g., neck movement) is not always clear. The age of the patient, his or her work activity, the presence of anxiety, intelligence, and the attitude of the family are some factors that influence the presentation. Repeated embolism or thrombosis may cause chronic or evolving clinical signs and symptoms—stable or progressive vertebrobasilar insufficiency. The condition may be worsened by systemic factors such as hypotension or cardiac arrhythmia.

The clinical examination should include a cardiovascular evaluation with auscultation of the heart and arteries (special attention to the supraaortic arteries), palpation of pulses (special attention to the carotid and brachial arteries) and bilateral blood pressure measurement. It is essential that generalized arterial disease, arrhythmia, and valvular lesions be detected at this point. If related to specific movements of the head and neck, signs and symptoms due to the possible vertebral artery compression can be evinced with a provocation test. This test should be performed with utmost care and very gradual movements. If a positive result is evinced, the test must be stopped immediately and the patient observed until recovery. If done properly the provocation test is priceless in identifying both compression and its functional consequences. Rotational provocation can provide important information about the mechanism involved if lateralized neurologic signs develop. The findings should be correlated with the results of imaging studies.

It is clear that the neurologist, vascular surgeon, and spinal surgeon or physician should cooperate closely from this clinical stage onward.

Differential Diagnostic Issues

Vertebrobasilar signs and symptoms are caused by temporary or lasting ischemia of the posterior territories. To correlate this with possible or documented spinal disease, one must rule out the other possible causes. Cardiac and vascular disease is so widespread, so much more frequent than the very narrow subject of the present chapter. Suspicion must not be directed primarily at extrinsic vertebral artery compression, but the possibility should be kept in mind. If suggestive elements were to be found, one must be aware that extrinsic compression is not restricted to inflammatory or degenerative disease of the spine. The most frequent causes are tumor and constitutional factors, such as fibrous, muscular, or nervous bands, as pointed out earlier. Recurrent symptoms clearly associated with specific head and neck movements should raise suspicion. Vertigo in itself is nonspecific (4). Apart from vestibular and ocular problems, proprioceptive derangement is likely to produce vertigo and ocular symptoms with many cervical spinal conditions, such as degenerative or posttraumatic disorders (e.g., whiplash), disease, or aging. Dizziness and uncertain stance and gait often are associated with jerky movements or sudden rising from a sitting or recumbent position. In an aging population the first diagnosis to consider is postural hypotension with or without antihypertensive medication such as β-blockers.

A patient with vertebrobasilar symptoms may seek treatment from or be referred to general practitioners, neurologists, otorhinolaryngologists, ophthalmologists, cardiologists, and vascular or spinal specialists or surgeons, depending on the primary symptoms and referral pathways in the medical community or institution. The initial clinical and technical approaches therefore may be quite different. True multidisciplinary discussion is mandatory before performing a large number of technical investigations.

Diagnostic Techniques

If sufficient clinical evidence has been accumulated about the extrinsic vertebral origin of the problem, technical investigations must be aimed at three successive targets—defining the spinal lesion, demonstrating arterial compression, and localizing the level of compression. Cervical radiography, computed tomography (CT), and magnetic resonance imaging (MRI) are routinely used to define spinal lesions. CT and MRI (9) can also be used to document the vertebral arteries. It may be useful to delay these examinations until a vertebral color duplex scanning has been performed (see later) and to ask the radiologist to combine spinal and arterial imaging. Thin slices can be obtained for a cervical level suspected through e.g. findings on plain radiography.

Demonstrating arterial compression calls for provocation. This must again be done with great care under clinical supervision. State-of-the-art color duplex ultrasound examination is gaining recognition (14,23). It depicts the vertebral artery (often with one or two veins) beneath its point of entry in the transverse canal and between consecutive transverse processes. Enhanced color algorithms provide better and better images. Flow can be nicely assessed with pulsed-wave Doppler technique. Volume flow is calculated by means of integrating the velocity curve against time and cross-sectional area (Fig. 7.7). The Doppler gate must then be set at the complete width of the artery and the scroll speed set to minimum. The cross section of the artery is considered to be a circle constructed on its measured diameter. Complete absence of flow in a vertebral artery may be caused by thrombosis or aplasia. In our duplex laboratory we found no difficulty keeping the probe targeted during rotation and extension or flexion of the neck. Extrinsic compression is signaled by a sharp decrease in flow velocity and volume flow (10) with the possible appearance of symptoms. Duplex scanning has many advantages. It is noninvasive and inexpensive and can be used to document the conditions of both the carotid and the vertebral arteries.

COLOUR DUPLEX ECHOGRAPHY OF THE VERTEBRAL ARTERY

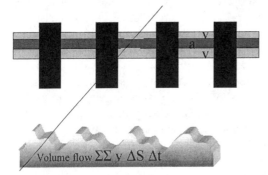

Volume flow $\Sigma\Sigma$ v ΔS Δt

FIG. 7.7. Volume flow is calculated by means of integrating the velocity curve against time and cross-sectional area.

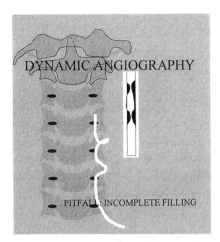

FIG. 7.8. A tandem lesion or compression is possible, and partial filling can be responsible for missing the second element.

Selective dynamic (i.e., with provocation) contrast angiography is necessary for precise determination of the compression level. It carries a general and a vascular risk (18), and the patient should be informed of this. CT can be useful to exclude important atherosclerotic irregularities of the aortic arch, which contribute to the risk of catheterization. The need for angiography should be questioned if the color duplex examination of the vertebral arteries does not show abnormality in the neutral position and with provocation. Angiographic images should be acquired in the neutral position and under provocation. A tandem lesion or compression is possible, and partial filling can be responsible for missing the second element (7) (Fig. 7.8).

Medical Therapy

Conservative measures can be considered at all times and often are useful in mild cases and for temporary relief. On the other hand, progressive vertebrobasilar deficiency under maximal therapy is a serious problem. If a good surgical solution is available, it is probably to be preferred over further contemplation of ischemic destruction of brain tissue. Bed rest, limitation of head and neck motion by means of instruction or with a collar can be effective (20) in reducing the severity of acute events and the frequency of intermittent symptoms. Antiinflammatory drugs may relieve some of the compression by diminishing edema. For intrinsic arterial lesions, primary or secondary platelet function inhibitors such as aspirin or anticoagulant drugs are important. In the absence of such intrinsic lesions, use of these therapies is not rational. Cardiac dysrhythmia must be controlled. The dose of antihypertensive medication should be adapted and postural hypotension minimized (1).

Surgical Therapy

If conservative therapy fails (7) and in the presence of a precisely defined lesion or compression site and after careful weighing of potential benefit against operative risk, a surgical option may be taken. As in so many other fields, a direct attack on the problem is the best policy: extrinsic compression should be relieved by decompression or bypass, not fusion (3,7,21). Compression by an unstable cervical element, on the other hand, should be managed by means of stabilization and fusion. If important primary or secondary intrinsic arterial lesions exist, vascular bypass is needed. Carney (1) states that, in general, the development of bypass procedures has reduced the number of indications for decompression. He emphasizes that fixed secondary lesions are frequent.

For direct vertebral decompression an anterolateral route often is chosen up to C3 and posterior access for C1-2. The experience and personal preference of the surgeon is important. The anterolateral approach advocated by George and Laurian (7) offers large and expandable access to the entire cervical region. The skin incision can be carried to the mastoid process to reach the highest level. The dissection is performed between the jugular vein and the sternocleidomastoid muscle down to the transverse processes. Care is taken not to harm blood vessels, lymphatic vessels, and nerves. Unroofing of the transverse canal is done with rongeurs after subperiosteal dissection and the vertebral vessels are left in their sheath, although some surgeons prefer to open the sheath (15). The vertebral canal usually is opened at the exact level of compression and the levels immediately above and below it.

Vascular bypass is performed with an autologous vein as close as possible to the rotation axis of the cervical spine—from the common carotid artery to the C1-2 level of the vertebral artery. Techniques and results are reviewed by Carney (1). Venous bypass carries a risk of late complications. Patients should be observed accordingly.

IATROGENIC VERTEBRAL ARTERY INJURY

The vertebral artery can be injured during surgery. Disc herniation itself does not pose a direct threat to the artery, but surgery for hernia does (22). Uncontrolled lateral drilling and the substantial tortuosity of the artery are distinct risk factors (16,22). Surgery on the smaller, more cephalic vertebrae can be more hazardous than operations on the other vertebrae (6).

The risk during direct decompression is probably related most to the experience of the surgeon. Particular techniques are promoted by certain authors and criticized by others. High-speed drilling, for example, is considered hazardous by some (6) and reported successful by others (2).

Manipulation of the spine by physical therapists and chiropractors carries risk. It is probably a low risk in view of the number of manipulative actions, but a survey of neurologists in California (13) found 55 cases of stroke after chiropractic spinal manipulations over a period of 2 years. Fifty-three cases (96%) occurred in the vertebrobasilar territory. Arterial dissection was proved angiographically in 25 (45%) patients. Forty-eight patients (87%) had a lasting deficit at 3 months. A literature review (5) covering 1925 to 1997, disclosed 177 separate cases with a mortality of 18%. Arterial dissection and spasm were the most common causes. The author of the review stated that physical therapists were involved in only 2% of all cases.

CONCLUSION

Extrinsic compression of the vertebral artery in degenerative and inflammatory spinal disease is uncommon. When it is suspected, a thorough clinical examination by a multidisciplinary team should be followed by a rational imaging program. Therapy is based on a good understanding of the mechanisms involved and on realistic prognostic data.

REFERENCES

1. Carney AL. Pathology, hemodynamics, and technique. In: Robicsek F, ed. *Extracranial Cerebrovascular Disease.* New York: Macmillan, 1986:395–424.
2. Citow JS, et al. Posterior decompression of the vertebral artery narrowed by cervical osteophyte: case report. *Surg Neurol* 1999;51:495–499.
3. Dan NG. The management of vertebral artery insufficiency in cervical spondylosis: a modified technique. *Aust N Z J Surg* 1976;46:164–165.
4. Daroff RB. Dizziness and vertigo. In: Wilson, Braunwald, Isselbacher, et al., eds. *Principles of Internal Medicine,* 12th ed. New York: McGraw-Hill, 1991:140–142.
5. Di Fabio RP. Manipulation of the cervical spine: risks and benefits. *Phys Ther* 1999;79:50–65.
6. Ebraheim NA, Lu J, Brown JA, et al. Vulnerability of vertebral artery in anterolateral decompression for cervical spondylosis. *Clin Orthop* 1996;322:146–151.
7. George B, Laurian C. Impairment of vertebral artery flow caused by extrinsic lesions. *Neurosurgery* 1989;24:206–214.
8. Hill EG. Surgical anatomy of the extracranial vessels. In: Robicsek F, ed. *Extracranial Cerebrovascular Disease.* New York: Macmillan, 1986:19–35.
9. Inui H, et al. Four cases of vertebrobasilar insufficiency. *Acta Otolaryngol Suppl (Stockh)* 1998;533:46–50.
10. Jargiello T, et al. Power Doppler imaging in the evaluation of extracranial vertebral artery compression in patients with vertebrobasilar insufficiency. *Eur J Ultrasound* 1998;8:149–156.
11. Kiwerski J. Decompression of the vertebral arteries in patients with arterial insufficiency syndrome in degenerative changes in the cervical spine. *Neurol Neurochir Pol* 1985;19:452–425.
12. Kuether TA, et al. Rotational vertebral artery occlusion: a mechanism of vertebrobasilar insufficiency. *Neurosurgery* 1997;41:427–433.
13. Lee KP, et al. Neurologic complications following chiropractic manipulation: survey of California neurologists. *Neurology* 1995;45:1213–1215.
14. Licht PB, et al. Vertebral artery volume flow in human beings. *J Manipulative Physiol Ther* 1999;22:363–367.
15. Nagashima C. Surgical treatment of vertebral artery insufficiency caused by cervical spondylosis. *J Neurosurg* 1970;32:512–521.
16. Oga M, et al. Tortuosity of the vertebral artery in patients with cervical spondylitic myelopathy: risk factor for the vertebral artery injury during anterior cervical decompression. *Spine* 1996;21:1085–1089.
17. Prescher A. Anatomy and pathology of the aging spine. *Eur J Radiol* 1998;27:181–195.
18. Redmond PL, et al. Principles of angiography. In: Rutherford RB, ed. *Vascular Surgery.* Philadelphia: WB Saunders, 1989:149–157.
19. Sakai F, et al. Regional cerebral blood flow during an attack of vertebrobasilar insufficiency. *Stroke* 1988;19:1426–1430.
20. Sheehan S, et al. Vertebral artery compression in cervical spondylosis. *Neurology* 1960;10:968–986.
21. Smith DR, et al. Cervical spondylosis causing vertebrobasilar insufficiency. *J Neurol Neurosurg Psychiatry* 1971;34:388–392.
22. Smith MD, et al. Vertebral artery injury during anterior decompression of the cervical spine: a retrospective review of ten patients. *J Bone Joint Surg Br* 1993;75:410–415.
23. Strek P, et al. A possible correlation between vertebral artery insufficiency and degenerative changes in the cervical spine. *Eur Arch Otorhinolaryngol* 1998;225:437–440.

SECTION 3

Diagnosis

The Degenerative Cervical Spine,
edited by Marek Szpalski and Robert Gunzburg
Lippincott Williams & Wilkins, Philadelphia © 2001.

8

Cervical Imaging: Dynamic Aspects and Clinical Significance

Jan T. Wilmink

Department of Neuroradiology, Academisch Ziekenhuis Maastricht,
6202 AZ Maastricht, The Netherlands

DYNAMIC IMAGING STUDIES
    Abnormal Spinal Narrowing • Abnormal Kyphotic Angulation
CLINICAL SIGNIFICANCE OF IMAGING FINDINGS IN CERVICAL NERVE ROOT COMPRESSION
CONCLUSION

This chapter is concerned with two aspects of diagnostic imaging in the evaluation of cervical degenerative disease. Flexion-extension movements of the spine affect the dimensions of the bony and ligamentous spinal canal and of the spinal cord. In addition, the spinal cord moves within the canal during flexion-extension. Dynamic imaging studies are helpful in understanding the various mechanisms of spinal cord involvement in degenerative disease, as well as in postoperative and posttraumatic conditions.

Modern high-resolution imaging techniques have the disadvantage that they frequently depict degenerative disc, joint, and canal abnormalities when the patient does not have symptoms, sometimes even when there is spinal cord involvement. When degenerative changes in the spine are depicted at magnetic resonance imaging (MRI) or computed tomographic (CT) myelography, it is important to be able to assess the clinical relevance in terms of potential for production of symptoms. The second part of this chapter discusses identification of imaging features that have a high likelihood of being associated with clinical signs and symptoms, as opposed to those unlikely to have much clinical relevance.

DYNAMIC IMAGING STUDIES

When the cervical spine moves from flexion (anteflexion or kyphosis) to extension (retroflexion or lordosis), the following anatomic changes normally occur:

The spinal canal shortens because it is posterior to the center of rotation of the vertebral motion segments (3).

The spinal canal narrows because of infolding of the ligamentum flavum as the vertebral laminae approach one another. This ligamentous infolding produces dorsolateral en-

croachment on the spinal canal. The posterior disc surface also may bulge somewhat, and the superior vertebra moves backward, adding to narrowing of the spinal canal (6).
The spinal cord shortens and thickens somewhat (3). Transverse measurements of cord area in flexion and extension obtained with in vivo CT myelography (Fig. 8.1) show an increase in extension of approximately 10%.
The spinal cord moves caudally and dorsally (Fig. 8.1).

The net effect of cervical extension is to produce a somewhat thicker spinal cord in a somewhat narrower spinal canal. When the spine goes from extension to flexion, the opposite occurs: the spinal canal becomes elongated and more capacious, and the spinal cord is drawn forward (9) and upward (7), becoming more slender. In the normal cervi-

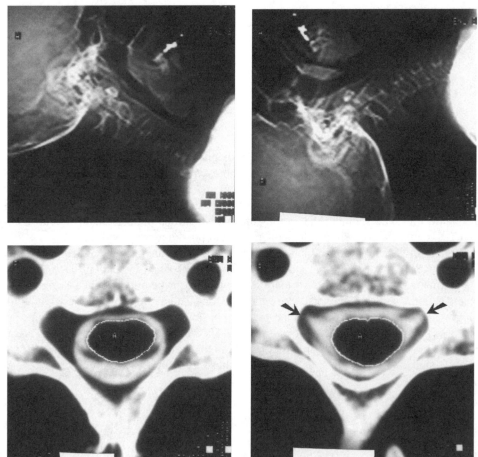

FIG. 8.1. Computed tomographic (CT) myelogram in flexion **(A)** with support under the occiput and extension **(B)** with support under the shoulders and head hanging down. Similar postures can be achieved at magnetic resonance imaging. Axial 3-mm CT sections at pedicular level in cervical flexion **(C)** and extension **(D)**. Forward movement of cord is evident in flexion and backward movement in extension. Root sleeves are above level of the section in flexion and fill the lateral recess in extension (*arrow*). Transverse cord area (*A*) measures approximately 80 mm² in flexion and 90 mm² in extension.

cal spine these posture-related changes do not cause problems. In certain conditions, however, posture-related changes cause spinal cord embarrassment.

Abnormal Spinal Narrowing

Persons with a congenitally narrow spinal canal can have further narrowing later in life owing to dorsal degenerative hypertrophy of the ligamentum flavum and ventral osteophyte formation at the posterior end-plate level (Fig. 8.2). The spinal cord, which was initially not at risk, undergoes pinching in cervical extension by the posture-dependent changes discussed earlier. The cross-sectional area of the cord gradually becomes eroded as the cord is molded to the shape and dimensions of the spinal canal in extension. In flexion the spinal canal becomes more capacious, but the cord remains deformed and diminished (Fig. 8.3). This mechanism explains the posture-dependent myelographic block and inconsistent Queckenstedt test result (abnormal in extension, normal in flexion) found in classic cases (6).

Cord deformation initially causes either no symptoms or irradiating pain somewhat resembling the brachialgia associated with cervical nerve root compression. After a certain point, long-tract cord signs occur, such as disturbances of gait and micturition, increased tendon jerks, and abnormal plantar responses. Cord measurements of persons with cervical spinal narrowing indicate that long-tract signs do not begin until the transverse cord area has been reduced by about one third (from a normal value of approximately 90 mm^2 to less than 60 mm^2) (8).

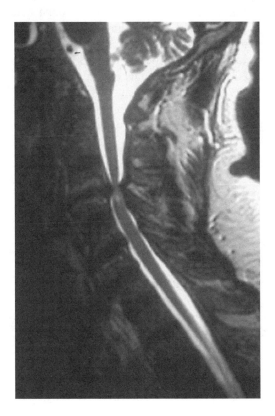

FIG. 8.2. T2-weighted midsagittal magnetic resonance section shows degenerative narrowing of the spinal canal at C3-4 caused by anterior osteophyte formation and posterior infolding of the ligamentum flavum. The combined effect is to pinch the cord, and this effect is aggravated in cervical extension. A lesion with high signal intensity is present within the cord at the site of compression. Degenerative changes of high signal intensity are present at the end plates at C3-4 and C5-6.

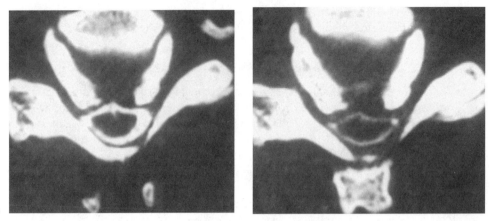

A   B

FIG. 8.3. Computed tomographic myelographic sections show compressive myelopathy due to narrowing of spinal canal. **A:** In cervical flexion the spinal canal is narrow, but the cord is surrounded by cerebrospinal fluid (CSF) and not actually compressed. **B:** In cervical extension, ligamentous borders of the spinal canal bulge inward and almost obliterate the CSF space around the cord. The spinal cord has been molded and deformed to adapt to the shape of the narrowed spinal canal in extension. In flexion, cord deformation persists.

Abnormal Kyphotic Angulation

Whereas abnormal spinal narrowing is associated with cervical extension, abnormal kyphotic angulation occurs with cervical flexion. Normal necks have mild kyphosis even in maximal hyperflexion. After cervical trauma or multilevel laminectomy, abnormal kyphosis may occur, frequently with local angulation. The cord is drawn firmly against the ventral wall of the spinal canal by the abnormal kyphosis, and further flexion of the spine increases traction on the cord over the angulation. At the level of angulation, the cord may be severely deformed and diminished (Fig. 8.4). This mechanism explains the course of symptoms among some patients with cord involvement due to cervical spinal narrowing. Progressive long-tract signs at first are caused by cord compression in extension. When decompressive laminectomy has been performed, progression of symptoms halts for months or years until abnormal kyphotic angulation causes renewed cord deterioration, now caused by traction in flexion.

CLINICAL SIGNIFICANCE OF IMAGING FINDINGS IN CERVICAL NERVE ROOT COMPRESSION

MRI is a sensitive method for detecting degenerative spinal abnormality and its effect on the spinal cord. The specificity of some MRI findings is questionable, however, because numerous degenerative cervical spinal features have been found among persons without neck symptoms, such as volunteers (2) or patients undergoing MRI for evaluation of a vocal cord disorder (10). The spines were completely normal in only a few cases, and changes such as disc-space narrowing, disc bulging and protrusion, and osteophyte formation were frequently found in varying degrees. This is not surprising considering the frequency with which plain radiographs of the spine show similar degenerative changes (5). More striking are the findings of cord involvement and sometimes substantial cord compression among persons without symptoms. Considerable compression and deformation of the cord may occur before signs of long-tract involvement begin.

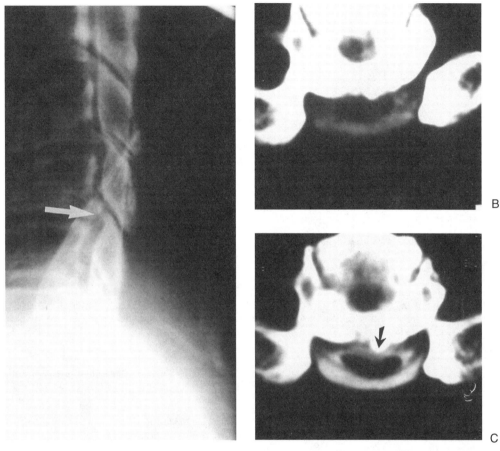

FIG. 8.4. Traction myelopathy due to postlaminectomy angulation and osteophyte formation. Conventional myelogram **(A)** shows angulation at C4-5 and C5-6 and osteophytes at the posterior end plates causing indentations in the dural sac and spinal cord (*arrow*). Computed tomographic myelographic sections of a similar case in flexion **(B)** and extension **(C)** show anteroposterior movement of the cord against an osteophyte, which has locally eroded the ventral cord surface (*arrow*).

The reports of the two studies mentioned (2,10) do not describe the signs of nerve root compression among the subjects who did not have symptoms. The MRI techniques used during the study period suffered from a lack of resolution with regard to depiction of nerve root compression. More recent developments have made it possible to produce a detailed MR myelogram (1). Conventional myelographic studies in the past have shown, however, that the presence of cervical nerve root and root sleeve deformation does not prove that clinically significant nerve root involvement exists (4). In a myelographic and CT myelographic study, my colleagues and I (8) found the following patterns of morphologic cord and root involvement with differing clinical associations:

1. Complete occlusion of the entrance to the intervertebral foramen by a laterally migrated mass of herniated disc material (soft disc) had the strongest association with clinical signs of radicular involvement (Fig. 8.5).

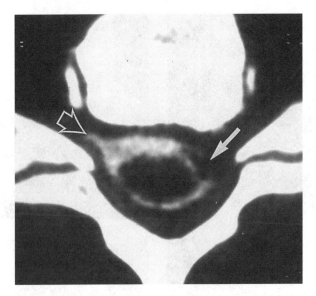

FIG. 8.5. Computed tomographic myelographic scan shows disc herniation that has migrated laterally to occlude the entrance to the intervertebral foramen. Normal root sleeve is present at right (*open arrow*) and a nonfilling root sleeve at left. A swollen intradural root also is evident (*solid arrow*).

2. Narrowing of the foramen by osteophytes (hard disc) caused only nerve root swelling at the foraminal entrance and was less reliably associated with clinical signs of root involvement.
3. The poorest occurred when disc herniation was present, sometimes displacing or compressing the cord (but not enough to cause cord signs) and not completely oc-

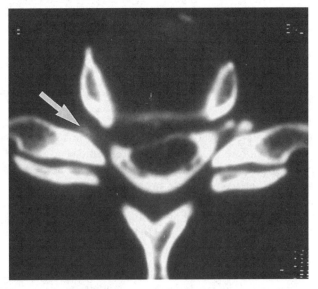

FIG. 8.6. Computed tomographic myelogram shows right disc herniation causing mild impression on cord and not fully occluding foraminal entrance. Filling of root sleeve is evident (*arrow*). The patient had no cord signs but had pain in the neck and contralateral arm.

cluding the foraminal entrance, thus not completely compressing the nerve root (Fig. 8.6). In these cases clinical symptoms were as likely to be present on the "wrong" side (opposite the side of radiologic signs of disc herniation) as on the "correct" side ipsilateral to the herniation.

We concluded that CT myelography can present a sometimes striking picture of disc herniation apparently not responsible for clinical signs and symptoms. Because neck and arm pain can have many causes besides soft or hard discs, critical interpretation of high-quality root and root sleeve images is essential to prevent false-positive interpretation. Myelography and CT myelography provide the highest resolution for imaging the nerve root and root sleeve and can be regarded as the radiologic standard of reference.

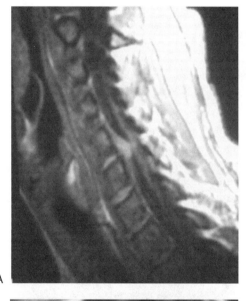

A

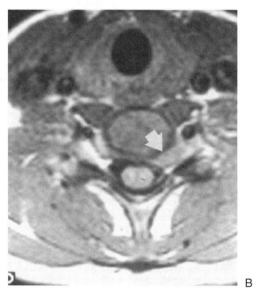

B

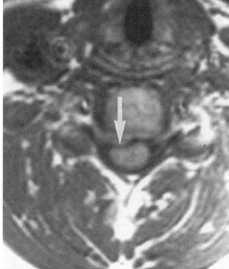

C

FIG. 8.7. A: T1-weighted magnetic resonance images of cervical herniations. Sagittal section lateral to the midline shows C5-6 herniation occluding the lateral canal and foraminal entrance. This is usually better assessed on axial sections. **B:** Image of the patient in **A** shows complete occlusion of left foramen (*arrow*). Normal foraminal fat at right. **C:** Image shows deformation of the cord and incomplete occlusion of foramen by small right disc herniation (*arrow*). Findings are similar to those in Fig. 8.6.

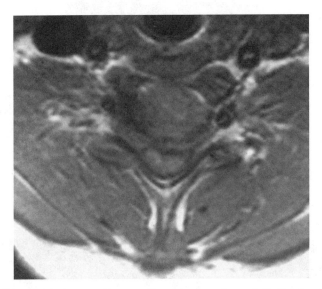

FIG. 8.8. Axial T1-weighted magnetic resonance image shows left disc herniation or osteophyte causing cord deformation, patent left intervertebral foramen, and unclear findings in right foramen.

The necessity of cerebrospinal fluid (CSF) puncture and intradural injection of contrast material for myelography has led to the widespread use of MRI to evaluate neck and arm pain. A standard MRI examination of the cervical spine usually comprises T1- and T2-weighted imaging sequences in the sagittal and axial planes. Quite frequently the images produced depict a soft or a hard disc (there is some difficulty in differentiating the

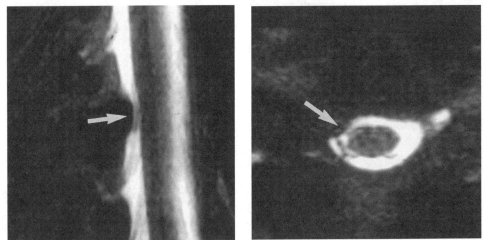

A   B

FIG. 8.9. A: Heavily T2-weighted oblique coronal magnetic resonance myelographic image shows compression of a single root sleeve and adjacent dural sac (*arrow*). Normal root sleeves and intradural roots are visible at adjacent levels. **B:** Axial heavily T2-weighted thin section from three-dimensional volume acquisition for patient in A shows compression of right root sleeve (*arrow*) compared with normal root sleeve at left. Because of the heavy T2 weighting of these images, only the dural sac and contents are depicted.

two) and allow assessment of the effects on the nerve root (Fig. 8.7). Disc protrusion is present sometimes while assessment of root compression is not possible (Fig. 8.8). In these cases, specialized imaging sequences can be used (Fig. 8.9). A heavily T2-weighted oblique coronal sequence produces an image strongly resembling a conventional x-ray myelogram with good depiction of the emerging roots and root sleeves. An axial thin-section three-dimensional volume acquisition, also heavily T2-weighted, provides an image most resembling a CT myelogram. Such MR myelographic sequences can be helpful when conventional MRI shows degenerative changes but the effect on the nerve root is not clear. The result of heavy T2 weighting of the myelographic sequences is that only the CSF within the dural sac produces a bright signal, and thus only the contents of the dural sac can be studied, not the extradural structures (11).

Conventional MR examination and MR myelography provide complementary information. The former is especially useful for detecting the cause (disc herniation or osteophyte formation) and the second for assessing the effect (nerve root compression). The best MR myelographic images are produced for persons with a normally capacious spinal canal. When the canal is narrow, there is not enough CSF present in the area of interest to provide myelographic contrast.

CONCLUSION

What is the value of dynamic imaging studies in daily clinical practice? Should these studies be routinely performed? Cervical dynamic imaging studies are a tool that aids in the understanding of the mechanisms of spinal cord involvement under conditions of abnormal spinal narrowing or abnormal kyphotic angulation. Dynamic studies are not necessary to establish the diagnosis of actual cord involvement. This can easily be done by studying the shape and cross-sectional area of the cord at the level of suspected involvement. The spinal cord is not elastic; it retains evidence of deformation in extreme flexion or extension, even when imaged in the neutral position. Acquiring additional images in cervical flexion and extension does not improve the sensitivity of the imaging study (be it myelography, CT myelography, or MRI) and is not without risk of cord damage from forced hyperextension in a patient with cervical spinal narrowing or forced hyperflexion in a patient with abnormal kyphotic angulation.

How reliable is MRI in the diagnosis of suspected cervical root compression syndromes, given the necessity of obtaining high-resolution images of the nerve roots and root sleeves and the sometimes disappointing results of MRI? My colleagues and I have found that MRI can be used as first modality in evaluation of these patients. It provides better diagnostic images than noncontrast CT and is less invasive than myelography and CT myelography. Most MRI studies have definitively normal findings or show unequivocally symptomatic abnormalities. In a few cases, an abnormality is seen, such as dural impression by a soft or hard disc the effect of which on the nerve root is uncertain. In these cases myelographic MRI often allows better assessment of the state of the nerve root.

Some situations necessitate additional imaging studies. When a dural impression is seen and it is unclear whether the cause is disc protrusion (soft disc) or an osteophyte (hard disc), noncontrast CT aimed at the disc level in question. When there is doubt about nerve root involvement, and the myelographic MR images are inadequate because of lack of CSF in a narrowed spinal canal, the patient needs cervical myelography followed by CT myelography.

In the diagnosis of cervical nerve root compression, MRI has considerably more pitfalls and problems than it has in the diagnosis of disorders of the lumbar region. Nevertheless, with the strategy described herein, the number of invasive cervical myelographic procedures performed can be reduced substantially—at my institution to less than one per month.

ACKNOWLEDGMENTS

The help of the secretarial staff of the radiology department in preparation of the manuscript is gratefully acknowledged. The work presented is largely the result of a long and fruitful collaboration with Lourens Penning, now emeritus professor of neuroradiology and still active in the field.

REFERENCES

1. Balériaux D, Metens T, Edal A, et al. Cervical MR myelography: an optimized technique. *Neuroradiology* 1996;38[Suppl 2];S83:(abstract).
2. Boden SD, Mc Cowin PR, Davis DO, et al. Abnormal magnetic resonance scans of the cervical spine in asymptomatic subjects. *J Bone Joint Surg Am* 1990;72:1178–1184.
3. Breig A. *Biomechanics of the central nervous system.* Stockholm: Almqvist & Wiksell, 1961.
4. Fox AJ, Lin JP, Pinto RS, et al. Myelographic cervical nerve root deformities. *Radiology* 1975;116:355–361.
5. Friedenberg ZB, Miller WT. Degenerative disc disease of the cervical spine. *J Bone Joint Surg Am* 1963;45:1171–1178.
6. Penning L. Functional pathology of the cervical spine. Amsterdam: Excerpta Medica, 1968.
7. Penning L, Wilmink JT. Biomechanics of the spinal canal. *Clin Biomech (Bristol, Avon)* 1986;1:28–232.
8. Penning L, Wilmink JT, van Woerden HH, et al. CT myelographic findings in degenerative disorders of the cervical spine. *AJNR Am J Neuroradiol* 1986;7:119–126.
9. Reid JD. Effects of flexion-extension movements of the head and spine upon the spinal cord and nerve roots. *J Neurol Neurosurg Psychiatry* 1960;25:214–218.
10. Teresi LM, Lufkin RB, Reicher MA, et al. Asymptomatic degenerative disc disease and spondylosis of the cervical spine: MR imaging. *Radiology* 1987;164:83–88.
11. Wilmink JT, Hofman PAM. MR imaging of cervical nerve root filaments: comparison of three acquisition techniques. In: Proceedings of the XVI Symposium Neuroradiologicum, Philadelphia, May 15-17,1998:270(abstract).

The Degenerative Cervical Spine,
edited by Marek Szpalski and Robert Gunzburg
Lippincott Williams & Wilkins, Philadelphia © 2001.

9

Computed Tomography and Magnetic Resonance Imaging

P.C. Seynaeve, B.P. Mortele

Magnetic Resonance Unit, Department of Radiology, AZ OLV Groeninghe, B 8500 Kortrijk, Belgium

---

Computed tomography (CT) and magnetic resonance imaging (MRI) are powerful techniques in the evaluation of degenerative disease of the cervical spine. CT is fast and reliable and provides high-resolution images of all bony structures around the spinal canal and the intervertebral foramina. However, CT does have limitations. The main disadvantage of CT is its inherent low-contrast resolution when it comes to evaluation of soft tissues. Many authors have advocated the use of CT myelography in the evaluation of disc disease to solve the problem of low-contrast resolution, which is particularly bothersome when it comes to the evaluation of the exact extent of small disc herniations or the exact extent of disc herniation in the intervertebral foramina. CT myelography is still considered the standard of reference. The aim of this chapter is to demonstrate that MRI can reliably replace CT myelography in evaluations of almost all patients when appropriate imaging sequences are used.

COMPARATIVE STUDY OF COMPUTED TOMOGRAPHY VERSUS MAGNETIC RESONANCE IMAGING

Materials and Methods

In the clinical setting of degenerative disease, MRI or CT are frequently requested. Many reports have been published about the comparison between CT or CT myelography and MRI (2,6,13). We started a prospective study to evaluate the ability of MRI to replace CT myelography in routine clinical use. The MRI examinations were performed on a 0.5 T whole-body imager equipped with a phased-array cervicothoracolumbar (CTL) coil. The following sequences were used: sagittal T1-weighted spin echo (SE) (repetition time [TR] 520 ms, echo time [TE] 22 ms) with a field of view (FOV) of 200 mm, 4 mm section thickness, 1 mm gap, and 256 × 192 matrix. Axial imaging was performed with axial two-dimensional gradient images (TR 923 ms, TE 28 ms) FOV 200 mm, 3-mm section thickness, 1-mm gap, 256 × 192 matrix. We examined 31 patients and compared three levels in each examination with the CT myelographic findings. Three MRI examinations were classified inadequate because of movement artifacts, which gave a total of 84 intervertebral foramina.

Results

A semiquantitative grading scale was used. Disc herniation was classified as medial, mediolateral, or foraminal and graded as mild, moderate, or severe. The degree of foraminal stenosis was classified as normal, slightly narrowed, significantly narrowed, or critically narrowed. The results of the semiquantitative data were analyzed by two readers. All disc herniations were seen with both imaging modalities (Fig. 9.1). Axial gradient images showed an artifactual narrowing of the intervertebral foramina of 10% to 15% (Fig. 9.2). However, because we used a semiquantitative scale, no foraminal stenosis was misclassified.

Taking into account the 18 intervertebral foramina that could not be evaluated, we obtained an accuracy of 82%. These results were in concordance with findings published by Youssem et al. (12), who found an accuracy of 86% for MRI in a comparison with CT myelography in the evaluation of degenerative disc disease. Another advantage of MRI over CT and CT myelography is that it depicts pathologic changes beneath the level of a total cerebrospinal fluid (CSF) block and that MRI is not prone to shoulder artifacts (2).

Discussion

The results of past comparisons between MRI and CT myelography have been contradictory, mainly because different authors have used different pulse sequences. For this reason, we believe that a short overview of all possible pulse sequences and their advantages and limitations is mandatory.

Magnetic Resonance Imaging Pulse Sequences

Sagittal T1-Weighted Pulse Sequence

Little discussion remains about the fact that the first sequence in evaluating degenerative disease of the cervical spine is a sagittal T1-weighted pulse sequence. This series allows a general overview of the cervical spine and evaluation of vertebral body alignment, the craniocervical junction, and the exact dimension of the cervical canal at all levels in the anteroposterior direction. The sagittal diameter of the spinal canal is smaller from C3 toward C6 with a minimum at C4 (12.9 ± 1.3 mm). The sagittal diameter of the cord decreases gradually' in the caudal direction (5).

The main advantage of the sagittal T1-weighted pulse sequence is that it allows differentiation of disc disease from osteophytes. A herniated disc has an intermediate signal intensity and is continuous with normal disc tissue. The central portion of osteophytes has a higher signal intensity than does disc tissue, and most osteophytes have a dark outline, which represents cortical bone and periosteum. A calcified osteophyte has a homogeneous low signal intensity and can be recognized as a bony spur.

The conventional spin echo (SE) sequence has been replaced in many institutions by a fast spin echo (FSE) sequence. In a conventional SE sequence, the initial 90-degree pulse is followed by a 180-degree pulse to obtain rephasing. For every line in the k space, this experiment has to be redone. In FSE sequences, the initial 90-degree pulse is followed by

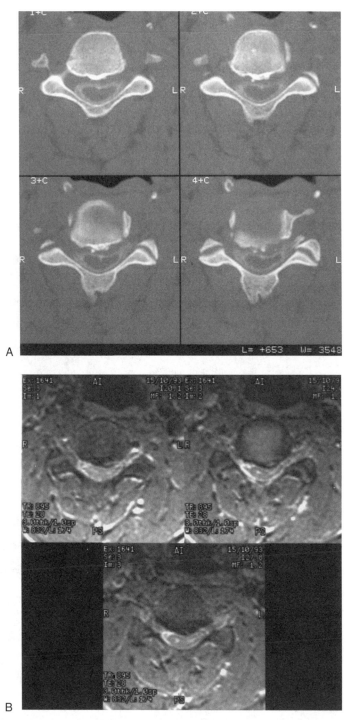

FIG. 9.1. A: Axial computed tomographic (CT) myelogram shows moderate mediolateral disc herniation with calcifications. Posterior rim osteophytes and bilateral slight uncarthrosis are present. **B:** Axial two-dimensional gradient magnetic resonance image at the same level as **A** shows the same disc herniation. The posterior osteophytic rim and the minimal degenerative disease at the level of the uncinate processes are visible. The resolution is less than that of the CT image because of the greater section thickness and the lower matrix used. This illustrates the shortcomings of two-dimensional gradient imaging compared with state-of-the-art CT myelography.

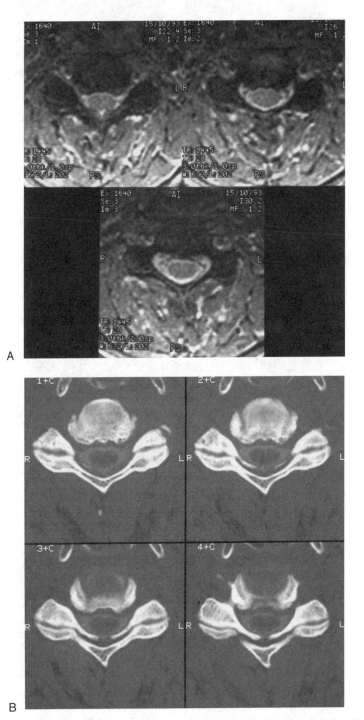

FIG. 9.2. A: Axial two-dimensional gradient image shows bilateral uncarthrosis with severe narrowing of the intervertebral foramina. **B:** Axial computed tomographic myelogram shows bilateral prominent uncarthrosis but without critical stenosis. This case illustrates artifactual narrowing of the intervertebral foramina, to which axial gradient imaging is prone. This problem can be overcome by using thin-section three-dimensional gradient imaging and accurate settings.

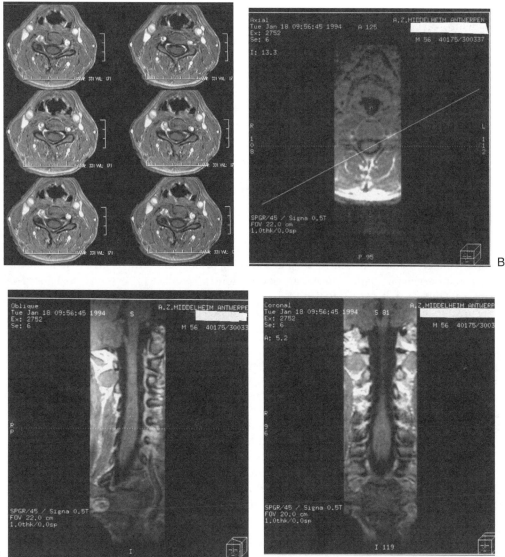

FIG. 9.3. Three-dimensional T1-weighted gradient echo images obtained with intravenous gadolinium injection. **A:** Axial reformatted images from a sagittal 3DTI wighted GRE set of images. **B:** Axial reformatted image with the indication of the obliquity of the reformations in **(C)**. **D:** Coronal reformatted image. The use of three-dimensional imaging allows reformatting in multiple planes. Some authors advocate the use of these reformations to better visualize the proximal part of the nerve roots. The main differences from T2-weighted images is the low signal intensity of the CSF and the high signal intensity of the peridural veins. In all T2-weighted sequences, both cerebrospinal fluid and the peridural veins and venous plexuses remain hyperintense.

many 180-degree pulses. The number of 180-degree pulses can be chosen by the operator within certain limits and is called the *echo train length* or *turbo factor.* This sequence allows filling of many k-space lines for every 90-degree pulse. For T1-weighted images an echo train of 3 to 6 generally is used. The time gain can be used to obtain higher resolution or for faster imaging. Some authors (8) have reported positive results with a single three-dimensional gradient T1-weighted gradient echo series with injection of gadolinium. Although this approach has its advantages, it makes the examination more expensive because of the extra cost of the intravenous contrast agent (Fig. 9.3).

Comparison Between Spine Echo and Fast Spin Echo Sequences

The main difference between SE and FSE sequences is the reduction in acquisition time for the latter. FSE imaging does have problems, however. It suffers from phase-encoded blurring, truncation artifacts, reduced magnetic susceptibility, and a high susceptibility to motion artifact. Most of these problems have been overcome in more recent FSE pulse sequences. However, there remains a difference in tissue contrast: fat is brighter on FSE images than on conventional SE images (4). In T2-weighted imaging, a long echo train length (16 to 32) and short echo spacing partially compensate for CSF flow and produce the best myelographic effect (9). Gillams et al. (4) found that FSE sequences are far superior to conventional SE sequences. In their study 20% of cord lesions were missed on conventional SE images; in 40% of cases, thecal sac compression was exaggerated on conventional SE images.

Sagittal T2-Weighted Sequences

In the literature a sagittal T2-weighted sequence generally is not used for the sole purpose of evaluating disc disease. In older studies T2-weighted images had low signal to noise ratios and had very low spatial resolution. For this reason they were used only to evaluate higher interstitial water content in medullary disease. Today T2-weighted FSE images are routinely obtained with a 512 matrix and have the same spatial resolution as T1-weighted images. Medullary processes are not within the scope of this discussion, but at this time T2-weighted FSE images have better contrast resolution than do T1-weighted FSE images but with the same spatial resolution.

Short Tau Inversion Recovery

The short inversion time (τ) inversion recovery (STIR) sequence is an older sequence but is still generally accepted as the most sensitive sequence in the detection of bone edema within the vertebral bodies. It allows acquisition of very heavily T2-weighted images with homogeneous fat suppression. In the recent literature the STIR and fast or turbo inversion recovery (FIR-TIR) sequence has been shown to be extremely sensitive in the detection of fluid in the facet articulations and in the detection of medullary abnormalities (3).

Axial Imaging

Imaging in the axial plane has long been and still is a matter of discussion, especially in the evaluation of the cervical spine. Because of the high pulsatility of CSF at the cervical level, almost all axial images have flow artifacts that cause focal signal loss and can easily be mistaken for abnormalities. Especially in the region just posterior to the cervical disc, pulsation artifacts frequently cause dephasing artifacts, which can be mistaken for disc disease.

Two-dimensional versus Three-dimensional Imaging

There remains little argument that axial cervical spinal imaging has to be performed with axial gradient-recalled echo (GRE) imaging with very short echo times and ultra-thin section thickness to minimize susceptibility artifacts. For this reason, state-of-the-art imaging is performed with axial three-dimensional GRE imaging, which allows thinner sections without any gap between sections and a higher signal to noise ratio. It also allows reformatting in multiple planes. However, a study by Atlas et al. (1) showed that reformatting in multiple planes does not increase diagnostic accuracy. In a study by Youssem et al. (12) axial high-resolution MRI was found to be accurate in delineating narrowing of the intervertebral foramina of the cervical spine. The accuracy was found to be almost equal to the rate of concordance of double readings of the accepted standard of reference—CT myelography (85%).

COMPARATIVE STUDY OF AXIAL TWO-DIMENSIONAL FAST SPIN ECHO VERSUS THREE-DIMENSIONAL GRADIENT IMAGING

We performed a comparative study in which we compared axial two-dimensional FSE images (TR 5,500 ms, TE 97 ms, echo train 16, section thickness 2.5 mm, matrix 384 × 256, field of view 240 mm, zero interpolation filling 512) with axial three-dimensional gradient images (TR 69, TE 12, flip angle 5 degrees, section thickness

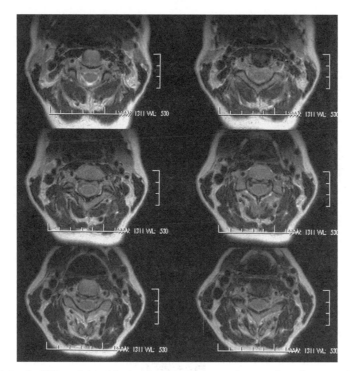

FIG. 9.4. Axial set of T2-weighted fast spin echo images shows a hypointense rim posterior to the disc caused by spin dephasing from flow artifacts. This can easily be mistaken for disc disease.

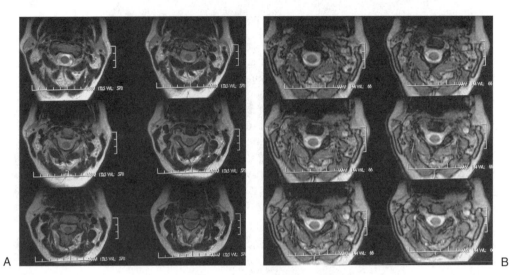

FIG. 9.5. A: Axial set of T2-weighted fast spin echo (FSE) images at the same level as B. **B:** Axial set of three-dimensional T2-weighted gradient images with 1.6-mm section thickness and accurate settings to minimize artifacts. Although gradient images usually have a lower resolution, the diagnostic yield is higher than that of FSE imaging because gradient images do not contain the flow artifacts common in FSE sequences (see Fig. 9.4).

1.6 mm, matrix 256 × 192, field of view 240 mm) with magnetization transfer. Melhem et al. (7) found magnetization transfer to be beneficial for three-dimensional gradient imaging and to have low spatial distortion and good soft-tissue contrast. We compared three levels in 10 patients with degenerative disc disease using a 1.5 T superconductive magnet. The flow artifacts on the axial T2-weighted FSE images were minimal and did not cause misreading or inconclusive interpretation (Fig. 9.4).

FSE images have a higher signal to noise ratio than gradient images and allow a better evaluation of the soft tissues of the anterior neck. Interpretation of one set of FSE images led to the diagnosis of lymphoma; the lymph nodes in the anterior neck were missed on the axial gradient images. Gradient images are not susceptible to flow artifacts. This makes a gradient sequence ideal for axial imaging of the cervical spine. Gradient images have a lower signal to noise ratio than FSE images, which explains the lower resolution generally used (Fig. 9.5). A major disadvantage is the sensitivity to magnetic susceptibility in gradient imaging. In cervical spinal disease, magnetic susceptibility can cause artifactual narrowing of the foramina. The degree of stenosis is related directly to the echo time (TE) and the flip angle. It ranges from 8% with a TE of 11 ms to 27% with a TE of 22 ms (10).

MAGNETIC RESONANCE MYELOGRAPHY

MR myelography of the cervical region is challenging because of the high-velocity pulsatility of the CSF. Especially in examinations of patients with a narrow spinal canal, MR myelography remains challenging and is therefore not widely used (11).

CONCLUSION

Sagittal FSE and axial high-resolution, high-signal-intensity CSF MRI techniques are as accurate as CT myelography in the evaluation of degenerative disc disease. State-of-the-art imaging in many institutions involves axial three-dimensional GRE imaging. However, axial high-resolution two-dimensional FSE sequences can be used if flow artifacts can be minimized. Sagittal or coronal STIR imaging is mandatory in the evaluation of bone edema, intraarticular fluid collections, or myelopathy.

REFERENCES

1. Atlas SW, Youssem DM. High-resolution three dimensional Fourier transform gradient echo MR imaging of the cervical spine: diskogenic disease—comparison of interpretations with axial acquisition alone versus reformatting in combination with axial images. In: Proceedings of the Annual Meeting of the Radiological Society of North America, Chicago, 1990:233.
2. Breidahl WH, Low V, Khangure MS. Imaging of the cervical spine: a comparison of MR with myelography and CT myelography. *Australas Radiol* 1991;35:306–314.
3. Clarysse J, Demondion X. IRM du Rachis et du canal rachidien: quelles séquences dans quels plans? In: Presented at the 9th Congress, February 2–4, 2000, at Groupe de Recherche sur les Applications du Magnétisme en Médecine (GRAMM), Lille, France.
4. Gillams AR, Soto JA, Carter AP. Fast spin echo vs. conventional spin echo in cervical spine imaging. *Eur Radiol* 1997;7:1211–1214.
5. Inoue H, Ohmori K, Takatsu T, et al. Morphological analysis of the cervical spinal canal, dural tube and spinal cord in normal individuals using CT myelography. *Neuroradiology* 1996;38:148–151.
6. Larsson EM, Holtas S, Cronqvist S, et al. Comparison of myelography, CT myelography and magnetic resonance imaging in cervical spondylosis and disk herniation. *Acta Radiol* 1989;30:233–239.
7. Melhem ER, Benson ML, Beauchamp NJ, et al. Cervical spondylosis: three-dimensional gradient echo MR with magnetization transfer. *AJNR Am J Neuroradiol* 1996;17:705–711.
8. Ross JS, Ruggieri PM, Tkach JA, et al. Gd-enhanced 3D MR imaging of cervical degenerative disk disease: initial experience. *AJNR Am J Neuroradiol* 1992;13:127–136.
9. Sze G, Kawamura Y, Negishi C, et al. Fast spin echo MR imaging of the cervical spine: influence of echo train length and echo spacing on image contrast and quality. *AJNR Am J Neuroradiol* 1993;14:1203–1213.
10. Tsuruda JS, Remley K. Effects of magnetic susceptibility artifacts and motion in evaluating the cervical neural foramina on 3D FT gradient-echo MR imaging *AJNR Am J Neuroradiol* 1991;12: 237–247.
11. Wilmink JT. MR imaging of the spine: trauma and degenerative disease. *Eur Radiol* 1999;9:1259–1266.
12. Youssem DM, Atlas SW, Goldberg HI, et al. Degenerative narrowing of the cervical spine neural foramina: evaluation with high resolution 3DFT gradient echo MR imaging. *AJNR Am J Neuroradiol* 1991;156:229–236.
13. Youssem DM, Atlas SW, Hackney DB. Cervical spine disk herniation: comparison of CT and 3D FT gradient echo MR scans. *J Comput Assist Tomogr* 1992;16:345–351.

The Degenerative Cervical Spine,
edited by Marek Szpalski and Robert Gunzburg
Lippincott Williams & Wilkins, Philadelphia © 2001.

10

Electrophysiologic Examination

A. Müller, Jiri Dvorak

Spine Unit, Department of Neurology, Schulthess Clinic, CH-8008 Zurich, Switzerland

SOMATOSENSORY EVOKED POTENTIALS
  Stimulation and Recording Techniques • Median Nerve SEPs
MOTOR EVOKED POTENTIALS
NEUROGRAPHY AND ELECTROMYOGRAPHY
  Nerve Conduction Studies • F-wave Studies • Electromyographic Studies • Sensitivity,
  Specificity, and Predictive Value
INDICATIONS FOR NEUROPHYSIOLOGIC INVESTIGATIONS
CONCLUSION

Electrophysiologic examinations should help in answering the following questions in the care of patients with cervical spinal disorders such as spinal stenosis: Which neural elements are involved? Which spinal segment is responsible for mechanical or other irritation? Is the lesion chronic, acute, or progressing? Has neural function improved?

Table 10.1 lists the neurophysiologic tests and the neural structures they are used to evaluate. Whereas somatosensory evoked potentials (SSEPs) and motor evoked potentials (MEPs) are most helpful in evaluation of the central nervous system pathways, electromyography (EMG), conventional neurography, and F-wave studies are most useful for evaluation of the peripheral segments of the sensory and motor pathways.

Sophisticated SSEP techniques allow for scrutiny of the neural elements of the sensory pathways: the dorsal roots, the root entry zone, the dorsal horns, the dorsal columns, the dorsal column nuclei, the lemnisci fibers, and the thalamus and its projections to the primary and secondary sensory areas of the cortex. MEPs allow assessment of lesions that affect the upper motor neuron and lesions that affect the motor root, plexus fibers, or peripheral nerve segments of the lower motor neuron. EMG of limb and paraspinal muscles allows differentiation between abnormalities of motor roots and those of more peripheral nerve elements. EMG allows evaluation of peripheral nerve disease and provides information about the age of the lesion. Neurography and F-wave studies also allow differentiation between proximal root and peripheral nerve disease. Fractionated peripheral nerve stimulation helps to localize a circumscribed peripheral lesion. Malfunction of the autonomic nervous system is difficult to assess. The sympathetic skin response has proved helpful in the evaluation of autonomic peripheral neuropathy (27) and in the differential diagnosis of erectile dysfunction (20).

TABLE 10.1. *Neurophysiologic techniques used for evaluation of different neural structures*

Neurophysiologic technique	Neural structures evaluated
Somatosensory evoked potentials	Sensory nerve fibers and dorsal roots, spinal cord dorsal columns
Motor evoked potentials	Corticospinal tract (lateral spinal cord), motor roots, motor nerve fibers
Neurography	Motor and sensory nerve fibers
F Wave	Motor roots, motor nerve fibers
Electromyography of limb muscles	Motor roots, motor nerve fibers
Electromyography of paraspinal muscles	Motor roots

From Dvorak J. Neurophysiologic tests in diagnosis of nerve root compression caused by disc herniation. *Spine* 1996;21[Suppl 24]:395–445, with permission.

SOMATOSENSORY EVOKED POTENTIALS

In the context of spinal cord and nerve root evaluation, only so-called short latency SSEPs are relevant. These are potentials recorded from the cervical spine and the first components of scalp recordings. Mid- and long-latency components of scalp-recorded potentials show great inter- and intraindividual variability that is highly dependent on alertness and psychological factors.

Stimulation and Recording Techniques

SSEPs generally are recorded after electric stimulation of peripheral nerves. The nerves usually used are the median or ulnar nerves of the upper limbs. In radicular and in spinal disease, several nerves supplied by different segments must be stimulated for a level diagnosis. Dermatomal stimulation and motor point stimulation have been proposed by several authors (2,7,29), but even without technical problems, these procedures have had inconsistent results.

For clinical purposes it is necessary to concentrate on components that can be consistently recognized in all healthy persons (2,7). Upper limb testing (median, ulnar, or radial nerve) has been most helpful in establishing the existence of lesions in the spinal roots, posterior columns, and brainstem in disorders such as cervical spondylosis, spinal stenosis, multiple sclerosis, and Guillain-Barré 82 syndrome, even when the clinical and radiological data are not definitive.

Median Nerve Somatosensory Evoked Potentials

The median nerve is stimulated in a typical position over the median nerve and the wrist. Electrodes should be placed over the Erb point, over C7 and C2, and in the scalp over the parietal somatosensory cortex opposite C_3 or C_4. The technique consists of applying painless electrical stimuli at a rate of 5 per second over the median nerve. The impulses generated in general touch fibers with 500 or more stimuli, which are averaged with a computer. The response can be traced through the peripheral nerves, spinal roots, and posterior columns of the nuclei of Burdach and Goll in the lower medulla, through the medial lemniscus to the contralateral thalamus, and then to the sensory cortex of the parietal lobes. Normal waveforms are designated by the symbol P (positive) or N (negative), with a number indicating the interval of time in milliseconds from stimulus to recording.

The waveforms are usually named Erb point N10 (brachial plexus component); cervical components C7, cervical entry N13, C2, and lower medullary component N13b; and scalp component, Cz' N20. Delay between the stimulus and Erb point indicates peripheral nerve disease. Delay from Erb point to C2 implies an abnormality in the appropriate nerve roots or in the posterior columns. The presence of lesions in the medial lemniscus and thalamoparietal pathway can be inferred from delays of subsequent waves recorded from the parietal cortex (Cz', scalp, N20). SSEP results are influenced by body size (29), body temperature, and the presence of peripheral neuropathy, especially demyelinating neuropathy.

MOTOR EVOKED POTENTIALS

The method of painless magnetoelectric transcranial stimulation of the cerebral cortex was introduced in 1985 by Barker et al. (4). They applied short magnetic pulses to the scalp. The pulses were produced by a device designed to stimulate the peripheral nerves. The device recorded muscle action potentials from upper and lower limb muscles—the motor evoked potentials. Stimulating currents within the nervous tissue are induced by a time-varying magnetic field (25) generated by a brief high-voltage current pulse conducted through a copper coil (3,6,16).

Figure 10.1 shows the sites at which the stimulating coil is placed to stimulate the motor cortex, the cervical nerve roots, the lumbar nerve roots, and the sciatic nerve. The muscles usually used for recording MEPs are the biceps brachii, abductor pollicis brevis, and the abductor digiti minimi. The tibialis anterior is used as a control. The segmental innervation of these muscles is used for consistent diagnosis in comparison with the segmental distribution of the afferent nerves stimulated for SSEPs. During transcranial stimulation, upper limb muscles are preferentially activated with the center of the coil positioned above the vertex (16).

The threshold of the resting muscle is determined by means of applying magnetoelectric stimuli of successively increasing strengths. It has proved most practical to use magnetic stimuli of an intensity 50% above threshold for data collection. The subject is instructed to perform a slight voluntary contraction of the muscles being recorded. This

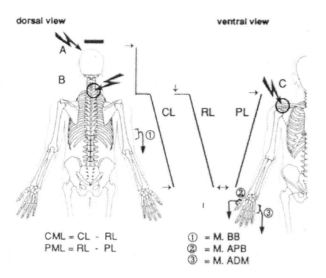

FIG. 10.1. Sites of magnetic stimulation. **A:** Motor cortex. **B:** Cervical nerve roots. **C:** Brachial nerve. *CL,* cortical latency; *PL,* peripheral latency; *RL,* root latency; *CML,* central motor latency.

procedure is called *facilitation* (15). Facilitation increases the amplitude and reduces the latency of MEPs.

For motor root stimulation over the cervical spine, the intensity of the stimulator is adjusted so that a potential with a steep negative rise can be recorded. With this adjustment, the onset latency is not critically dependent on the positioning of the coil or the stimulation strength (5). The excitation site of the nerve root is most likely in the region of the root exit from the intervertebral foramen (5) and does not differ from that suggested for electric stimulation over the spine (24). This is probably the effect of "channelling" of the current flow within the foramina, which produces depolarizing currents (6).

MEPs after motor root stimulation are analyzed for onset latency (root latency; RL) only. To assess MEP waveforms it is necessary to obtain an M-wave recording by means of conventional neurography. F-wave recordings allow determination of total peripheral conduction time (peripheral latency; PL) from the anterior horn cell to the muscle, which includes conduction over the motor root to its exit from the intervertebral foramen.

Latencies and amplitudes of MEPs after cortical or root stimulation are measured the same was as those in peripheral nerve conduction studies. Onset latency is measured at the point of first deflection of the trace from the baseline. If several sweeps have been recorded, the shortest reliable latency measurement is taken. Central motor latency (CML) is calculated in two ways:

1. CML minus RL using MEPs after magnetoelectric stimulation only (CML-M)
2. CL minus PL using transcranial magnetoelectric stimulation and the F-wave technique (CML-F)

MEPs after cortical (transcranial) stimulation are analyzed for amplitude, duration, and number of phases. Because of the sometimes unstable baseline during facilitatory preinnervation for cortical stimulation, amplitudes are measured peak to peak rather than baseline to peak. This becomes obvious in severely abnormal MEPs. The highest reliable amplitude is used. Amplitude and duration are expressed as ratio of the M-wave amplitude and duration after supramaximal electric peripheral nerve stimulation.

Dvorak et al. (9) examined 73 patients with cervical spinal disorders (37 women, 36 men 20 to 87 years of age, mean age ± SD 59 ± 16 years). As were healthy subjects, pa-

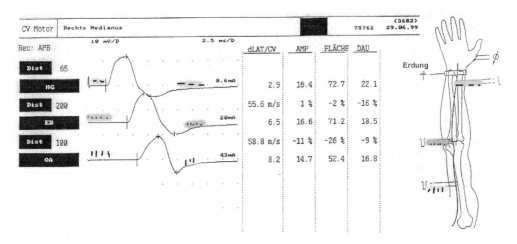

FIG. 10.2. Median nerve motor nerve conduction. Technique and normal result.

tients were grouped according to age (young, n = 7; old, n = 66) and size (short, n = 55; tall, n = 18). According to clinical and radiologic findings, the diagnoses were having spinal stenosis (n = 43) and nerve root compression syndrome (n = 30).

Twenty-eight of 43 patients with spinal stenosis (65%) had significantly increased CML-M to at least one muscle of at least one leg. Ten of 32 patients for whom MEPs were recorded from muscles of both lower limbs had bilaterally increased CML-M. Clinical examination showed a significant motor or sensory deficit in 11 lower limbs of 8 patients. CML-M to the muscles of 9 of these limbs (82%) were markedly increased. For 35 patients, clinical examination did not reveal appreciable motor or sensory deficit. Among these patients MEP showed increased CML-M in 29 of 64 limbs examined (45%). F-wave recordings were obtained from 16 muscles to which increased CML-M had been determined. The calculated CML-F was normal in 12 cases. Thus the conduction slowing was localized within the proximal segment of the lower motor neuron, that is, the cauda fibers, in 75% of these patients.

NEUROGRAPHY AND ELECTROMYOGRAPHY

Seddon (26) defined three degrees of nerve injury—neurapraxia, axonotmesis, and neurotmesis. This classification can be applied to nerve root injuries within the cervical spinal canal. *Neurapraxia* is characterized by conduction failure without structural changes in the axon. Fibers usually regain function promptly. Short-term changes in nerve conduction within the affected nerve segment (reduced conduction velocity by as much as 30% and finally complete conduction block) are probably caused by anoxia due to ischemia. The prognosis for complete recovery is excellent, and there are generally no EMG changes. Voluntary innervation of reduced interference is temporary. There are no signs of denervation, such as spontaneous activity.

Axonotmesis causes loss of continuity of the axons and immediate conduction block across the site of nerve injury. There is subsequent wallerian degeneration of the distal segment. Four or 5 days after acute interruption, the distal segment becomes inexcitable. Before conduction failure, there is no change in the maximal conduction velocity of the efferent motor potential or of the afferent sensory nerve action potential, nor is it possible to differentiate axonotmesis from neurapraxia on the basis of distal nerve excitability. Recovery depends on regeneration of nerve fibers, a process that occurs at a rate of 1 to 3 mm/d, therefore taking months, perhaps years.

Neurotmesis is the state of transection of the entire nerve, including myelin sheath and connective tissue. The nerve must be sutured. Regeneration often is poorly oriented, and regenerating nerve fibers do not regain their original number or diameter. Initial neurographic findings are identical to those in axonotmesis. In both axonotmesis and neurotmesis, EMG shows positive sharp waves 8 to 14 days and fibrillation potentials 14 to 20 days after nerve injury. Whereas reduced voluntary activity may be preserved in axonotmesis, this is not the case in neurotmesis.

Nerve Conduction Studies

Traditional nerve conduction studies consist of electrical stimulation of the nerve and recording of the evoked potential, either from the muscles, as in the study of motor nerves, or from the nerve itself as in the study of sensory nerves. Measuring the time between stimulation and response at two stimulation sites and the distance between the stimulation site allows easy calculation of the conduction velocity (Fig. 10.2). Although the methods are relatively simple, several technical factors influence the result and can lead to misinterpretation of the findings. The goals of nerve conduction studies are to assess the number of functioning axons and the state of the myelin of the functioning axons. This is a accomplished through study of conduction velocity, amplitude of the evoked response, and duration of the evoked response. Nerve root stimulation with needle electrodes is one technique that can be performed, but it is not commonly used.

F-wave Studies

Motor conduction of cervical fibers can be assessed more directly by means of measurement of the F-wave first described by Magladery and McDougal (23). It is a late compound muscle action potential caused by backfiring of antidromically activated anterior horn cells after supramaximal peripheral stimulation of a motor nerve. This concept was first explored in detail by Kimura (17) in studies involving patients with Charcot-Marie-Tooth neuropathy.

Recurrent activation of anterior horn cells occurs in only a small number of alpha motor neurons, preferentially in the larger motor neurons with faster conducting axons. Thus the minimal F-wave latency is a measure of the fastest conducting fibers. However, the latency variability of consecutive F waves is high because with successive supramaximal stimuli, recurrent discharges occur in different groups of motor neurons.

The conduction time from the spinal cord to the muscle (total PL) can be calculated with the following formula (17):

$$PL \text{ in milliseconds} = [(\text{Minimal F-wave latency in milliseconds} + \text{M-wave latency in milliseconds}) - 1 \text{ ms}] / 2$$

One millisecond is the estimated delay in turnaround time of the antidromic volley at the anterior horn cell. The F wave usually is normal in mild cases of radiculopathy. Distinct delay of the F wave or a reduced number of clearly distinguishable F waves after a given number of supramaximal peripheral stimuli yet normal results of distal motor conduction studies is a sign of a proximal lesion.

Electromyographic Studies

EMG must be considered an extension of the physical examination rather than simply a laboratory procedure. The muscles to be tested are selected according to clinical findings. Knowledge of the physiologic mechanisms underlying normal muscle contraction is a prerequisite for understanding the electrophysiologic abnormalities that occur in various disorders of the motor system. Electromyographers must be thoroughly familiar with the numerous factors that can affect the outcome of recordings (18).

Needle myography is not free of pain. However, an experienced examiner learns to perform this technique in a manner that is well tolerated by most patients. Care should be taken in examinations of patients with coagulopathy those at high risk of recurrent systemic infection.

The following are the main steps in an EMG examination:

1. Insertional activity is evaluated with placement and repositioning of the needle electrode in the muscle.
2. After stationary and stable positioning of the needle electrode, the recording is evaluated at rest for detection of spontaneous activity.

3. Single motor unit action potentials (MUAPs) are recorded with mild voluntary contraction of the muscle and examined with respect to amplitude, duration, and number of phases.
4. Motor unit recruitment and the interference pattern are recorded with a gradual increase in voluntary muscle contraction and maximal voluntary contraction, respectively.

Because a needle electrode registers MUAPs in a limited area close to surface, it is necessary to record in many different sites within the muscle by means of repositioning the needle. The tip is moved at least 2 mm perpendicular to the muscle fibers each time. Ten distinct areas should be sampled.

In evaluations of persons with cervical spinal disorders, EMG studies are aimed at delineating damage to the lower motor neuron, that is, axonotmesis or neurotmesis of the motor roots with muscular denervation. Denervated muscle fibers become unstable, because they no longer are under neural control, and individual muscle fibers fire in the absence of neural stimuli. This uncontrolled activity causes increased insertional activity, increased end-plate activity, and spontaneous activity. These EMG signs of denervation can be spotted at the earliest about 8 days after the injury. Analysis of single MUAPs also may reveal changes typical of but not specific for lower motor neuron damage, such as radiculopathy. The changes include increased amplitude, increased number of phases, and increased duration. These changes are seen only after reinnervation or sprouting of unaffected fibers. They are therefore considered chronic signs.

Localization of the lesion with respect to the motor roots affected is supported by examination of a variety of muscles innervated by different motor roots. If motor roots on the intraspinal course or the spinal nerve trunks within the intervertebral foramen are affected by the lesion, the paraspinal musculature, which is supplied by the posterior ramus from the spinal nerve, may have the typical EMG changes otherwise found only in limb muscles or muscles of the anterolateral body wall supplied by the anterior ramus.

In central paralysis, voluntary activity is reduced or absent, although the muscle can be activated through reflexes. Reduced voluntary activity produces an incomplete interference pattern. If voluntary activity is completely lost, the basic low-frequency discharges at rest are unchanged during maximal effort to contract the muscle and may also remain unchanged during attempts at defecation, thereby prohibiting normal defecation.

In incomplete peripheral paralysis caused by lesions in the cauda equina, few motor units with polyphasic potentials of long duration can be volitionally activated to discharge at high frequency. If axonal degeneration occurs, fibrillation potentials, positive sharp waves, or complex repetitive discharges can be seen.

Sensitivity, Specificity, and Predictive Value

Only a few studies address sensitivity, specificity, and predictive value—important measures of the diagnostic capability of neurophysiologic assessment of nerve root compression syndromes (8,13,31,32), and most of the studies have been aimed at lumbar and lumbosacral disorders. EMG performed with concentric needle electrodes is the oldest neurophysiologic method in the diagnosis of nerve root compression syndrome (28). Shea et al. (28) found EMG to be the most sensitive among EMG, neurography, and F-wave studies, but the sensitivity was only 20%, which must be considered poor. This finding is contrary to those of previous studies in which the sensitivity of EMG was 54% (21), 67% (22), and even 78% (19). However, the poor sensitivity of 20% was related to prediction of exact level of a root lesion. The sensitivity of abnormal EMG findings unrelated to level was 45% and possibly is explained by the pleurisegmental innervation of the extremity muscles.

The sensitivity of F-wave studies in the evaluation of root lesions has been found to be 35% (1,11,12,30); however, the results are poor in terms of predicting the exact level of a lesion. Tullberg et al. (31) found dermatomal SSEPs to have a sensitivity of 40%, but the correct level was determined in only 15% of cases, as it was in a study by Aminoff et al. (1). Tullberg et al. (31) concluded that of the three neurophysiologic methods evaluated alone or in combination, none was a reliable predictor of anatomic level even if more than one test is performed.

INDICATIONS FOR NEUROPHYSIOLOGIC INVESTIGATIONS

Neurophysiologic studies should be performed for the evaluation of suspected cervical radiculopathy or spinal stenosis, if radiologic results and clinical symptoms are conflicting or inconclusive. Patients with normal neurophysiologic test results are not considered as candidates for surgery (18). To predict surgical outcome, a complete neurophysiologic evaluation should be performed, including tests of both motor and sensory function.

Vohanka and Dvorak (32) analyzed the sensitivity of neurophysiologic methods in evaluations of patients with cervical spinal disorders, such as spinal stenosis and radiculopathy due to disc herniation or foraminal bone stenosis. Quantitative and qualitative EMG examinations were performed to look for signs of denervation signs and to analyze the mean duration of motor action potentials (average of 20 motor units per muscle). F-wave studies, MEPs, and dermatomal SSEPs also were obtained from the peroneal and tibial nerves. This complex investigations took 3 to 4 hours to obtain reproducible results.

There are generally accepted for an abnormal test result. For MEP, normal values within 3 standard deviations adjusted for body size have been used (10,14). Vohanka and Dvorak (32) correlated the neurophysiologic findings with computed tomographic or magnetic resonance imaging findings, which were not confirmed at surgery. Quantitative analysis of motor unit potentials showed 30% sensitivity among patients with radiculopathy but without motor deficit. The MEPs and SSEPs reached sensitivities of 55%, and the MEPs had 75% false-negative findings. If all neurophysiologic tests were used, a nerve root lesion would be suspected in 73% of 29 patients with radiculopathy. On the other hand, 53% of patients with objective clinical signs of nerve root compression had false-negative SSEP findings, 59% had signs of denervation at EMG, 65% had polyphasic reinnervation potentials, and 75% had normal MEP findings. The high incidence of false-negative findings indicates that neurophysiologic tests have a low reliability in confirming clinical findings. It is important that in the study Vohanka and Dvorak (32), a correlation was made between clinical, neurophysiologic, and neuroradiologic assessments only; the diagnoses were not confirmed at surgery.

CONCLUSION

On the basis of the results of a few studies, mostly conducted to evaluate lumbosacral disorders, it can be concluded that for patients with cervical radiculopathy due to nerve root compression or spinal stenosis, the overall sensitivity and specificity of neurophysiologic assessment are low. Neurophysiologic assessment of spinal stenosis is justified in following situations:

To exclude distal nerve damage, such as neuropathy or nerve entrapment

To verify subjective muscle weakness by means of needle EMG for patients with pain inhibition due to lack of cooperation

To document preoperative muscle status before a reoperation on the spine, if difficult surgery is expected (medicolegal reasons)

REFERENCES

1. Aminoff MJ, Goodin DS, Parry GJ. Electrophysiologic evaluation of lumbosacral radiculopathies: electromyography, late response, and somatosensory evoked potentials. *Neurology* 1985;35:1514–1518.
2. Anziska B, Cracco RQ. Short latency somatosensory evoked potentials: studies in patients with focal neurological disease. *Electroencephalogr Clin Neurophysiol* 1980;49:227–239.
3. Barker AT, Freeston IL, Jalinous R, et al. Magnetic stimulation of the human brain and peripheral nervous system: an introduction and the results of an initial clinical evaluation. *Neurosurgery* 1987;20:100–109.
4. Barker AT, Freeston IL, Jalinous R, et al. Magnetic stimulation of the human brain. *J Physiol* 1985a;369:3P.
5. Britton TC, Meyer BU, Herdmann J, et al. Clinical use of the magnetic stimulator in the investigation of peripheral conduction time. *Muscle Nerve* 1990;13:396–406.
6. Cadwell J. Principles of magnetoelectric stimulation. In: Chokroverty S, ed. *Magnetic stimulation in clinical neurophysiology*. Boston: Butterworth-Heinemann, 1989:13–32.
7. Chiappa KH, Choi S, Young RR. Short latency somatosensory evoked potentials following median nerve stimulation in patients with neurological lesions. In: Desmedt JE, ed. *Progress in Clinical Neurophysiology*. Basel: Karger, 1980:264–281.
8. Dvorak J. Neurophysiologic tests in diagnosis of nerve root compression caused by disc herniation. *Spine* 1996;21 [Suppl 24]:39S–44S.
9. Dvorak J, Herdmann J, Janssen B, et al. Motor-evoked potentials in patients with cervical spine disorders. *Spine* 1990;15:1013–1016.
10. Dvorak J, Herdmann J, Theiler R, et al. Magnetic stimulation of motor cortex and motor roots for painless evaluation of central and proximal peripheral motor pathways: normal values and clinical application in disorders of the lumbar spine. *Spine* 1991;16:955–960.
11. Eisen A, Hoirch M. The electrodiagnostic evaluation of spinal root lesions. *Spine* 1983;8:98–106.
12. Fisher MA, Shivde AJ, Teixera C, et al. Clinical and electrophysiological appraisal of the significance of radicular injury in back pain. *J Neurol Neurosurg Psychiatry* 1978;41:303–306.
13. Haig AJ, LeBreck DB, Powly SG. Paraspinal mapping: quantified needle electromyography of the paraspinal muscles in persons without low back pain. *Spine* 1995;20:715–721.
14. Herdmann J, Dvorak J, Rathmer L, et al. Conduction velocities of pyramidal tract fibres and lumbar motor nerve roots: normal values. *Zentral bl Neurochir* 1991;52:197–199.
15. Hess CW, Mills KR, Murray NMF. Magnetic stimulation of the human brain: facilitation of motor responses by voluntary contraction of ipsilateral and contralateral muscles with additional observations on an amputee. *Neurosci Lett* 1986;71:235–240.
16. Hess CW, Mills KR, Murray NMF. Methodological considerations for magnetic brain stimulation. In: Barber C, Blum T, eds. *Evoked potentials III*. London: Butterworths, 1988:456–461.
17. Kimura J. F-wave velocity in the central segment of the median and ulnar nerves: a study in normal subjects and patients with Charcot-Marie-Tooth disease. *Neurology* 1974;24:539–546.
18. Kimura J. *Electrodiagnosis in diseases of nerve and muscle: principles and practice,* 2nd ed. Philadelphia: FA Davis, 1989.
19. Knuttsson B. Comparative value of electromyographic, myelographic and clinical-neurological examinations in diagnosis of lumbar root compression syndrome. *Arch Orthop Scand Suppl* 1961;49:1–135.
20. Kunesch E. Bedeutung von Quellenlokalisationstechniken evozierter Potentiale (Brain Electric Source Analysis, Magnetencephalographie) zur Untersuchung der sensiblen Kontrolle von Handbewegungen. 1991.
21. LaJoie WJ. Nerve root compression: correlation of electromyographic, myelographic and surgical findings. *Arch Phys Med Rehabil* 1972;53:390–392.
22. Lane ME, Tamhankar MN, Demopoulos JT. Discogenic radiculopathy: use of electromyography in multidisciplinary management. *NY State J Med* 1978;78:32–36.
23. Magladery JW, McDougal DB. Electrophysiological studies of nerve and reflex activity in normal man, 1: identification of certain reflexes in the electromyogram and the conduction velocity of peripheral nerve fibres. *Bull Johns Hopkins Hosp* 1950;86:265–290.
24. Mills KR, Murray NMF. Electrical stimulation over the human vertebral column: which neuronal elements are exited? *Electroencephalogr Clin Neurophysiol* 1986;63:582–589.
25. Polson MJR, Barker AT, Freeston IL. Stimulation of nerve trunks with time varying magnetic fields. *Med Biol Eng Comput* 1982;20:243–244.
26. Seddon HJ. *Surgical disorders of peripheral nerves,* 2nd ed. Edinburgh: Churchill Livingstone, 1975.

27. Shahani BT, Halperin JJ, Boulu P, et al. Sympathetic skin response: a method of assessing unmyelinated axon dysfunction in peripheral neuropathies. *J Neurol Neurosurg Psychiatry* 1984;47:536–542.
28. Shea PA, Woods WW, Werden DH. Electromyography in diagnosis of nerve root compression syndrome. *Arch Neurol Psychiatry* 1950;64:93–104.
29. Stöhr M. Somatosensible Reizantworten von Rückenmark und Gehirn (SEP). In: Stöhr M, et al., eds. *Evozierte Potentiale.* Berlin: Springer-Verlag, 1989:112–120.
30. Tonzola RF, Ackil AA, Shahani BT, et al. Usefulness of electrophysiological studies in the diagnosis of lumbosacral root disease. *Ann Neurol* 1981;9:305–308.
31. Tullberg T, Svanborg E, Isacsson J, et al. A preoperative and postoperative study of the accuracy and value of electrodiagnosis in patients with lumbosacral disc herniation. *Spine* 1993;18:837–842.
32. Vohanka S, Dvorak J. Motor and somatosensory evoked potentials in cervical spinal stenosis. Presented at the 40th Congress of the Czech and Slovak Neurophysiology, Brno, 1993.

SECTION 4

Conservative Treatment Modalities

The Degenerative Cervical Spine,
edited by Marek Szpalski and Robert Gunzburg
Lippincott Williams & Wilkins, Philadelphia © 2001.

11

Rheumatologic Treatments

Michel Benoist

Department of Orthopaedic Surgery and Section of Rheumatology
University of Paris VII, 75116 Paris, France

GENERAL CONSIDERATIONS
PHARMACOLOGIC TREATMENT
Simple analgesics • Nonsteroidal Antiinflammatory Therapy • Systemic Glucocorticoids
• Muscle Relaxants • Psychotropic Drugs • Anticonvulsants
THERAPEUTIC STRATEGIES
Axial Neck Pain • Cervical Radiculopathy • Cervical Chemonucleolysis • Cervical
Myelopathy
CONCLUSIONS

A wide range of arthropathies can affect the cervical spine. This chapter is limited to the medical management of the complications of cervical spondylosis. The efficacy of the various therapies is reviewed according to the pertinent data in the literature. Unfortunately, nonoperative care has no solid scientific foundation. In this era of evidence-based medicine, there are still many unanswered questions.

GENERAL CONSIDERATIONS

Stimulation of the nociceptive system is the most frequent pain-generating mechanism in acute and subacute neck and radicular pain syndromes. In the case of neck pain without a radicular component, the local receptors are located in the anulus, facets, ligaments, and muscles. In the case of arm pain due to radicular irritation, the nociceptive message starts from the inflamed nerve root and ganglion. In both cases, the nociceptive input is transmitted through the dorsal horn of the cord to the ascending pathways and high centers with the final cortical processing. In chronic neck pain, central sensitization, psychologic factors, and loss of physiologic inhibitory controls have a central role, often more important than the peripheral nociception.

Stimulation of the nociceptive system can be mechanical from trauma (excessive single load, repetitive microtrauma, or instability). It can also be of chemical origin related to inflammatory mediators as, for example, in degenerative discs or facets. Medical treatment is aimed at suppressing inflammation and pain with pharmacologic agents and at limiting mechanical constraints with rest, collars, physical therapy, posture education, and ergonomics.

PHARMACOLOGIC TREATMENT

The four major types of pharmacologic agents in current use are analgesics, nonsteroidal antiinflammatory drugs (NSAIDs), systemic glucocorticoids, and muscle relaxants.

Simple Analgesics

Use of simple analgesics is self-explanatory. Uncontrolled pain can induce abnormal conditions in the central nervous system and make subsequent control of pain more difficult. Salicylates in low dosages, less than 2 g a day, have an analgesic rather than an antiinflammatory effect. Aspirin is the least expensive of the group and can be administered in many forms, such as enteric coated, to minimize its gastric irritant effect.

Paracetamol (USAN, acetaminophen) is the most commonly prescribed analgesic. In doses of up to 1 g four times a day, this drug has few side effects. At a higher dosage, paracetamol can cause hepatic damage. The dose should be decreased in the presence of liver disease. To enhance the analgesic effect paracetamol can be combined with codeine or dextropropoxyphene (USAN, propoxyphene hydrochloride), each of which has a central mechanism of action. It is important, however, to be aware that paracetamol is found in many commercial mixtures and compounds. This concurrent therapy needs to be ascertained and the maximum dose of paracetamol from all potential sources most be explained to the patient.

The use of morphine or opioid analgesics is justified if neck and arm pain is severe. Use of these agents in the management of chronic pain is controversial because of the risk of addiction and adverse respiratory effects.

Nonsteroidal Antiinflammatory Therapy

Numerous NSAIDs are available. They have more or less the same mode of action—inhibition of formation of prostaglandins through the cyclooxygenase pathway. The large number of NSAIDs available reflects the facts that none of them is ideal and that all have potential toxicity. The main adverse effect is gastrointestinal problems. Gastric ulcers with or without bleeding represent the most important iatrogenic complication. The effect on the stomach is mediated through inhibition of the prostaglandins responsible for production of bicarbonate in the mucosal layer, which protects the gastric epithelium. Prophylactic use of ulcer-healing drugs should be considered for patients at risk, such as those with previous gastric ulcers, elderly patients, or those taking anticoagulants. Cyclooxygenase-2 (COX-2) antagonists seem to have less gastrointestinal toxicity than the other NSAIDs.

The kidney is another site of action of prostaglandins. Under the usual physiologic conditions and in healthy adults, prostaglandins play only a small part in regulation of the normal function. However, if renal blood flow is reduced, for example by vomiting, diarrhea, or concurrent therapy, normal renal vasodilatation is impaired and there is a risk of renal insufficiency. The risk is particularly high among older patients with existing renal impairment. Other adverse effects include skin, hepatic, hematologic, and central nervous system manifestations.

Efficacy of NSAIDS has been demonstrated empirically, and several clinical trials in the field of low back pain have demonstrated the pain-relieving effect (1,4). It seems that the new highly selective COX-2 antagonist NSAIDS such as celecoxib (Cerebrex) are effective in the management of degenerative osteoarthritic disorders and of rheumatoid arthritis (3,6,15). Celecoxib has sustained antiinflammatory and analgesic activity, which appears on a par with that of classic NSAIDS. An additional benefit is that the rate of adverse gastrointestinal effects is low, comparable with that among healthy, symptom-free volunteers, even with long-term use (6). If no other adverse effects appear in the future, COX-2 selective products will have an important place in the management of degenerative osteoarticular disorders, especially when long-term use is necessary.

Because there is little difference in efficacy between the numerous NSAIDs, the prescriber should become familiar with a few of these drugs and try to use the smallest dose to achieve the desired effect. There is variation in response among patients, and it is advisable to try an alternative drug if the first one is ineffective.

Systemic Glucocorticoids

Systemic glucocorticoids sometimes are used to manage acute pain. A high loading dose is necessary to obtain pain relief, which is sometimes spectacular. However, one has to bear in mind that even short-term glucocorticoid therapy can induce serious side effects, including osteonecrosis.

Muscle Relaxants

Therapy with muscle relaxants is aimed at suppressing muscle spasms and hypertonus. Excessive muscle contraction may activate the muscular nociceptors and aggravate the nociceptive input in the spinal cord (23). However, there is little evidence to support the efficacy of these agents controlling muscle spasm. In conventional oral doses, most of these drugs act centrally and produce sedation. If used for a long time, benzodiazepines are addictive.

Psychotropic Drugs

Tricyclic antidepressants are the main psychotropic agents to be considered. Patients with chronic pain often are depressed as a cause or a consequence of pain. Some patients with no evidence of depression benefit from use of tricyclics because of the analgesic effect. Tricyclics have a stimulating effect on the normal physiologic inhibitory descending system through action on the dorsal horn of the spinal cord. Different tricyclic preparations are available, and most clinicians have their favorites. Amitriptyline is commonly prescribed at doses lower than those used in depressive syndromes, except in the treatment of patients with major depression. The starting dose is usually 25 mg at night and can be increased gradually up to 75 mg (9).

Anticonvulsants

Anticonvulsants such as carbamazepine or phenytoin have limited indications. However, they can be useful in the management of chronic radicular pain, especially among patients with postlaminectomy deafferentation syndrome, which generates constant and shooting pains.

THERAPEUTIC STRATEGIES

Therapy must be adapted to various factors such as age, severity of pain, and stage of evolution (acute, subacute, or chronic). Previous trauma and presence of litigation also are important factors. Nonoperative care is discussed according to the clinical complications of spondylosis—neck pain, cervical radiculopathy, and myelopathy—with the accompanying imaging abnormalities.

Axial Neck Pain

Most acute sprains and strains resulting from an awkward position or activity respond quickly to treatment, often without relapses. Patients need only a short course of analgesics or NSAIDs. Patients with acute neck pain after an automobile accident may benefit from a high dose of intravenous methylprednisolone administered within 8 hours of the injury (19). A controlled, double-blind study has assessed the effect of tenoxicam on pain and motion in the acute early phase of whiplash injury and has shown a beneficial effect on both pain and motion (22).

Subacute Axial Neck Pain

Despite early pharmacologic intervention, pain may persist over a few weeks and become subacute, especially after an injury (8). Grade 1 and 2 whiplash injuries are good examples of subacute axial neck pain without a neurologic component. Medical treatment includes drugs, infiltration, orthotic devices, physical therapy, and education. The use of analgesics and antiinflammatories is self-explanatory, but the efficacy in the management of subacute neck pain has not been validated. Efficacy and tolerance of various devices such as collars, methods of physical therapy, and injections are discussed in Chapters 12 through 16. A few studies have indicated that exercise and normal activity are more beneficial than rest and immobilization for these patients (16,17). Prolonged rest and sick leave may cause anxiety, depression, muscular atrophy, and loss of mobility. My therapeutic approach is summarized in

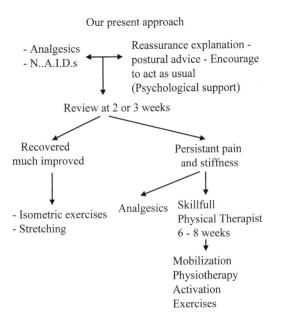

FIG. 11.1. Rheumatologic management of subacute axial neck pain.

Fig. 11.1. The main objective is to avoid chronic pain. This strategy is not always successful, and the patient may be referred for therapy after the pain has entered the chronic phase.

Chronic Axial Neck Pain

The major causes of chronic axial neck pain in the degenerative cervical spine are listed in Table 11.1. Poor posture and psychosocial difficulties are aggravating factors. Most data in the literature indicate that late whiplash syndrome is a combination of severe organic lesions and secondary psychologic factors. Therapy should be structured accordingly to manage the physical problem and the psychologic consequences of the injury. No controlled trial of medications, physical therapy, traction, or manipulation has demonstrated the efficacy of these modalities at this stage of pain. Intraarticular injection of glucocorticoids is not effective (2). Percutaneous radiofrequency neurotomy for chronic facet joint pain has proved beneficial in a controlled study (13). Chronic pain in late whiplash often is accompanied by depression. A combination of psychotherapy and antidepressant medications often is needed. In some cases, a multidisciplinary approach and behavioral strategies, as provided in pain clinics, are useful.

Osteoarthritis in the aging cervical spine is a frequent cause of chronic pain among elderly persons. The source of nociceptive input may be mechanical owing to instability or chemical through inflammatory mediators, as in the peripheral joints. Therapy for spondylotic chronic neck pain includes oral medications, collars, and physical therapy. However, the therapeutic strategy is totally empiric and is based on the patient's response to treatment. This is true for the type of medications used, the doses, and the regimen. The efficacy of orthoses and physical therapy has not been scientifically validated.

Chronic neck pain is a frequent feature of fibromyalgia. This syndrome includes widespread musculoskeletal pain and stiffness associated with poor sleep, muscular fatigue, and the presence of numerous tender points. Tricyclic antidepressants aid sleep and relieve pain for 25% to 30% of patients. Tramadol seems to be the most useful analgesic. Management of fibromyalgia has been reviewed (12).

Myofascial pain syndrome primary or secondary to disc or facet lesions has no proven pathologic lesion. Myofascial pain may respond to massage, stretching, or trigger point injections. No controlled study has substantiated the efficacy of these modalities.

Chronic neck pain can be aggravated by poor posture, sometimes work related. Poor posture induces abnormal forces and strains on the muscles. The ensuing excessive muscle contraction may activate the nociceptors in muscles and tendons. Exercise, postural reeducation, and workstation ergonomics are part of the rehabilitation program.

Cervical Radiculopathy

Two types of lesions may compress and irritate the cervical nerve root: (a) a lateral soft disc, which is a posterolateral herniation of nucleus pulposus into the intervertebral fora-

TABLE 11.1. *Causes of chronic neck
pain without neurologic involvement*

Posttraumatic disorder (late whiplash)
Degenerative osteoarthritis
Fibromyalgia
Myofascial pain syndrome
Aggravating factors
  Psychosocial problems
  Poor posture

men, or (b) a lateral hard disc, which is a bony proliferation at the posterolateral margins of the intervertebral disc that encroaches on the nerve in the foramen. Initial management of radicular pain is identical for both conditions but remains pragmatic, as in axial discogenic neck pain. Treatment includes analgesics, narcotics in the acute phase, NSAIDs, and muscle relaxants. In some cases, addition of high doses of glucocorticoids is necessary. Some authors recommend perineural or epidural injection of glucocorticoids. The efficacy and complications of this procedure are discussed in Chapter 16. No controlled study has proved the efficacy of this treatment, and it carries substantial risks of complications (5,21). Rest, use of a cervical collar, manual and mechanical traction, physical therapy, and isometric exercises are part of the management program. An algorithm of medical management of cervical radiculopathy is presented in Fig. 11.2. The outcome of such a program was prospectively studied by Saal et al. (21). After 2 years of follow-up study, 20 of 26 patients had good or excellent results. Two patients were not available for follow-up evaluations. Two patients underwent cervical surgery, and two patients had poor results. Twenty-one patients returned to the same job. The best outcomes were obtained in the care of patients with disc extrusion (21).

Bush et al. (5) conducted a prospective study with 13 consecutive patients who had cervical radiculopathy. All patients had substantial posterolateral discal herniation. All patients were treated with medications and serial periradicular and epidural glucocorticoid injections. They were evaluated after an average of 12 months by an independent clinician. Twelve of 13 patients had good or excellent results.

Despite the lack of a randomized clinical trial, the aforementioned studies and personal experience indicate that appropriate medical therapy is successful among most patients with cervical radiculopathy. However, these studies have been conducted with patients with cervical discal herniation, which has been shown eventually to regress (5,14,18). The efficacy of nonoperative treatment has not yet been investigated in the care of patients with pure bony compression of the nerve root. Further controlled investigations are clearly needed to appreciate the specifically effective component of medical treatment and to determine the reasonable time after which operative management should be con-

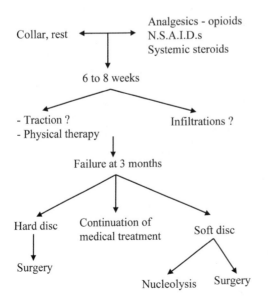

FIG. 11.2. Rheumatologic management of cervical radiculopathy.

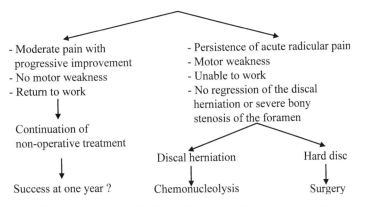

FIG. 11.3. Cervical radiculopathy. Failure after 3 months of nonoperative treatment.

sidered for these two pathologic conditions. Fig. 11.3 shows my present approach of more aggressive treatment. The decision to continue medical treatment in the hope of complete healing is empiric. The few data in the literature (5,21) and personal experience seem to indicate that most patients recover after 1 year. But the proportion of those who have relapses or chronic symptoms is not known. A retrospective study (10) showed that after an average of 5 years (range 4.6 months to 10.6 years) radicular pain had disappeared among all 39 conservatively treated patients. Additional prospective, controlled studies similar to that of Weber for sciatica are needed. The choice of 3 months of evolution before radical treatment is provided is arbitrary. The point at which failure of conservative therapy is recognized depends on many factors, such as severity of pain, severity of the pathologic condition, and socioeconomic considerations.

Persistence of an acute pain and motor weakness after 3 months of appropriate medical management justifies radical treatment. At my institution patients with a pure discal herniation undergo chemonucleolysis. Those with a bony compression or a combination of discal and osseous proliferation receive a surgical treatment. Techniques and results of surgery are discussed in Chapters 17 through 29. Intradiscal injection of chymopapain is the ultimate stage of medical treatment.

Cervical Chemonucleolysis

Nucleolysis with chymopapain in the management of cervical discal herniation has been performed in a few European centers (7,8,20; Guigui P, Abiad R, Benoist M, et al., unpublished data, 2000). In the United States it was considered contraindicated because of potential neurologic complications. A pilot study has been conducted at my institution. It was started in 1990, and since then 141 patients have been enrolled. The mean age at chemonucleolysis was 41 years, and the mean follow-up period was 4.5 years (range 6 months to 8 years). Patients were evaluated by an independent observer. The outcome was appreciated on a global functional score, a visual analog scale, and a degree of satisfaction questionnaire. Table 11.2 shows the clinical results at long term. In this series no complication was observed. Identical results were obtained in three published series. They are presented in Table 11.3. Two cases of infectious discitis and one of meningeal hemorrhage, which healed without sequelae, were described in one series (11).

It can be argued that the good results obtained after 5 years of follow-up study are similar to those observed with the evolution of pain as previously described. However, the

TABLE 11.2. *Long-term clinical results of cervical chemonucleolysis*

Result	Percentage of patients
Exellent	58
Good	34
Poor	8

Patients treated at author's institution; N = 141; mean follow-up period 4.5 years.

TABLE 11.3. *Clinical results of cervical chemonucleolysis*

Study	No. of patients	Percentage of excellent or good results	Complications
Richaud et al. (20)	38	83	None
Krause et al. (11)	190	86	Discitis (2 cases) Meningeal hemorrhage (1 case)
Gomez Castrasena et al. (7)	87	92	None

results of these studies show the safety of the procedure and the persistence of good results at long term. Moreover and most important, in the four series described, radicular pain disappeared rapidly within the first 2 weeks among more than 80% of the patients. Reactive axial neck pain was rare and usually was mild or moderate.

Chemonucleolysis can accelerate the course of discal herniation and of the radiculopathy among patients who after appropriate conservative treatment still suffer from intractable neck and arm pain. On average the patient can resume work after 2 to 4 weeks. In summary, if the indications and contraindications listed in Tables 11.4 and 11.5 are used, cervical nucleolysis appears likely to replace or redefine the indications for surgery. The efficacy of the procedure is similar to that of surgery with minor risk of complications. For patients with radiculopathy caused by osseous compression or a combination of disc and osseous tissue, cervical disc surgery through an anterior approach has a high success rates.

Cervical Myelopathy

There is no medical therapy for cord compression caused by central discal herniation or bony spurs. The efficacy of rest, collars, and traction has never been validated. If dis-

TABLE 11.4. *Indications for cervical chemonucleolysis*

Severe radiculopathy not responding to at least 2 months of conservative treatment
Good correlation of clinical signs and symptoms with clear evidence of posterolateral discal herniation

TABLE 11.5. *Contraindications to cervical chemonucleolysis*

Myelopathy
Severe motor deficit
Combination of discal and osseous
   compression
Pure axial neck pain
Pregnancy
Known allergy to chymopapain

cal herniation occurs, the decision for surgery must be made rapidly. In the case of spondylotic myelopathy, close medical and neurologic surveillance is mandatory. The techniques of and indications for surgery are discussed in Chapter 20.

CONCLUSIONS

The therapeutic strategies presented are for a large part empiric and lacking in scientific validation. Further investigation is needed to define the components of nonoperative treatment that may be specifically efficacious in management of the various conditions. Therapy for subacute or chronic axial neck pain has limited scientific foundation and is still based on data obtained through tradition or empiricism. In this age of evidence-based medicine, interventions such as periradicular or epidural injections in the management of radiculopathy must be analyzed in prospective, controlled studies. Results of well-conducted studies will define the exact place of cervical nucleolysis.

REFERENCES

1. Amile E, Weber H, Holm I. Treatment of acute low-back pain with pyroxicam: results of a double-blind placebo controlled trial. *Spine* 1987;12:473–476.
2. Barnsley L, Lord SM, Wallis BJ, et al. Lack of effect of intra-articular steroids for chronic pain in the cervical zygapophyseal joints. *N Engl J Med* 1994;330:1047–1050.
3. Bensen WG, Fiechner JJ, McMillen JI, et al. Treatment of osteoarthritis with celecoxib, a cyclooxygenase-2 inhibitor: a randomized controlled trial. *Mayo Clin Proc* 1999;74:1095–1105.
4. Berry H, Bloom B, Hamilton EBD, et al. Naproxen sodium, diflunisal and placebo in the treatment of chronic back pain. *Ann* Rheum Dis 1982;41:129–132.
5. Bush K, Chaudhuri R, Hillier S, et al. The pathomorphologic changes that accompany the resolution of cervical radiculopathy. *Spine*, 1997;22:183–187.
6. Emery P, Zeidler H, Kvien TK, et al. Celecoxib versus diclofenac in long-term management of rheumatoid arthritis: randomized double blind comparison. *Lancet* 1999;354:2106–2111.
7. Gomez Castresana FB, Vazquez H, Baltes H. Cervical chemonucleolysis. *Orthopedics* 1995;18:237–242.
8. Gore DR, Sepic SB, Gardner GM, et al. Neck pain: a long term follow up of 205 patients. *Spine* 1987;12:1–5.
9. Hameroff SR, Weiss JL, Lerman JC, et al. Dexopin effects on chronic pain and depression: a controlled study. *J Clin Psychiatry* 1984;45:45–52.
10. Heckmann JG, Lang C, Zobebein L. Herniated cervical intervertebral discs with radiculopathy: an outcome study of conservatively or surgically treated patients. *J Spinal Disord* 1999;12:396–401.
11. Krause D, Drape JL, Jambon F, et al. Nucléolyse cervicale: indications, technique et résultats. *J Neuroradiol* 1993;20:42–59.
12. Leventhal LJ. Management of fibromyalgia. *Ann Intern Med* 1999;131:850–858.
13. Lord SM, Barnsley L, Wallis BJ, et al. Percutaneous radiofrequency neurotony for chronic cervical zygapophyseal joint pain. *N Engl J Med* 1996;335:1721–1726.
14. Maigne JY, Deligne L. Computed tomographic follow up study of 21 cases of non-operatively treated cervical intervertebral soft disc herniation. *Spine* 1994;19:189–191.
15. Manek NJ, Lane NE. Osteoarthritis: current concepts in diagnosis and management. *Am Fam Physician* 2000;61:1795–1804.
16. McKinney LA. Early mobilisation and outcome in acute neck sprain of the neck. *BMJ* 1989;299:1006–1008.
17. Mealy K, Brenman H, Fenelon CC. Early mobilisation of acute whiplash injuries. *BMJ* 1986;292:656–657.
18. Mochida K, Komori H, Okawa A, et al. Regression of cervical disc herniation observed on magnetic resonance images. *Spine* 1998;23:990–997.
19. Pettersson K, Toolanen G. High dose methylprednisolone prevents extensive sick leave after whiplash injury: a prospective double blind study. *Spine* 1998;23:984–989.
20. Richaud J, Lazorthes Y, Verdie JL, et al. Chemonucleolysis for herniated cervical disc. *Acta Neurochir (Wien)* 1988;91:116–119.
21. Saal JA, Saal JS, Yurth EF. Nonoperative management of herniated cervical intervertebral disc with radiculopathy. *Spine* 1996;21:1877–1883.
22. Szpalski M, Gunzburg R, Sceur M, et al. Pharmacologic interventions in whiplash: associated disorders. In: Gunzburg R, Szpalski M, eds. *Whiplash injuries.* Philadelphia: Lippincott-Raven, 1997:175–181.
23. Weber H. Lumbar disc herniation. A controlled, prospective study with ten years of observation. *Spine* 1998;8:131–140.
24. Zimmermann M. Pain mechanisms and mediators in osteoarthritis. *Semin Arthritis Rheum* 1989;18:22–29.

The Degenerative Cervical Spine,
edited by Marek Szpalski and Robert Gunzburg
Lippincott Williams & Wilkins, Philadelphia © 2001.

12

Combination Treatment for Nonspecific Neck Pain

Margareta Nordin, Markus Pietrek, Manny Halpern

*Occupational and Industrial Orthopaedic Center, Hospital for Joint Diseases,
Mount Sinai NYU Health, New York, New York 10014*

EVALUATION
PROGNOSIS FOR RECOVERY
TREATMENT
 Education • Exercise • Ergonomics
CONCLUSIONS

Neck pain is fairly common among adults in industrialized societies. It is often associated with shoulder and/or upper extremity pain. The point prevalence of neck disorders among the general population ranges from 13% to 22% (7,31), the 1-year prevalence from 34% to 46% (5,7,22), and the lifetime prevalence from 67% to 71% (7,20), depending on the sex and age of the population and the definition of pain. Chronic neck pain is highly prevalent among adults (5) and disables approximately 5% of the adult population (7). Neck pain increases with age (5) and is more common among women than among men (5,7,20).

The origin of neck pain can be traumatic or nontraumatic. More information is becoming available about prognostic factors and treatment efficiencies in traumatic neck pain, the so-called whiplash-associated disorders (WAD). In the nontraumatic degenerative and inflammatory cervical spine, the prognosis is less well known. As for treatment efficiency, the importance of physical therapy and exercise should not be underestimated. The evidence of successful outcome can be questioned, however. Few randomized, controlled studies have been conducted, patient classification is often poor, and the success criteria lack stringent definitions. This chapter suggests and presents a combination treatment of education, exercise, and ergonomics for nonspecific degenerative and mechanical neck pain.

EVALUATION

A standardized clinical evaluation and classification is mandatory. If the origin of neck pain is traumatic, the Quebec Task Force classification (WAD grade 0 through IV) can be used (25). If a nontraumatic origin is the cause of neck pain, the classification must address the cause of the pain origin—mechanical, inflammatory, or other (e.g., cervical spinal stenosis, torticollis, or tumor). For almost all patients with nontraumatic neck pain, the exact anatomic source of the pain is difficult to locate. This nonspecific neck pain often has a slow onset and becomes exacerbated during specific tasks. These patients are the focus of this chapter. There is no globally accepted classification of nonspecific neck pain. No task force has attempted to review existing literature about neck pain at large and thereby suggest a classification system.

A history that includes onset, characteristics, radiation, and duration of pain, exacerbating tasks, type of job, and preferred activity must be documented. The clinical evaluation must include musculoskeletal and neurologic examinations (8). A pain drawing, a clinical screening tool (2), and a questionnaire about perceived function such as the Neck and Upper Limb Index (NULI) (26) or Disabilities of the Arm, Shoulder, and Hand (DASH) (15) can be helpful. Neck pain often is part of cumulative trauma disorders (CTD), also called repetitive strain injuries (RSI) (16). Patients with nonspecific neck pain should be referred for physical therapy and exercises with a possible combination treatment of stress and pain management and ergonomic evaluation. The goal is to identify risk of chronicity and disability at an early stage.

PROGNOSIS FOR RECOVERY

Prognostic factors for delayed recovery and chronicity in less severe WAD (WAD grades I through III) (25) are neck pain on palpation, muscle pain, radiating pain or numbness, and headache. Female sex and older age also contribute to slower recovery from WAD (27,28). Prognostic factors in non-WAD-associated neck pain are less known. In a systematic review of the sparse literature on prognostic factors for delayed recovery from nonspecific neck pain, Borghouts et al. (4) concluded that a higher severity of pain and a history of previous neck pain seem to be associated with a worse prognosis. In a longitudinal epidemiologic study to estimate the 1-year predictive role of several medical and nonmedical factors for neck disorders, Leclerc et al. (19) found female sex, older age, headaches or pain in the head, psychologic distress, and psychosomatic problems to be predictors of both the occurrence and persistence of neck pain. Burdorf et al. (6) stated that the presence of neck or shoulder pain among male welders and metal workers contributed significantly to work absence due to neck or shoulder pain (relative risk 3.3; 95% confidence interval 1.7–6.5). This indicates that the neck or shoulder should be evaluated in relation to work and activity demands. Prolonged work absence was associated with job title, which points to the fact that the type of task may influence the possibility of returning to work (6).

TREATMENT

The most successful treatment outcomes for many nonspecific musculoskeletal conditions, which do not require surgery or more invasive care, have been obtained with combination treatments. Success is hereby defined as return to work and activity and a decrease in or relief from pain. The combination treatment suggested for nonspecific neck pain is education (an informed consumer), range of motion and muscle endurance training (exercise), and ergonomic workstation evaluation (low-cost adjustment). Priority is given to active treatment. Passive physical modalities such as heat, ultrasound, electrical stimulation, and massage should be used only temporarily as an adjunct. If stress or pain management by a psychologist is necessary, it is to be provided early. Treatment sessions are limited; progress should be obtained after five to eight therapy visits. Extensions of treatment or referrals to a psychologist are decided within the therapist team. If the patient does not respond to the proposed treatment, he or she is referred to a specialty evaluation by a psychologist or physician. Further nonsurgical treatment, such as drugs, manual therapy, acupuncture, or injections, are discussed in Chapters 11 and 13 through 16. The suggested combination treatment consists of the following elements.

Education

The patient has to be an informed consumer. The aim is to educate the patient about the condition and its mostly benign nature, to discuss the treatment options, and to set a common goal. Return to normal activity should be promoted. Compliance with treatment must be discussed at the first encounter. Information given should be evidence based. If no evidence of efficacy about a treatment exists, the patient should be informed as such. Neck schools have not had the expected effect (18), but individual instruction and information with reinforcement through brochures, videotapes, interactive CD-ROMs, and Internet websites may be helpful. Education should begin at the first contact with the health care provider. Discussion with the treating physician is most valued by the patient.

Exercise

Exercise programs can be tailored to the individual patient (30) and are low cost. There is one caveat: compliance or adherence to exercise is low. Only approximately 50% of the patients to whom exercises are recommended adhere to the program (1,23). Silverman et al. (24) in a cross-sectional study reported significantly weaker anterior neck muscles among patients (n = 30; age 48 ± 12 years) with mechanical neck pain than among a control group (n = 30; age 42 ± 12 years). The investigators postulated that weakness of the anterior neck muscles can cause neck pain. This observation is interesting. For the first time, a study quantified the weakness of this muscle group. However, the authors did not discuss whether the findings may have been related only to pain inhibition during testing, which is an intrinsic problem with all the muscle effort tests of patients with musculoskeletal pain.

Berg et al. (3) conducted a study with middle-aged female workers (n = 17; age 40 ± 12 years) in an outcome study. The investigators reported a significant decrease in neck pain and an increase in maximal isometric neck torque as great as 35% after a 12-minutes specific strength training twice a week for 8 weeks. The results of this study indicated a fast response of the neck muscles to specific training. They also indicated pain reduction with exercise. Dyrssen et al. (9), Highland et al. (14), and Jordan et al. (17) reported similar or better results.

Only three randomized, controlled trials have been conducted to study the effect of neck exercises (10,17,23). None of these studies had a control or placebo group, and therefore the results have to be interpreted with caution. Jordan et al. (17) compared the effectiveness of intensive training of the neck muscles, an individual physical therapy treatment, and a cervical spine manipulative treatment. One hundred nineteen patients were randomized. A blinded physician performed a global assessment. There was no significant difference in any of the clinical outcome measures for the three groups. All groups improved in strength and endurance, and all three groups reported a decrease in pain. One interpretation of the results may be that all three groups used some form of exercises and that all groups also received neck school where exercises were taught. The differences in type of treatment between the options were not distinct. Another interpretation may be that there is no difference. The future will tell.

Randlov et al. (23) randomized 77 patients (mean age 39 years, range 18 to 61 years) with chronic neck and shoulder pain (duration of pain 6 to 348 months) to an intensive neck and shoulder training program or a program with lesser intensity but of similar duration. Fifty percent of the patients reported reduced pain, and improved neck muscle strength and endurance were measured. The results showed no significant differences between the two groups in almost all of the outcome measures. Unfortunately, the study had an almost 50% dropout rate.

Har-El (10) randomized 64 patients with chronic neck pain either to neck exercises and the Chace technique of dance therapy or to the same neck exercises combined with an aerobic training. Both patient groups reported reduced neck pain, an elevation of mood, and an increased neck range of motion as measured by an independent evaluator. No significant differences were found between the two groups.

Only a few randomized, controlled trials have examined the effect of exercise and activity on neck pain among patients with acute or chronic nonspecific cervical spinal problems. A cautious conclusion from the above studies is that exercise does not harm and is as effective as other treatments, such as individualized physical therapy and cervical spinal manipulation. The treating clinician can expect 50% compliance with exercise. Patients who comply perceive decreased pain, increased muscle strength and endurance, and improved mood and better function. Should we expect more from an exercise regimen for patients? Again, the future will tell.

Ergonomics

Using several criteria for assessing epidemiologic evidence, the National Institute for Occupational Safety and Health (NIOSH) reviewed the literature to determine the work-relatedness of musculoskeletal disorders of the neck (21). The review concluded that there is evidence of a causal relation between highly repetitive work or forceful exertion and the occurrence of neck disorders. There is also strong evidence that working groups with high level of static contraction, prolonged static loads, or extreme working postures involving the neck and shoulder muscles are at increased risk of neck and shoulder disorders.

To the extent that neck disorders are caused or aggravated by physical activity during work, daily living, or recreation, it would seem logical to control exposure to the risk factors found in the epidemiologic studies. The few prospective studies that have included interventions to decrease workplace exposure—decreasing repetitive work and less extreme working postures—showed a decrease in the incidence of neck disorders and improvement in symptoms among affected workers (21). These strategies apply to primary as well as secondary prevention.

Because more people are interacting with computers at work and at home, the effects of prolonged visual and precision tasks have become a public concern. Three ergonomic interfaces need to be considered—the viewing conditions, the manipulative requirements, and the positioning of the body. All three may affect posture and the forces exerted by the neck and shoulder muscles (13).

Viewing conditions depend on the quality of the image displayed for a task and the visual acuity of the exposed person. Improper viewing conditions can occur when the viewer is located too far away from the display on a monitor screen or source document. The viewing distance is directly affected by the person's eyesight. Low contrast between the image and the background occurs when the ambient lighting is too strong, the source document is not sufficiently illuminated, or light sources are reflected from the display surfaces, causing glare. In these cases, the user tends to bend forward and get closer to the display. In addition to static strain, the neck and shoulder may be engaged repetitively when the visual displays are placed far apart. For example, when a source document is placed on a desk far away from the monitor screen, the user's head and neck need to be rotated repeatedly while the eye gazes shift.

Manipulations involve the hands and arms operating keyboards or other implements, as well as assembly or precision tasks at work or in recreational activities. Maintaining the weight of the upper extremities alone generates a moment around the shoulder joint, engaging the neck and shoulder muscle complex in forceful exertions. Even higher forces are needed to counter the moments produced when the arms manipulate heavy objects or engage in forceful actions such as drilling. Some objects are manipulated with the direct assistance of the head, neck, and shoulder. An extremely awkward posture is adopted, for example, when cradling a telephone handset between the shoulder and the head.

Performing tasks in a seated or standing position indirectly affects the posture maintained by the neck and head or the forces exerted by the neck and shoulder muscles. The viewing conditions and the manipulative requirements are different when a task is performed standing or seated. For example, someone sitting in a chair with the back rests set at angles larger than 110 degrees increases neck flexion to compensate for deteriorating conditions in reading from a monitor screen (12).

Forethought and resourcefulness help control the cost of intervention. The adjustments of the interfaces in visual and precision tasks may not entail expensive equipment. Tilting a monitor may remove glare; repositioning a monitor or chair may improve viewing distance. Placing a copy holder close to the monitor may reduce repetitive neck rotation. Active short breaks for stretching may bring relief from static exertion of the neck, or at least help maintain productivity levels (29).

The concept of "neck hygiene" includes ergonomics at least on a empiric clinical basis. It can be translated to the following set of empowering actions for the patient:

1. Be aware of your posture and change position regularly.
2. Avoid extreme postures of the neck (11).
3. Avoid maintaining the neck in a fixed position (prolonged static work).
4. Adjust the work bench or station to your size, eyesight, and task.
5. Learn and use relaxation and stretching exercises for the neck.

Although no definitive studies have provided evidence to support every recommendation, cumulative knowledge from the epidemiologic and ergonomic literature is enough to suggest that no harm is likely to occur in applying common sense to reduce exposure to risk of neck disorders and consequently to relieve discomfort.

CONCLUSIONS

Nonspecific degenerative neck pain is highly prevalent among adults. Unlike whiplash-associated disorders, nonspecific degenerative neck pain does not have a globally accepted classification system. A careful evaluation is necessary to ascertain whether a patient is at risk of chronicity and to refer the patient for appropriate treatment. Despite a lack of strong evidence, combination treatment including education, range of motion and endurance exercises, and ergonomic evaluation is suggested.

REFERENCES

1. Alexandre NM, Nordin M, Campello M, et al. Compliance with back pain treatment. Submitted for publication.
2. Barr AE, Badenchini IT, Forsyth-Bee M, et al. Development of a physical examination for a company-based

management program for work-related upper extremity cumulative trauma disorders. *J Occup Rehabil* 1999; 9:63–77.

3. Berg HE, Berggren G, Tesch PA. Dynamic neck strength training effect on pain and function. *Arch Phys Med Rehabil* 1994;75:661–665.

4. Borghouts JA, Koes BW, Bouter LM. The clinical course and prognostic factors of non-specific neck pain: a systematic review. *Pain* 1998;77:1–13.

5. Bovim G, Schrader H, Sand T. Neck pain in the general population. *Spine* 1994;19:1307–1309.

6. Burdorf A, Naaktgeboren B, Post W. Prognostic factors for musculoskeletal sickness absence and return to work among welders and metal workers. *Occup Environ Med* 1998;55:490–495.

7. Côté P, Cassidy JD, Carroll L. The Saskatchewan health and back pain survey: the prevalence of neck pain and related disability in Saskatchewan adults. *Spine* 1998;23:1689–1698.

8. Dvořák J. Epidemiology, physical examination, and neurodiagnostics. *Spine* 1998;23:2663–2673.

9. Dyrssen T, Svedenkrans M, Paasikivi J. Muskelträning vid besvär i nacke och skuldror: effektiv behandling för att minska smärtan. *Lakartidningen* 1989;86:2116–2120.

10. Har-El RB. *Influence of neck exercises, combined with either the Chace technique of dance therapy or aerobic training, on pain perception, mood state, and cervical range of motion of adults with chronic mechanical neck pain* [doctoral thesis]. New York: New York University, 1999.

11. Harms-Ringdahl K, Ekholm J. Intensity and character of pain and muscular activity levels elicited by maintained extreme flexion position of the lower-cervical–upper-thoracic spine. *Scand J Rehabil Med* 1986;18:117–126.

12. Harms-Ringdahl K, Schuldt K. Maximum neck extension strength and relative neck muscular load in different cervical spine positions. *Clin Biomech (Bristol, Avon)* 1988;4:17–24.

13. Haslegrave CM. What do we mean by a "working posture"? *Ergonomics* 1994;37:781–799.

14. Highland TR, Dreisinger TE, Vie LL, et al. Changes in isometric strength and range of motion of the isolated cervical spine after eight weeks of clinical rehabilitation. *Spine* 1992;17:S77–S82.

15. Hudak PL, Amadio PC, Bombardier C. Development of an upper extremity outcome measure: the DASH (disabilities of the arm, shoulder, and hand). The Upper Extremity Collaborative Group. *Am J Ind Med* 1996;29: 602–608.

16. Jackson R. Cervical trauma: not just another pain in the neck. *Geriatrics* 1982;37:123–126.

17. Jordan A, Bendix T, Nielsen H, et al. Intensive training, physiotherapy, or manipulation for patients with chronic neck pain: a prospective, single-blinded, randomized clinical trial. *Spine* 1998;23:311–319.

18. Kamwendo K, Linton SJ. A controlled study of the effect of neck school in medical secretaries. *Scand J Rehabil Med* 1991;23:143–152.

19. Leclerc A, Niedhammer I, Landre MF, et al. One-year predictive factors for various aspects of neck disorders. *Spine* 1999;24:1455–1462.

20. Mäkelä M, Heliövaara M, Sievers K, et al. Prevalence, determinants, and consequences of chronic neck pain in Finland. *Am J Epidemiol* 1991;134:1356–1367.

21. National Institute for Occupatinal Safety and Health. Musculoskeletal disorders and workplace factors: a critical review of epidemiologic evidence for work-related musculoskeletal disorders of the neck, upper extremity, and low back. NIOSH publication no 97-141; 1997.

22. Rajala U, Keinänen-Kiukaanniemi S, Uusimäki A, et al. Musculoskeletal pains and depression in a middle-aged Finnish population. *Pain* 1995;61:451–457.

23. Randlov A, Ostergaard M, Manniche C, et al. Intensive dynamic training for females with chronic neck/shoulder pain: a randomized controlled trial. *Clin Rehabil* 1998;12:200–210.

24. Silverman JL, Rodriquez AA, Agre JC. Quantitative cervical flexor strength in healthy subjects and in subjects with mechanical neck pain. *Arch Phys Med Rehabil* 1991;72:679–681.

25. Spitzer WO, Skovron ML, Salmi LR, et al. Scientific monograph of the Quebec Task Force on whiplash-associated disorders: redefining "whiplash" and its management. *Spine* 1995;20:S1–S73.

26. Stock SR, Streiner D, Tugwell P, et al. Validation of the neck and upper limb index (NULI), a functional status instrument for work-related musculoskeletal disorders. In: Proceedings of the International Commission on Occupational Health 1996 Conference, Stockholm, September 15-20, 1996.

27. Suissa S, Harder S, Veilleux M. The Quebec whiplash-associated disorders cohort study. *Spine* 1995;20: S12–S20.

28. Suissa S, Harder S, Veilleux M. The effect of initial symptoms and signs on the prognosis of whiplash. Proceedings of the Whiplash Associated Disorders World Congress 1999, Vancouver, British Columbia, Canada, February 7–11, 1999:149.

29. Swanson NG, Sauter SL. The effects of exercise on the health and performance of data entry operators. In: Luczak H, Cakir A, Cakir G, eds. *Work with display units.* Amsterdam: Elsevier Science, 1993:288–291.

30. Tan JC, Nordin M. Role of physical therapy in the treatment of cervical disk disease. *Orthop Clin North Am* 1992;23:435–449.

31. Van der Donk J, Schouten JS, Passchier J, et al. The associations of neck pain with radiological abnormalities of the cervical spine and personality traits in a general population. *J Rheumatol* 1991;18:1884–1889.

The Degenerative Cervical Spine,
edited by Marek Szpalski and Robert Gunzburg
Lippincott Williams & Wilkins, Philadelphia © 2001.

13

A Role for Manipulative Management of the Degenerative or Inflammatory Cervical Spine?

Tim McClune, A. Kim Burton

Spinal Research Unit, The University of Huddersfield, Huddersfield HD1 2SP, United Kingdom

WHY? THE BACKGROUND
WHAT? - EPIDEMIOLOGY AND PATHOLOGY
HOW? CLINICAL CONSIDERATIONS
    Acute • Chronic
WHO? THE EVIDENCE
WHEN NOT? CONTRAINDICATIONS AND DANGERS
SUMMARY

WHY? THE BACKGROUND

This brief chapter is included to present some salient features of a common, though somewhat controversial, therapy for neck disorders. It is not presented as a comprehensive review; rather the role of manipulation in the management of the degenerative and inflammatory cervical spine is outlined from a pragmatic perspective. Manipulation is a common therapeutic approach to musculoskeletal disorders, including those of the cervical spine, and many patients with cervical abnormalities by default receive treatment from manipulative practitioners.

Manipulation traverses several clinical specialities—chiropractic, manual medicine, osteopathy, and physiotherapy. These professions, generally operating in private practice, have similar aims and objectives, but their specific technical procedures and theoretical concepts vary considerably. The term *manipulation* is used here to refer to the therapeutic techniques common to all four groups, including but not limited to soft-tissue massage and stretching, myofascial techniques, neural mobilization, joint articulation and mobilization, and high-velocity thrust techniques. In addition to hands-on treatment, these practitioners tend to give advice on matters such as sports and ergonomics and prescribe specific exercise regimens. Explanations of the presenting problem, the aims of the treatment, and the likely outcome probably are addressed in some detail. Indeed, therapeutic benefit may well arise from the time taken by these clinicians during consultation, particularly when compared with the usual state health service or managed care provision, which is compromised by limitations on available time allocated for each visit or consultation. It is likely that the patient groups seeking care from the various manipulative professions are very similar and that they approximate clinically those in conventional primary health care environments (5,6,19). They may differ, however, with respect to certain social variables and differ from hospital outpatient populations on clinical criteria (7).

Although this book is concerned with both the degenerative and inflammatory cervical spine, the focus of this chapter is the degenerative element. It is difficult to consider the inflammatory cervical spine to be compatible with manipulative treatment.

WHAT? EPIDEMIOLOGY AND PATHOLOGY

The cervical spine undergoes age-related "degenerative" changes starting at the end of the second decade and increasing during following decades. The result is that by the sixth decade, such changes are evident in almost all (86% to 89%) cervical spines (16). These changes are variable with regard to pathologic extent and severity, yet the symptoms do not necessarily reflect the physical changes (2,16).

The detailed descriptions of degenerative changes can be read elsewhere in the book, but some details relevant for manipulative clinicians and their clinical decision making can be reiterated. Stated briefly, the effects of the degenerative process reasonably may be expected to produce signs and symptoms of musculoskeletal dysfunction, predominantly stiffness and pain, but this is not necessarily the case. However, if the structural changes are sufficiently severe, more serious and potentially life-threatening consequences may develop.

In addition to simple symptoms and signs of musculoskeletal dysfunction, the structural changes consequent to the degenerative process can lead to radiculopathy and less commonly myelopathy. These effects may result from osteophytic growth and loss of disc height, which lead to foraminal encroachment or canal narrowing. In rare instances, osteophytes may compress the vertebral artery and cause vascular insufficiency of the hindbrain and cerebellum. It is now thought that radiculopathy in particular can be caused by nonphysical factors such as chemical inflammatory effects on nerve roots. Uncritical reliance on the findings from imaging may lead to inappropriate conclusions, particularly when deliberating over the advisability of surgical intervention. For a conclusion that the symptomatic effects are most likely caused by structural changes, the clinical symptoms must correspond exactly to the imaging findings, and electrodiagnostic tests may be needed.

Structural changes due to the degenerative process may not necessarily be the cause of the presenting symptoms (18,20). Musculoskeletal symptoms, particularly pain, occur among the general population with no specific pathologic cause. Neck pain is a common experience for all age groups. The lifetime prevalence of neck pain among the general population has been estimated to be as high as 34% (4,9,15). The proportion of patients with symptoms lasting more than 1 month is higher among women than among men. The prevalence tends to increase with age, as do the duration and chronicity of pain. Approximately 14% of a randomly selected population can meet the criteria for chronic neck pain (9). Surveys of manipulative practice have shown that approximately 30% of consultations are for neck-related problems, and the patients frequently are middle-aged (5,6,21).

As with low back pain, these symptoms may resolve without recourse to therapeutic intervention, but recurrence is common. Structural changes may be present without any signs or symptoms (2), and symptoms may persist even at quite a severe level without any structural changes, for example, symptoms following whiplash-type trauma (3,22). This picture presents a dilemma for the practitioner, particularly when giving prognostic advice and more specifically in a medicolegal context.

HOW? CLINICAL CONSIDERATIONS

A patient with degenerative changes in the neck often seeks treatment with symptoms and signs of musculoskeletal dysfunction. These may include one or a number of the following: pain in the neck, upper extremity, headaches, paraesthesia, anesthesia, paresis in the upper extremity, upper motor neuron symptoms in the spinal levels distal to the neck (spastic weakness, paresthesia, anesthesia, pain), vertigo, and neck stiffness. The onset may be gradual and insidious, or may be a sudden result of trauma—physical or psychologic.

A detailed case history is necessary to identify red flags for systemic disease, serious pathologic changes in the spine, or comorbidity that may preclude manipulative treatment. The psychosocial aspects of neck trouble have not been as clearly described as they have for low back pain. However, when the symptom is considered a pain state, avoiding the specific of *cervical,* then issues such as psychologic distress and illness behavior (17) can be entertained, and assessment of psychosocial factors considered appropriate. This may allow early identification of the potential for chronicity, and traditional musculoskeletal assessment can be followed within the context of a biopsychosocial model (14). A patient with chronic symptoms may need a more detailed psychologic assessment. The persistence of symptoms may be more likely in the presence of distress and cognitive or behavioral influences than because of specific physical tissue damage. The treatment of patients with intractable cervical pain is complex and requires specific approaches, which may not be within the capability of most manipulative practitioners. Some experts argue that the chronic nature of symptoms can be explained largely on the basis of the pathologic state—the presence of degenerative changes; however, there is no firm evidence to support this view in most cases.

Throughout this section we assume that patients with serious radiculopathy, myelopathy, or vascular signs have been referred to the appropriate experts. (During a course of treatment radicular symptoms may increase, or indeed signs or symptoms of myelopathy, or more rarely vascular compression, may develop and should trigger referral.) What remains is the group of patients with neck pain, a high proportion of whom have degenerative changes.

It is not the intention here to describe in detail the various manual techniques used by the various disciplines; rather they are discussed generically. Stated briefly, they comprise techniques targeted at soft tissues together with techniques that ostensibly focus on joints. The latter group has two important variants: the *thrust techniques* that involve application of high velocity, low amplitude movement to the joint and the *mobilizing techniques* that involve gradual application of forces of varying magnitude. The degree of force used in these maneuvers varies between professions and between practitioners within the same profession, but most practitioners would use only low-force techniques when there are known to be moderate or substantial degenerative changes.

The manipulative practitioner undertakes a normal clinical routine of detailed case history, clinical musculoskeletal examination including functional and palpatory assessment of the thoracic spine, the glenohumeral joint, and the scapulothoracic complex as well as the cervical spine. There also is a standard neurologic and orthopedic assessment. The eventual diagnosis is likely to be specific to one or more cervical segments or muscle groups, this being based largely on the findings from the palpatory examination. Although there is no scientific evidence to show that this highly specific approach systematically guides treatment decisions, it is a common feature throughout the manipulative professions.

Acute

Patients who visit manipulators often have the benefit of early access, which means that manipulators see a high proportion of acute cases. Because acute symptoms can occur with or without degenerative pathologic changes, it follows that manipulators see many patients with cervical degenerative changes. The focus of treatment, though, is on symptoms and function rather than the pathologic condition.

Manipulative treatment consists of one or more of the following: joint mobilization, joint thrusts and soft-tissue stretch and massage. Advice on cervical, thoracic, and shoulder exercises, muscular conditioning, increasing activity, and decreasing fear of activity or further damage. Specific advice related to sport or work activities, such as avoidance of cervical extension during computer work, may be given to maintain normal activity levels.

The treatment program most likely comprises a number of treatments, although some manipulators claim that only one treatment is needed. Typically four to eight treatment sessions over a period of up to 2 to 3 months are given. Reassessment and referral would normally be considered if adequate improvement has not taken place or if activity levels are not improving after 4 weeks of treatment; in our view, prolonged treatment regimens cannot be justified.

Chronic

Chronicity is defined herein as a symptomatic episode that lasts more than 3 months, although symptoms that do not improve during the first 3 weeks after onset may be an early indication of a possible chronic course. Despite the availability of rapid access, presentation of chronic neck trouble to manipulators is not unusual. The treatment regimen entails a range of techniques similar to that for acute cases, although the focus probably is more on higher amplitude, lower velocity maneuvers, and there may be greater use of exercises and advice.

A difference in the treatment of patients with chronic neck pain is that physical tissue damage (or degenerative changes) may not be considered the most important factor. The finding of asymptomatic abnormal structural changes provides evidence that degeneration does not necessarily equate with pain. This brings us back to the consideration that what is being managed is (chronic) pain as opposed to degenerative changes.

Manipulators traditionally have suggested that chronic symptoms can be accounted for by some measure of physical musculoskeletal dysfunction or degenerative pathologic changes. However, in the absence of clear evidence supporting the physical nature of chronic symptoms, current theories about pain mechanisms suggest that an alternative model is needed. The biopsychosocial model is an attractive concept that helps to explain what is observed better than the traditional biomedical model (14). This is not to say that physical (manipulative) treatment cannot be helpful in the management of chronic neck pain, but any beneficial influences are unlikely to result from purely mechanical effects. We caution against giving patients alarmist diagnoses that focus on degenerative changes or physical damage. These messages can be readily misinterpreted and may be counterproductive by inducing negative psychologic sequelae.

The manipulative professions need to address the question of which aspect of manipulative practice is most likely to be effective. Is it the physical manipulative techniques, the advice on lifestyle and exercise, the reassurance and time spent explaining, or simply that someone cares and seems to understand? As for acute problems, we caution that prolonged treatment programs cannot be justified, and they may have a detrimental effect by maintaining a sense of dependence on the therapy or therapist.

WHO? THE EVIDENCE

There is surprisingly little scientific evidence for manipulative therapy for neck pain, and none specifically related to the degenerative cervical spine. On balance, the evidence suggests that manipulative therapy for neck pain (with or without referred upper extremity symptoms) can have a positive influence on clinical outcomes, but the strength of that evidence is limited (11,12). There is little doubt that many of the patients in clinical trials have had some degree of degenerative change, and there is some evidence that manipulation can provide benefit in the management of chronic neck pain (13,23). However, there is no specific information concerning the response of patients with degenerative changes compared with those without such changes. In the present climate, all that can be said is that manipulation may be considered as a treatment option if musculoskeletal signs or symptoms are present with or without minimal or nonprogressive radiculopathy.

WHEN NOT? CONTRAINDICATIONS AND DANGERS

Gross structural changes with marked or progressive radiculopathy, myelopathy, and vascular compression are contraindications to manipulative treatment of the cervical spine. Substantial caution should be exercised in the presence of osteoporosis, long-term glucocorticoid therapy, and history of carcinoma. Manipulative practitioners do not usually have direct or easy access to imaging, so they tend to rely on careful assessment of clinical features when considering the possibility of contraindications. Although most patients who visit manipulative practitioners have conditions suitable for treatment, this is clearly an unsatisfactory situation and one we suggest be addressed by the professions concerned. If marked or progressive radiculopathy is present, manipulation is contraindicated, and referral should be made for imaging and possibly for a surgical opinion. If myelopathy or vascular symptoms are present, referral for imaging and surgical opinion is mandatory.

In our opinion, inflammation of the cervical spine (defined as the presence of evidence of rheumatoid arthritis or other types of seronegative arthropathy or related conditions) is not compatible with manipulative treatment. Although some manipulators may claim that gentle soft-tissue massage does help reduce discomfort in the neck and shoulder muscles, there is no scientific evidence to support this view, and the potential dangers should not be underestimated.

Manipulation of the cervical spine is not without risk. Catastrophic events (stroke and death) do occur, albeit relatively rarely (1). Although provocative tests of vertebral artery stability generally are recommended, the results are unreliable. Authors of a review (10) concluded that it is not possible to ascertain whether a patient is at risk of vertebrobasilar artery dissection. The question has been raised whether the benefits outweigh the risks (8). In our opinion the catastrophic events are sufficiently rare not to abandon cervical manipulation on the grounds of safety, assuming careful clinical assessment and treatment are performed by a properly trained practitioner. We strongly recommend, however, that rotational thrust techniques on the upper cervical segments be avoided altogether, that such techniques not be used in the presence of marked degeneration, and that they be used only with great caution in the presence of moderate degenerative changes.

SUMMARY

The epidemiologic characteristics of symptoms related to the cervical spine and common patterns of care seeking dictate that manipulators frequently treat patients with cervical degenerative changes. If the predominant symptom is considered pain, which can be unrelated to any underlying pathologic change, there is limited evidence that manipulative treatment can be considered a management option that offers modest benefit, at least for patients expressing a preference for this form of treatment. Treatment is aimed at improving musculoskeletal function and reducing symptoms. There is no reason to suppose that it affects the structural changes of degeneration. The use of exercises, advice, and reassurance normally supplements the manipulative procedures. It is uncertain which of these components contributes most to clinical outcome.

Inflammatory or systemic disease and marked degenerative changes with severe or progressive neurologic signs are specific contraindications. Manipulative treatment of the cervical spine carries a small risk of catastrophic events, which are exceedingly difficult to predict. Risk can be partly controlled by means of careful clinical assessment and the avoidance of rotatory thrust techniques.

The paucity of evidence makes these conclusions tentative. There seemingly is some potential, but a need remains for further carefully conducted, randomized clinical trials of manipulative therapy for neck trouble to determine the subgroups of patients who may do well and to identify the optimal features of the discipline.

REFERENCES

1. Assendelft WJJ, Bouter LM, Knipschild PG. Complications of spinal manipulation: a comprehensive review of the literature. *J Fam Pract* 1996;42:475–480.
2. Boden SD, McCowin PR, Davis DO, et al. Abnormal magnetic-resonance scans of the cervical spine in asymptomatic subjects: a prospective investigation. *J Bone Joint Surg Am* 1990;72:1178–1184.
3. Borchgrevink GE, Kaasa A, McDonagh D, et al. Acute treatment of whiplash neck sprain injuries: a randomized trial of treatment during the first 14 days after a car accident. *Spine* 1998;23:25–31.
4. Bovim G, Schrader H, Sand T. Neck pain in the general population. *Spine* 1994;19:1307–1309.
5. Breen AC. Chiropractors and the treatment of back pain. *Rheumatol Rehabil* 1977;16:46–53.
6. Burton AK. Back pain in osteopathic practice. *Rheumatol Rehabil* 1981;20:239–246.
7. Burton AK, Getty CJM. Differences between "orthopaedic" and "osteopathic" patients with low back trouble: implications for selecting patients for rehabilitation. In: Roland MO, Jenner JR, eds. *Back pain: new approaches to rehabilitation and education.* Manchester: Manchester University Press, 1989:166–173.
8. Di Fabio RP. Manipulation of the cervical spine: risks and benefits. *Phys Ther* 1999;79:50–65.
9. Dvorak J. Epidemiology, physical examination, and neurodiagnostics. *Spine* 1998;23:2663–2673.
10. Haldeman S, Kohlbeck FJ, McGregor M. Risk factors and precipitating neck movements causing vertebrobasilar artery dissection after cervical trauma and spinal manipulation. *Spine* 1999;24:785–794.
11. Hurwitz EL, Aker PD, Adams AH, et al. Manipulation and mobilization of the cervical spine: a systematic review of the literature. *Spine* 1996;21:1746–1758.
12. Kjellman GV, Skargren E, Oberg B. A critical analysis of randomised clinical trials on neck pain and treatment efficacy: a review of the literature. *Scand J Rehabil Med* 1999;31:139–152.
13. Koes BW, Assendelft WJJ, van der Heijden GJ, et al. Spinal manipulation and mobilisation for back and neck pain: a blinded review. *BMJ* 1991;303:1298–1303.
14. Main CJ, Watson PJ. Psychological aspects of pain. *Man Ther* 2000;4:203–215.
15. Makela M, Heliovaara M, Sievers K, et al. Prevalence, Determinants, and consequences of chronic neck pain in Finland. *Am J Epidemiol* 1991;134:1356–1367.
16. Matsumoto M, Fujimura Y, Suzuki N, et al. MRI of cervical intervertebral discs in asymptomatic subjects. *J Bone Joint Surg Br* 1998;80:19–24.

17. McIntosh G. Prognostic factors for illness behaviour in low back pain. Presented to the International Society for the Study of the Lumbar Spine, Brussels, June 9-13, 1998.
18. Modic MT. Degenerative disc disease and back pain. *Magn Reson Imaging Clin N Am* 1999;7:481–491.
19. Pedersen P. A survey of chiropractic practice in Europe. *Eur J Chiropract* 1994;42:3–28.
20. Penning L, Wilmink JT, van Woerden HH, et al. CT myelographic findings in degenerative disorders of the cervical spine: clinical significance. *AJR Am J Roentgenol* 1986;146:793–801.
21. Pringle M, Tyreman S. Study of 500 patients attending an osteopathic practice. *Br J Gen Pract* 1993;43:15–18.
22. Ronnen HR, de Korte PJ, Brink PR, et al. Acute whiplash injury: is there a role for MR imaging? a prospective study of 100 patients. *Radiology* 1996;20:93–96.
23. Skargren EI, Oberg BE. Predictive factors for 1-year outcome of low-back and neck pain in patients treated in primary care: comparison between the treatment strategies chiropractic and physiotherapy. *Pain* 1998;77: 201–208.

The Degenerative Cervical Spine,
edited by Marek Szpalski and Robert Gunzburg
Lippincott Williams & Wilkins, Philadelphia © 2001.

14

The Role of Cervical Orthoses in Degenerative and Inflammatory Disorders of the Cervical Spine

Tim Pigott

Walton Centre For Neurology and Neurosurgery, Liverpool L9 7LJ, United Kingdom

---

NORMAL MOTION IN THE CERVICAL SPINE
WHAT ARE COLLARS USED FOR?
WHAT IS THE EVIDENCE THAT COLLARS RESTRICT MOTION?
TYPES OF COLLARS
WHAT IS THE EVIDENCE OF THE BENEFIT OF COLLARS?
DO COLLARS HAVE HARMFUL EFFECTS?
RATIONALE FOR USE OF COLLARS
CONCLUSION

Various methods for the restriction of movement of the neck have been used over the last century. Despite the number of articles in the literature, there is little in the way of substantive evidence for their use as compared with other treatment modalities, such as medication or physical therapy (2–5,9,15,17,19–21,23,24,27,30,36). The available literature on use of collars in the management of degenerative and inflammatory disease tends to compare the results of surgery with those of conservative management, rather than the role of cervical orthoses on their own against other nonsurgical treatments (1,32–34,37). A large number of reports refer to the use of collars to manage traumatic injury (both accidental and after surgery) rather than to manage degenerative or inflammatory disease (11,27,29,35,36,39). In one major textbook of spinal surgery (14), which runs to 1,143 pages, there are only five references to cervical collars, two of which occur in a chapter on inflammatory disease.

NORMAL MOTION IN THE CERVICAL SPINE

A number of authors have analyzed the movement of the cervical spine, both segmental and as a whole (2,6,10,13,16). Lysell (26) has discussed the anatomic features of the cervical spine and the range of motion at segments of the cervical spine. Most flexion and extension occur at C5-6 and at C4-5; the least occurs at C2-3 and C7-T1. Lysell (26) also describes maximal rotation with lateral flexion at C4 and C2 and minimal motion at C7 (26). Clearly a major component of rotation occurs at C1-2. The range of normative values has been produced for motion in the cervical spine (2,6,10,13,16,40). Chapter 2 describes the biomechanics of the cervical spine.

WHAT ARE COLLARS USED FOR?

Most patients with inflammatory and degenerative conditions of the cervical spine respond to conservative management. Only a small percentage need any form of surgical intervention. It is relevant therefore to look at the role of cervical orthoses, because they constitute an important component of the cost of conservative management of these conditions. Askins and Eismont (4) estimated that revenues from the sale of cervical collars, including extrication collars, in the United States will exceed $40 million by the end of the year 2000.

Lusskin and Berger (25) in 1975 suggested that collars should act as a reminder for the patient to restrict head and neck movement, to mechanically restrict flexion, extension, lateral flexion, and rotation and to partially relieve the effect of cranial weight on the neck muscles. The suggestion was that the collar reduced the load-bearing function of the neck (5). Caillet (8) held that the collar should hold the head in a slightly flexed position. This was said to separate the posterior facet joints and open the foramina. Caillet contended that this minimized the need for muscle splinting, restricted excessive motion, and gave warmth to the neck. The evidence for all these contentions is not strong. Certainly there is good evidence that a neck scarf provides just as much warmth to the neck surface (5). Carter et al. (9) suggested that cervical orthoses be used to decrease inflammation, pain, and spasm; to control instability; to support the cervical spine; and to immobilize the cervical spine after surgery or trauma. Sandler et al. (36) proposed similar uses of cervical orthoses. In conclusion, a number of authors have proposed reasons for using cervical collars in the care of patients with cervical inflammatory and degenerative diseases (1,3–5,8,9,14,18,21,23,25,27,30,32–34,36,37). There does not seem to be any convincing evidence of scientific validity for the use of cervical collars.

WHAT IS THE EVIDENCE THAT COLLARS RESTRICT MOTION?

The choice of collar used to treat individual patients seems capricious and based on folklore rather than hard medical evidence. Much of the existing work on motion relates to collars used for trauma and the extrication of accident victims at the scene of the accident (27,35,39). Studies of motion restriction have been performed with a wide range of materials, including radiographs, goniometers, and overhead photographs, among others (2,4,5,7,9,11,15–17,19–22,24,25,27,29,35,36,39). The first reports of use of the CA-6000 motion analyzer by Johnson and Schuit (22,38) suggested that this may be an objective test for range of motion in the cervical spine as a whole. The advantage of this system is that it can record three movements (flexion-extension, axial rotation, and lateral bending) simultaneously in real time and has been shown to produce reliable and reproducible data (12,13). Other studies with different methods have problems with reproducibility and reliability. Some methods also necessitate a considerable degree of exposure to x-rays (2,7,10,15,16,19,20,23,24,27).

It is sensible to look at the studies that have the most objective measure of cervical motion to assess the effect of cervical orthoses on motion. Sandler et al. (36) used the CA-6000 motion analyzer to determine the effect of cervical orthoses on motion among healthy persons. The subjects compared with previously described age- and sex-matched controls (13). The investigators compared a soft collar, Philadelphia collar, Philadelphia collar with extension, and the sternal occipital mandibular immobilizer (SOMI) brace. The investigators found that all collars restricted neck motion but that no collar restricted motion to a mean value less than 50 degrees, the soft collar allowing more than 75 degree in all motions. The authors commented that if a greater degree of restriction were required then none of these collars would be effective and a more substantial orthosis would be needed. The conclusion from this work must be that collars provide a degree of restriction of motion in the cervical spine, but they must be targeted to the specific purpose. Simmons in his comment on the article (36) makes the valid point that the study examined movement of the entire cervical spine rather than segmental motion.

Carter et al. (9) examined a specific issue: the effect of a soft collar, used as normally recommended or reversed, on three planes of cervical range of motion. They used the CA-6000 system and found that a soft cervical collar produced statistically significant reduction in motion over wearing no collar, whichever way it was worn. Studies investigating restriction of motion in halo jacket devices suggest that these devices provide a considerable degree of restriction of movement (29). However, despite common belief, none of the commercially available devices produces complete restriction of movement. There is good objective evidence that cervical collars reduce motion of the cervical spine with differing degrees of effectiveness for different collars. The least effective is the soft collar and the most effective the SOMI brace or halo jacket if a more invasive method is needed.

TYPES OF COLLARS

A large range of orthoses are available. They are of varying complexity and patient compatibility. Collars can be categorized as follows on the basis of the degree of restriction they provide:

1. Soft collar. Provides the least degree of restriction but has high patient compliance.
2. Hard collar. The most commonly used is the Philadelphia collar with or without the thoracic extension. More restrictive than the soft collar but less comfortable for the patient. The Philadelphia collar gives a mean reduction of movement in flexion-extension of 42 degrees (36).
3. SOMI. Provides a greater degree of motion restriction with extension onto the chest to provide more stability with a mean reduction in flexion-extension of a further 31 degrees over the Philadelphia collar (36).
4. Halo jacket. Requires pins in the head and is best restricted to care of trauma victims and postsurgical patients.

Within the categories it appears that there is little choice between the various collars. Individual patient and clinician preference will determine which collar is suitable.

WHAT IS THE EVIDENCE OF THE BENEFIT OF COLLARS?

Simmons in his comment on the article by Sandler et al. (36) suggests that the specific goals of treatment with a collar are usually to eliminate excessive motion that would strain an area of injury or surgery, to protect that portion of the spine from extremes of motion, to reduce any tendency of recurrent soft-tissue injury, to allow soft-tissue healing, or to provide a reminder to the patient. No randomized, controlled trial has been conducted to compare the use of a cervical orthosis with use of other conservative treatment modalities. Most of the arguments for use of these devices in the management of inflammatory and degenerative cervical disease are based on common practice.

Two studies by Persson et al. (32,33) compared a prospective trial of surgery for brachialgia with conservative treatment with a collar or physiotherapy. The outcome measures were pain intensity profile (including a visual analog scale), sickness impact profile, and a measure of patient mood. The results suggested that 1 year after treatment there was no difference between the groups but that surgery had a greater influence on pain relief at the 4-month review. It appeared that use of a cervical orthosis and physiotherapy were as effective as surgery in the long term.

Mealy and Fenelon (28) and Pennie and Agambar (31) found that use of a cervical collar in the management of whiplash was not supported by the evidence. Although not strictly applicable to the degenerative and inflammatory spine, this evidence does provide some weight to an argument against the use of collars. In conclusion, there is little objective evidence for the clinical benefit of use of a cervical orthosis in the treatment of patients with cervical inflammatory and degenerative disorders.

DO COLLARS HAVE HARMFUL EFFECTS?

Lusskin and Berger (25) have suggested that cervical orthoses might produce harmful effects. They described four potential adverse effects of cervical collar:

1. Muscle atrophy and weakness
2. Tightness and contracture of tissues
3. Psychological dependence
4. Aggravation of symptoms and progression of undiagnosed disorders

Clinicians practicing in this field have encountered the problem of psychologic dependence on an orthosis. This can be a real clinical problem and is one that has not been properly addressed in the literature. The literature contains no objective evidence of muscle atrophy or contracture, but there is evidence that movement continues to a marked degree in all collars, making this suggestion unlikely. It would be fair to conclude that there is only anecdotal evidence of harm from cervical orthoses.

RATIONALE FOR USE OF COLLARS

Arguments for the use of a cervical orthosis are described earlier. The most important decision for clinicians is to decide what they want to achieve with the orthotic device and for what diagnosis. There is no objective evidence for the use of an orthosis and there is some anecdotal evidence of harm. In this context, the device should not be used long term. The results must be reviewed. It should not be left for the patient to decide when and whether the device should be removed.

If the device is for pain relief, it seems reasonable to start with that which allows the least restriction of movement and to reassess the patient's response after a specified time. Medication can be used concomitantly and the collar withdrawn if symptoms come under control or if the device is having no effect.

Use of a collar after surgery is common. The collar most probably acts as an *aide memoire* for the patient and may have a role in the promotion of fusion, although there is no good evidence of this effect. It would be sensible to start with a more restrictive collar than in the management of pain and to limit the time used to an agreed schedule with the patient.

A patient with pain from instability is most likely to be helped by a restrictive, well-fitting collar before a decision is made about surgical intervention. A collar is not a good long-term measure and is not well tolerated by the patient. The goal of management should be the temporary relief of pain before definitive treatment.

CONCLUSION

The use of a cervical orthosis in the management of cervical inflammatory disease is based on poor evidence and folklore. There is a great need for a proper randomized trial of use of orthotic devices because there is anecdotal evidence of harm, and considerable resources are involved in the provision of orthoses. It is incumbent on the treating clinician to ensure that if a collar is prescribed, it is done so for a limited period and to achieve specific goals. Long-term use of a collar is to be deprecated.

REFERENCES

1. Agrillo U, Faccioli F, Fachinetti P, et al. Guidelines for the diagnosis and management of the degenerative diseases of cervical spine. *J Neurosurg Sci* 1999;43:11–14.
2. Alaranta H, Hurri H, Heliovaara M, et al. Flexibility of the spine: normative values of goniometric and tape measurements. *Scand J Rehabil Med* 1994;26:147–54.
3. Althoff B, Goldie I. Cervical collars in rheumatoid atlanto-axial subluxation: a radiographic comparison. *Ann Rheum Dis* 1980;39:485–489.
4. Askins V, Eismont F. Efficacy of five cervical orthoses in restricting cervical motion: a comparison study. *Spine* 1997;22:1193–1198.
5. Beavis A. Cervical orthoses. *Prosthet Orthot Int* 1989;13:6–13.
6. Bhalla SK, Simmons E. Normal range of intervertebral joint motion of the cervical spine. *Can J Surg* 1969;12: 181–187.
7. Boone DC, Lin CM, Spence C, et al. Reliability of goniometric measurements. *Phys Ther* 1978;58:1355–1360.
8. Caillet R. *Neck and arm pain.* 2nd ed. Philadelphia: FA Davis, 1981.
9. Carter V, Fasen J, Roman JJ, et al. The effect of a soft collar, used as normally recommended or reversed, on three planes of cervical range of motion. *J Orthop Sports Phys Ther* 1996;23:209–215.
10. Colachis S, Ganter E. Cervical spine motion in normal women: radiographic study of effect of cervical collars. *Arch Phys Med Rehabil* 1973;54:161–169.
11. De Lorenzo R. A review of spinal immobilisation techniques. *J Emerg Med* 1996;14:603–613.
12. Dvorak J VE, Panjabi M, Grob D. Normal motion of the Lumbar Spine as related to age and gender. *Eur Spine J* 1995;4:18–23.
13. Dvorak J AJ, Panjabi M, Loustalot D, et al. Age and gender related normal motion of the cervical spine. *Spine* 1992;17:393–398.
14. Findlay G OR. *Surgery of the spine: a combined orthopaedic and neurosurgical approach.* ed. Oxford, England: Blackwell Scientific Publications, 1992.
15. Fisher SV BJ, Awad EA, Gullickson G. Cervical orthoses effects on cervical spine motion. *Arch Phys Med Rehabil* 1977;58:109–115.
16. Gajdosik RL. Clinical measurement of range of motion: review of goniometry emphasising reliability and validity. *Phys Ther* 1987;67:1867–1872.
17. Garth G. Efficacy of five cervical orthoses in restricting cervical motion: a comparison study [letter; comment]. *Spine* 1998;23:961–962.
18. Hart DL, Simmons EF, Owen J. Review of cervical orthoses. *Phys Ther* 1978;58:857–860.
19. Hartman J, Hill B. Cineradiography of the braced normal cervical spine. *Clin Orthop* 1975;109:97–102.
20. Hughes S. How effective is the Newport/Aspen collar? a prospective radiographic evaluation in healthy adult volunteers. *J Trauma* 1998;45:374–378.
21. Hughes S. Efficacy of five cervical orthoses in restricting cervical motion: a comparison study [letter; comment]. *Spine* 1998;23:744.
22. Johnson RD, Petersen CM. Reliability of the OSI CA-6000 spine motion analysis system for active cervical range of motion measurement in normal subjects. *Phys Ther* 1993;72:S108.
23. Johnson RM, Simmons E, Ramsby G, et al. Cervical orthoses: a study comparing their effectiveness in restricting cervical motion in normal subjects. *J Bone Joint Surg Am* 1977;59:332–339.
24. Jones M. Cineradiographic studies of the collar-immobilised cervical spine. *J Neurosurg* 1960;17:633–637.
25. Lusskin R, Berger N. Prescription principles. In: American Academy of Orthopaedic Surgeons, eds. *Atlas of orthotics: biomechanical principles and application.* St Louis: Mosby, 1975:370–372.
26. Lysell E. Motion in the cervical spine: an experimental study on autopsy material. *Acta Orthop Scand* 1969; S123:5–61.
27. McCabe JB, Nolan D. Comparison of the effectiveness of different cervical immobilisation collars. *Ann Emerg Med* 1986;15:50–53.

28. Mealy K, Fenelon GCC. Early mobilisation of acute whiplash injuries. *Br Med J* 1986;292:656–657.
29. Mirza S, Moquin R, Anderson P, et al. Stabilising properties of the halo apparatus. *Spine* 1997;22:727–733.
30. Naylor J, Mulley G. Surgical collars: a survey of their prescription and use. *Br J Rheumatol* 1991;30:282–284.
31. Pennie BH, Agambar L. Whiplash injuries: a trial of early management. *J Bone Joint Surg Br* 1990;72:277–279.
32. Persson L, Carlsson C, Carlsson J. Long-lasting cervical radicular pain managed with surgery, physiotherapy, or a cervical collar: a prospective, randomised study. *Spine* 1997;22:751–758.
33. Persson L, Moritz U, Brandt L, et al. Cervical radiculopathy: pain, muscle weakness and sensory loss in patients with cervical radiculopathy treated with surgery, physiotherapy or cervical collar—a prospective, controlled study. *Eur Spine J* 1997;6:256–266.
34. Rechtine G. Nonsurgical treatment of cervical degenerative disease. *Instr Course Lect* 1999;48:433–435.
35. Rosen P, Arata M, Stahl S, et al. Comparison of two new immobilisation collars. *Ann Emerg Med* 1992;21:1189–1195.
36. Sandler A, Dvorak J, Humke T, et al. The effectiveness of various cervical orthoses: an in vivo comparison of the mechanical stability provided by several widely used models. *Spine* 1996;21:1624–1629.
37. Schimandle J, Heller J. Nonoperative treatment of degenerative cervical disk disease. *J South Orthop Assoc* 1996;5:207–212.
38. Schuit D, Peterson C, Johnson RD. Reliability and validity of the OSI CA-6000 spine motion analyser for sagittal and frontal plane motions. *Phys Ther* 1993;72:S62.
39. Solot J, Winzelberg G. Clinical and radiological evaluation of vertebrace extrication collars. *J Emerg Med* 1990;8:79–83.
40. White A, Panjabi M. The basic kinematics of the human spine: a review of past and current knowledge. *Spine* 1978;3:12–20.

The Degenerative Cervical Spine,
edited by Marek Szpalski and Robert Gunzburg
Lippincott Williams & Wilkins, Philadelphia © 2001.

15

The Use of Radiofrequency and Neuromodulation Techniques

Jean Pierre Van Buyten

Department of Anesthesia and Pain Management, Maria Middelares Hospital,
B-9100 St. Niklaas, Belgium

ALGORITHM FOR THE DEGENERATIVE CERVICAL SPINE
Cervical Zygapophyseal Joints • Segmental Nerve Block • Discogenic Pain • Sympathetically Maintained Pain
CERVICOGENIC HEADACHE
SPINAL CORD STIMULATION

In a pain clinic practice, many patients have pain of cervical origin. Most of the time the pain syndrome is caused by degenerative changes in the cervical spine, but whiplash and problems after cervical surgery also are common. The pain syndromes mostly are mixed neuropathic-nociceptive disorders and are sympathetically maintained. Treatment requires an algorithm. Pain management techniques should be attempted before major opioid therapy is begun.

Neuromodulatory and neuroablative techniques must be differentiated. Neuromodulation is dynamic functional inhibition of conduction through the pathways. Neuroablation is the physical interruption of the pathway. Neuromodulation can be performed electrically with spinal cord stimulation, deep brain stimulation, peripheral nerve stimulation, motor cortex stimulation, or medically by means of perspinal administration (epidural or intrathecal) of analgesics (e.g., opioids, clonidine, local anesthetics, calcium channel blockers, or N-methyl D-aspartate [NMDA] receptor antagonists). Neuroablation can be performed surgically by means of incision of the dorsal root entry zone, chordotomy, or sympathectomy; through radiofrequency thermocoagulation; or chemically with neurolytic agents such as alcohol or phenol.

In the management of cervicogenic pain, the first step is use of radiofrequency techniques. Whether these techniques are neuromodulatory or neuroablative is being argued. It probably depends on the temperature used. Percutaneous chordotomy for cancer pain is performed with a temperature of 90°C and is certainly neuroablative. Radiofrequency thremocoagulation of the zygapophyseal joints or the dorsal root ganglions is performed at 67°C and is probably less ablative. The pulsed radiofrequency generates a temperature of barely 40°C and cannot be defined as neuroablative (4).

ALGORITHM FOR THE DEGENERATIVE CERVICAL SPINE

Cervical Zygapophysial Joints

An approach to the zygapophysial joints is indicated in the management of degenerative cervical disease, postsurgical neck pain ("failed neck"), and whiplash syndrome (1). The indications are permanent unilateral or bilateral neck pain with limitation of extension or ipsilateral rotation.

A test block is performed with a small volume of local anesthetic with or without a sustained-released glucocorticoid. The target is the medial branch of the posterior ramus of the segmental nerve. If there is a positive response, percutaneous radiofrequency neurotomy is performed. The neurotomy must be performed on two or three levels because the zygapophysial joints have bisegmental innervation. The results are excellent if the patients are well selected. Treatment at C2-3 usually produces poor results because of technical difficulty. The best results are seen at C3-4 and C6-7.

Segmental Nerve Block

Segmental nerve block indicated when pain radiates to the head and shoulder (dorsal root ganglion of C3, C4), shoulder and arm (dorsal root ganglion of C4, C5, C6). Radiofrequency percutaneous partial rhizotomy is performed only after a test block has a positive result. The initial results are good for 75% of the patients, pain recurs among 44% of patients (5,6).

Discogenic Pain

The outer layer of the anulus fibrosus is richly innervated and can be a source of pain. The posterior part of the intervertebral disc is richly innervated by the recurrent nerve of Luschka. Radiofrequency to the cervical discs is performed after a positive result of a test block for patients with chronic nonspecific neck pain with axial pressure pain.

Sympathetically Maintained Pain

Sympathetically maintained pain manifests as diffuse, nonspecific, segmental pain, and sympathetic overactivity. It is managed with stellate ganglion blocks and eventually with a radiofrequency lesion to the stellate ganglion. The possibility of the existence of Horner syndrome has to be kept in mind.

CERVICOGENIC HEADACHE

Cervicogenic headache is a different problem and can be managed with the following algorithm:

1. If radiofrequency to the zygapophyseal joints does not produce sufficient pain relief, dorsal root ganglion blocks of C1 or C2 should be attempted.
2. Block at C1 is indicated when pain originates from the atlantoaxial or atlantooccipital joint. This type of pain includes neck, shoulder, and facial pain. Attacks can resemble migraine or cluster headache.
3. Block at C2 is indicated for occipital neuralgia because the ramus posterior of spinal nerve C2 is the main occipital nerve.

Weiner (7) obtained good results in the management of occipital neuralgia with subcutaneous placement of electrodes. Neuromodulation, such as spinal cord stimulation, is the next step in the algorithm for the management of cervicogenic pain.

SPINAL CORD STIMULATION

Cervical spinal cord stimulation is indicated in the management of typically neuropathic pain syndromes, that is, radiculopathy, mononeuropathy, deafferentation pain, peripheral neuropathic pain (posttraumatic, postsurgical), and postganglionic plexopathies (after brachial plexus elongation). The mechanism of spinal cord stimulation is not clear, but the clinical results validate the gate-control theory (8). The technique targets the ascending collaterals of the large gate-closing A beta fibers. An inhibitory system probably is being activated, facilitatory circuits blocked, and sympathetic efferent neurons influenced. Spinal cord stimulation does not increase levels of endorphins in the cerebrospinal fluid, and analgesia induced by spinal cord stimulation is not reversed by naloxone.

Cervical neurostimulation includes dorsal column stimulation, dorsal root entry zone stimulation, and dorsal root stimulation. It is difficult to stimulate the neck and higher cervical dermatomes (1,3). Nevertheless, the new dual-stimulation technologies and basic studies (Holsheimer model) enable one to steer paresthesia in a segmental way. These new technologies have made it possible to manage specific pain syndromes related to specific dorsal root ganglions (C2, C3).

Peripheral subcutaneous stimulation as described by Weiner (7) gives promising results in the management of refractory occipital neuralgia. The algorithm will be refined in the near future. At present, radiofrequency and neuromodulation techniques are powerful modalities in the management of pain syndromes of cervical origin and can be considered before surgery, especially before repeated surgical procedures.

REFERENCES

1. Barolat G. *J Neurosurg* 1993;78:233–239.
2. Bogduk N. *N Engl J Med* 1996;335:1721–1726.
3. Holsheimer J. *Neurosurgery* 1997;41:654–660.
4. Sluijter M, et al. Pulsed radiofrequency. *Pain Clin* 1998;11:109–117.
5. Van Kleef M, et al: *Neurosurgery* 1996;38:1127–1131.
6. Vervest, AC, Schimmel GH. *Pain* 1988;3:318–321.
7. Weiner R. *Neuromodulation* 1999;2:217–221.
8. Melzack R, Wall PD. *Science* 1965;150:971–979.

The Degenerative Cervical Spine,
edited by Marek Szpalski and Robert Gunzburg
Lippincott Williams & Wilkins, Philadelphia © 2001.

16

Pain Clinic Treatment and Injections

Charles Pither

Pain Management Unit, St. Thomas' Hospital, London SE1 7EH, United Kingdom

ASSESSMENT OF THE PATIENT WITH PAIN
PAIN CLINIC TREATMENTS
CERVICAL EPIDURAL INJECTION
    Technique • Risks • Efficacy
FACET JOINT INJECTION
    Technique • Risks • Efficacy
CERVICAL NERVE ROOT BLOCK
    Technique • Efficacy
INTERDISCIPLINARY TREATMENT AND PAIN MANAGEMENT PROGRAMS
FUNCTIONAL RESTORATION
PAIN MANAGEMENT

Although degenerative changes in the cervical spine are common, it is pain that takes people to their physicians. Pain in the neck is a common symptom. The prevalence was estimated to be 24% in one study; and in nearly 14% of the cases, pain was classified as chronic, with symptoms lasting more than 6 months (6). The problem is that symptoms of pain correlate very poorly with radiographic or magnetic resonance imaging changes (3). The sources and nature of pain arising from the cervical spine undoubtedly are complex. Although efforts to identify sources of nociception from the spine and surrounding tissues are of value, they are not the entire story. Two other aspects deserve mention. First are changes within the nervous system itself as a result of continued nociceptive input. It is now appreciated that chronic pain is very different from acute pain. The difference is related to the plastic changes not only within the dorsal horn but also within the entire central nervous system (23). These changes enhance the effects of peripheral nociceptive input and sensitize the sensory system. The result is an increase in pain for a given level of tissue damage or irritation.

Second, it is crucial to consider the whole person, not simply the cervical spine. The prediction of long-term problems after an episode of acute back pain does not depend on any measurable level of pathologic changes in the tissue or on findings at examination but rather a number of psychosocial variables (7). For this reason it is of paramount importance to view reports of pain in the context of the person's psychologic state and environment as well as other relevant variables, such as issues relating to work, litigation, or the benefits system. If such variables are to be taken into account, a thorough and broad assessment of a patient with pain is crucial.

ASSESSMENT OF THE PATIENT WITH PAIN

Pain is always a subjective perception experienced only by the individual. There will always be limits on the ability of a person with pain to convey exactly the nature of this experience. In a traditional medical setting, interpretation of symptoms leads to a diagnosis and the delivery of appropriate and curative treatment. However, pain of spinal origin is seldom if ever pathognomonic of a particular syndrome or lesion. Therapy has to be guided not only by the history, examination, and diagnostic tests, but also by the effect of the pain on the patient and the presence of external influences. For proper assessment, it is important that sufficient time is allowed and that appropriate disciplines are incorporated into the process. These would include psychology, physiotherapy, and various medical specialties. It is frequently helpful to use standard psychometric or other questionnaires, the answers to which can provide supportive information in decision making (34).

Assessment should focus on the following:

The nature of the symptoms (the illness)
The extent of the physical problem (the disease)
The degree of psychologic distress (depression and anxiety)
The patient's perceived decrement of function (disability)
The presence or absence of social reinforcement

It is important to differentiate the level of disability experienced by the patient and the level of impairment assessed at medical examination (31).

PAIN CLINIC TREATMENTS

Although many fields of medicine can offer specific therapies for diseases that produce complete or almost complete resolution of symptoms based on modifying the fundamental pathophysiologic processes involved, this is not possible for many chronically painful conditions. Pain is a multidimensional experience influenced by processes at all levels within the central nervous system. Seldom if ever is chronic pain relieved completely with manipulation of peripheral nociceptive input. For this reason, pain clinic therapy is usually multimodal and is aimed at symptomatic relief rather than disease management. Treatment is pragmatic in that the therapy with the greatest likelihood of relieving pain is initiated first. If this fails to provide benefit, other therapies are tried. The aim is not simply to cure the condition—pain clinic treatment seldom if ever provides a complete cure—but to improve the quality of life of the person with pain. In general, the following treatment modalities are available:

Drugs
Stimulation analgesia (transcutaneous electrical stimulation [TENS] and acupuncture)
Nerve blocks and injections
Psychologic techniques
Invasive implantation techniques

This review focuses on injections with some discussion of pain management approaches.

CERVICAL EPIDURAL INJECTION

Epidural injections have been used for many years to treat patients experiencing back and neck pain. The rationale has been based on considerable anecdotal evidence of efficacy, a theoretic basis for expectation of benefit, and a lack of other more effective therapies. Through injection into the epidural space, many potentially painful structures can be brought into contact with the injectate. This includes the internal facet capsule, the longitudinal ligament, the anulus of the disc, the nerve root itself, and other sensitive neural elements within the canal. If, as is likely, the sources of pain in radiculopathy and degenerative disc disease are multiple (1) and in part related to inflammation due to the presence of degenerative disc material in the epidural space, injection of antiinflammatory medications close to the source of pain is logical.

Most outcome data are related to the use of epidural agents in the lumbar region because there has been much more experience in that area. The lumbar epidural space is larger than the cervical space. As the spinal cord terminates at the upper lumbar level, injection is safer, at least as far as the likelihood of penetration of the spinal cord is concerned. Many practitioners have been reluctant either to perform or recommend cervical epidural injection on the grounds of safety. This reluctance is irrational, however, because the technique is safe and, with experience, injection can be performed simply and with minimal trauma or risk.

Technique

Numerous techniques exist for the performance of cervical epidural block, and it is neither possible nor desirable to suggest that one approach should be favored or is safer than any other. There are, however, some theoretic considerations that confer advantages to certain techniques.

The spinous processes of the cervical spine are more horizontally situated than those of the thoracic spine, and greater flexion is possible in the neck than in the chest. Thus the gap between adjacent vertebrae, especially in the lower cervical region, opens considerably with good neck flexion. This is best achieved when the patient is sitting with arms crossed in front and resting on a high table or support. This position also diminishes pressure in the epidural space and can be used advantageously for accurate localization of the space. The hanging drop technique with a winged needle works extremely well.

The patient is positioned in the sitting, arms crossed position. The nurse or assistant stands in front of the patient and can offer comfort, assistance, and aid in positioning. The skin is prepared in the usual way, and the most accessible space is identified. This is usually C7-T1. Local anesthetic is infiltrated. An 18-gauge Touhy needle is inserted in the midline. This is easy to identify given the position of the patient. The needle is advanced through the interspinous ligament with the trocar in situ. Once gripped firmly by the ligament, indicating the midline, the needle is advanced farther at an angle approximately 20 to 30 degrees above the horizontal. The trocar is removed, and a drop of saline solution is placed in the hub. Given the hydrophobic nature of the plastic cannula hub, a good drop can be obtained. The physician, both hands resting on the patient's back, advances the needle using the wings. Entrance into the epidural space is clearly marked by loss of the drop, which is sucked into the needle. When the needle is correctly placed, cardiac pulsation usually is visible in the meniscus. Correct placement can be confirmed with a glass or low-resistance syringe (Fig. 16.1). Bupivacaine 0.25% in a volume up to 7 mL is injected with a suitable glucocorticoid preparation, such as 80 mg depomedrone.

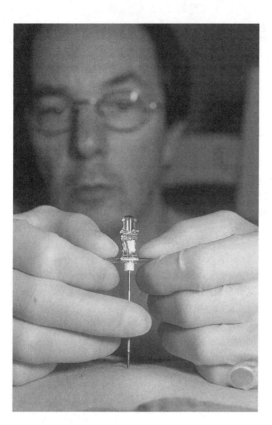

FIG. 16.1. Cervical epidural injection. Patient is sitting. The angle of needle insertion and positioning of the hands are important. This technique provides fine control of needle progression and considerable stability if the patient moves suddenly. The bulging meniscus of the hanging drop is evident.

Risks

Because of the danger of cord penetration, and the consequences of high neural blockade, the risks of cervical epidural injection inevitably are greater than those of injection by the lumbar route, but these are still very low. Reports of cord injury do occur (13,20). Respiratory and cardiovascular effects of the block can occur but seem to be of no clinical significance. In general, the complications are the same for any entry to the epidural space—dural puncture, hematoma, nerve injury, and infection.

Efficacy

Epidural injection both in the lumbar and cervical regions has been the subject of numerous studies but of all to few well-controlled trials. One study frequently cited is that of Bush and Hillier (8). This study examined the effects of serial injection in the treatment of 68 patients with cervical radiculopathy. All patients avoided surgery, and 76% were free of arm pain at telephone follow-up interviews a mean of 39 months after treatment. Grenier et al. (12) reported that 83% of patients gained benefit 3 months after a single injection of lignocaine and triamcinolone. Both of these studies were hindered by lack of control groups. Stav et al. (25) compared two groups of patients with neck and arm pain, one receiving epidural injections of lignocaine and glucocorticoid and the other the same dose into the muscles of the neck. Follow-up evaluation at 1 year suggested that the group receiving the epidural injections had less pain and a greater range of motion and were more likely to be working than the group who received intramuscular injections.

No metaanalyses or systematic reviews of epidural injection in the neck have been conducted, but given the clinical parallels between cervical and lumbar injection, it is reasonable to extrapolate from two recent studies of epidural injection in general. Koes et al. (17) in a systematic review examined the efficacy of epidural steroid injection for low back pain. Twelve randomized studies were identified, only four scoring more than 60 points on methodologic assessment. Of these four studies, two showed benefit and two did not. This pattern was repeated when the remaining 8 studies were included. Half of the studies indicated the treatment was more effective than the reference condition, and half showed the treatment was no better or worse. The authors concluded that there were flaws in the designs of most studies and that the efficacy of epidural steroid injection has not yet been established.

Watts and Silagy (33) undertook a metaanalysis to assess the benefit of epidural administration of glucocorticoids in the management of sciatica. The authors found 11 trials that included 907 patients. The analysis showed that the use of epidural steroids increased the odds ratio of short-term pain relief (>75%) to 2.61 (95% confidence interval [CI], 1.9–3.77). For longer-term relief (up to 1 year), the odds ratio fell to 1.87 (95% CI, 1.31–2.68). The conclusion was that the epidural administration of glucocorticoids is effective in the management of lumbosacral radicular pain. It should be noted that these two studies adopted different methods and examined different aspects of outcome. It has long been clinical wisdom that epidural injections are more effective for radicular or limb pain than for back pain, and this finding emerges from the metaanalyses. Both studies also showed the lack of serious side effects and the lack of long-term adverse consequences.

FACET JOINT INJECTION

Over the years the facet joint has been the subject of much controversy among spine specialists. Although most would agree that it is likely that the facet joint can be a cause of pain, identification of a clear-cut facet syndrome is not universally acknowledged (14). Degenerative changes in the cervical spine often cause changes in the architecture of the facet region, and arthritic changes frequently can be seen on computed tomographic scans. The problem is that such findings occur in the absence of pain in the healthy population (3). Dwyer et al. (10) found that injection into the cervical facet joint can produce a typical pattern of pain among healthy volunteers. Thus it is likely that the facet joint is the source of pain in some instances. Given the persistent and troublesome nature of neck pain, and the limited efficacy of most treatment options, diagnostic block of the facet joints can be a rational and indeed helpful treatment. There are, however, some problems with the conclusion that because a single facet joint injection with local anesthetic produces pain relief, it is definitely the facet joint complex that is the source of pain. This is because injectate spreads around the joint capsule to other pain-producing tissues, and one cannot eliminate nonspecific effects with a single injection.

Even if the facet complex is the source of pain, it is not the case that injection of steroid into or around the joint produces long-term benefit. In this situation enthusiasts recommend a denervation procedure in which a radiofrequency nerve lesion is used to destroy the nerves supplying the joint. Once again, it is mandatory to fully assess the effects of temporary block performed under blinded conditions before proceeding to the lengthy and complex procedure of denervation (19).

Technique

Injection into the cervical facets can be performed from the posterior or the lateral approach. Most practitioners adopt the posterior approach recommended in textbooks (9). The patient is positioned prone with the head supported by foam cushions. A degree of flexion of the cervical spine is helpful because this opens the joint. However, flexion is not easy in the prone position. Radiographic control with image intensifier is mandatory if accurate needle placement is to be achieved. Because the injection is painful, intravenous sedation is administered. On a lateral radiograph the angle of the facet joint can be seen and an appropriate insertion site chosen 2 to 3 cm from the midline. This position should be verified by means of screening. Insertion too near the midline runs the risk of epidural injection or penetration of the cord.

A skin wheal is raised 3 to 4 cm below the level to be injected. A 10-cm 22-gauge spinal needle is inserted through the skin wheal and through the paraspinal muscles toward the joint. It is not always possible to enter the joint space, but pericapsular injection is probably satisfactory because the capsule is richly innervated and is a likely source of inflammation and pain. Roy et al. (24) could detect no difference in outcome between patients receiving intraarticular versus periarticular injections. If the needle is in the joint, it is difficult to inject more than 0.5 mL of long-acting local anesthetic with steroid. A larger volume can be administered by means of pericapsular injection. It is possible to perform injection into several levels at one time, but clinical practice usually dictates it is either the upper or lower joints that are troublesome, and thus injection at more than three levels is unusual (Figs. 16.2, 16.3).

Cervical facet neurotomy by means of radiofrequency lesion is a much more complicated procedure. The facet joint is innervated from the posterior ramus of both the nerve above and below the joint (4); thus two lesions are needed for each joint. The tip of a radiofrequency lesion needle is inserted from the lateral onto the waist of the pedicle (28) (Fig 16.2).

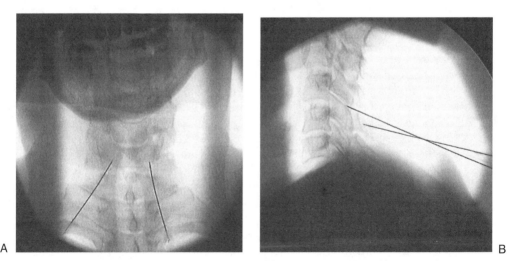

A

B

FIG. 16.2. Cervical facet joint injection. Anteroposterior **(A)** and lateral **(B)** radiographs show needles in C5-6 facet joint.

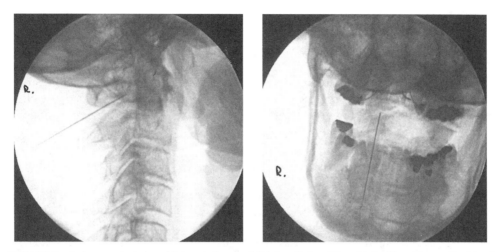

FIG. 16.3. Anteroposterior and lateral views of C1-2 unilateral facet injection. The patient had pain from unilateral degenerative disease of the atlantoaxial joint. This was managed successfully with intraarticular injection of a glucocorticoid.

Risks

There are very few reported side effects of simple facet joint injection. Needle malplacement can cause injection into the epidural space or dural penetration with resultant headache. Nerve damage is rare with small-diameter needles. Hemorrhage from unintentional puncture of the vertebral artery is a potential complication.

Efficacy

The main problem with attempting to assess the place of cervical facet joint injections in the management of degenerative and inflammatory conditions of the cervical spine is the lack of good quality-controlled studies. Injections frequently are performed because the person with pain continues to report pain and there is no definitive treatment, rather than because there is good evidence of efficacy. Although it is fair to say that there are few data to support a positive outcome from facet joint injections in the lumbar region, the case for injection into the cervical spine is even worse, with very few outcome studies of any type. Bovim et al. (5) examined a group of 14 patients with this condition and found that blockade of the cervical facets produced pain relief for only 2 of a subgroup of 9 patients. The authors were unsure of the mechanisms and mentioned that the injected local anesthetic may have spread to other structures.

Roy et al. (24) performed injection into the facet joints of 21 patients with facet joint syndrome. They found the blocks relieved the symptoms of 91% for variable lengths of time. The effects were acknowledged to be short lived. There was no difference between the results for intraarticular and those for periarticular injection. Barnsley et al. (2) reported that the addition of steroid to the injectate did not improve quality or duration of pain relief; there was minimal benefit beyond 2 weeks.

The most substantial body of literature on facet joint injection relates to the use of radiofrequency blockade of the posterior cervical rami supplying the facet joint. Much of these data concern whiplash injury and the use of diagnostic blocks to identify the source of pain, with subsequent ablation of the nerves if the block is shown to be of benefit

(18,32). Although these studies provide convincing data that pain after whiplash can be aided by appropriate interventions, the numbers involved have been small, and patients have always been carefully selected, leading to questions about ability to generalize the results of the studies (15).

The use of radiofrequency lesions is supported by a number of case reports and poorly controlled studies (29,30). Lord et al. (18), in one of the few double-blind, controlled studies, found that the use of these techniques can produce long-term pain relief of good quality (Fig 16.3).

CERVICAL NERVE ROOT BLOCK

Degenerative conditions in the cervical spine often cause nerve root irritation that produces pain that radiates into the arm or hand. Clear-cut nerve root compression frequently is not found in such cases, and there is difficulty ascertaining whether the symptoms are genuinely related to nerve root irritation or they are referred from other spinal or paraspinal tissues. In this situation nerve root block can be a useful diagnostic procedure. In cases of demonstrable nerve root irritation for which surgery is not the first-line therapy, the use of therapeutic nerve root block with steroid can be beneficial.

Technique

Two approaches are commonly used—posterior and lateral oblique. The use of radiographic screening is mandatory if accurate needle placement is to be achieved. The patient is positioned prone or in the lateral position. The relevant level is identified by means of counting up from the first rib or down from the occiput. In the posterior approach, a 22- or 25-gauge needle is inserted 2 cm lateral to the outer border of the relevant vertebra at the level of the intervertebral disc. The needle is directed slightly medially to pass the posterior elements and enter the intervertebral foramen from the rear. The position in the anteroposterior dimension is checked by means of screening in the lateral position.

In the alternative approach, the x-ray tube is swung into the oblique view until the intervertebral foramen is clearly seen. The needle is then inserted directly over the foramen and advanced in the line of the x-ray beam. Care has to be exercised as the vertebra is approached because severe paresthesia can be elicited, which can cause the patient to jolt and change position. With either technique the spread of the injectate can be ascertained by means of injection of a small amount of contrast material. Three to seven milliliters of local anesthetic is injected with or without glucocorticoid.

Efficacy

Most reports of the benefits of root blocks are anecdotal. No controlled studies have been conducted, and there are few reports in the literature.

INTERDISCIPLINARY TREATMENT AND PAIN MANAGEMENT PROGRAMS

Most patients referred to pain clinics in the United Kingdom have spinal pain. The epidemiologic characteristics of back and neck pain and studies of the factors that affect the development of chronicity clearly show the importance of psychosocial factors (4). After an episode of acute back pain, the likelihood of development of persistent pain and disability is not predicated by physical or disease related factors. The likelihood is related to reported pain level in the initial attack, perception of damage and illness, and psychologic distress measured with a depression inventory. Elucidation of this aspect of understanding of back pain has led to the description of so-called yellow flags or psychosocial risk factors (16).

Yellow flags cover areas such as attitudes and beliefs about pain, behaviors, compensation issues, diagnosis and treatment, emotions, family issues, and work. Assessment and management of low back pain increasingly are taking these factors into account. The need to address these issues must be recognized if effective treatment is to be provided. It follows that for a great many spinal pain problems, treatment needs to encompass broader dimensions than the purely biologic. It is not simply a case of substituting psychologic or psychiatric therapy for ineffective medical treatment. These patients are not psychotic, nor can their pain problems be cured with psychologic treatment. Psychologic therapies do have a place but only when combined with broader medical treatment. This has led to the provision of interdisciplinary therapy, whereby various disciplines work together to provide therapy to address the problems. Such disciplines include physiotherapy, psychology, medicine, nursing, occupational therapy, ergonomics, and fitness instruction. Many patients have undergone outpatient treatment from practitioners of one or many of these disciplines, often with little benefit.

The most commonly used psychologic treatment approaches adopt cognitive behavioral techniques. Cognitive behavioral principles are as follows:

- The way we feel about issues, events or bodily sensations depends on our evaluation of them.
- This internal evaluation is influenced by our knowledge and understanding of the causes, or meaning, of the symptom or event.
- The knowledge base we have is a complex repository of information (both correct and incorrect), views, beliefs, and experiences.
- When we do not have hard facts or information, we make inferences to fill in the gaps in our knowledge.
- Such inferences may not be correct.
- The conclusion we make about a symptom or issue, based both on the facts we have and the inferences we make, has emotional loading. This is the same regardless of the truth of the inference. For example, if the discovery of a lump in a breast implies cancer, the emotional experience is negative even before clinical confirmation of malignancy.
- Although such processes are normal and essentially human, the views we take can at times, and for certain persons, be too strongly held, too rigid, or erroneous. Given pain usually is a negative experience, it is not surprising that it can often become associated with a series of negative emotions.
- Patterns of negative thinking tend to become stereotyped and automatic. Thus persons with pain report that the same negative series of thoughts occur several times a day, often provoked by everyday situations. This process has been termed *catastrophization.* These thoughts provoke negative emotions, such as fear, low mood, anger, frustration, and despair.
- In the context of spinal pain, it is frequently the case that a person with pain has a catalog of negative or catastrophic views as to the cause, implications, and prognosis of the illness.

- Such inferences usually are erroneous, but this does not prevent them from having a considerable influence on the person with pain in terms of negative emotional load.
- Inferences alter behavior.
- A belief that back pain represents crumbling of the bones is not compatible with activities that provoke pain, because the increased pain signifies to the person with pain crumbling or worsening of the damage being done to the spine.
- This process has been called *fear avoidance* and is a common feature of chronic spinal pain.

Cognitive behavioral therapy aims to help the person by teaching ways to recognize these automatic negative thoughts when they occur and to challenge them with other ways of looking at things based in a more balanced and accurate representation. Alternative, less catastrophic ways of viewing problems produce less negative emotions and enable the person to feel better. These techniques are combined with practical approaches aimed at gradually reintroducing the person to feared activities, tasks, and movements. In practice this devolves to two areas—physiotherapist-led stretching and exercises in the gym and occupational therapist–led activity programming involving planning, goal setting, and pacing.

Usually this form of treatment is delivered in a group setting for a fixed length, such as 3 or 4 weeks. Programs differ depending on level of difficulty and the goals of therapy. The literature is replete with outcomes of various protocols delivered by differing disciplines in a multitude of settings. There is no agreed nomenclature for such programs, but in general *functional restoration* is the term given to a physically based rehabilitation program with psychologic input aimed at managing these illnesses. This would seem to be logical. Many patients return to normal function, including work. *Pain management programs* are aimed at more disabled and distressed patients, for whom normal function may not be a realistic expectation. Such programs are more psychologic in emphasis.

FUNCTIONAL RESTORATION

For patients not seriously disabled or excessively distressed, functional restoration is logical and effective. Suitable patients have back or neck pain that has persisted for at least 1 year and have undergone a number of therapies that have not been totally successful in alleviating the symptoms. Typical patients find the pain intrusive in daily activities and are struggling at work. They may have had some deterioration of mood as a result of the pain and its effects on lifestyle and would be worried and anxious about the future. In general the premorbid state was good with little in the way of serious pain-related problems or psychosocial dysfunction. Typical components of a functional restoration program are as follows:

- Information and education
- Stretching and exercise
- Fitness program
- Hydrotherapy
- Pacing
- Relaxation
- Stress management
- Cognitive training
- Postural retraining
- Biomechanics

The outcome of such programs shows that considerable improvement in physical performance and mood can be obtained with a high rate of return to work (21). Although most of the data refer to the lumbar spine or to general musculoskeletal problems not site specific, Wright et al. (35) compared the outcome from rehabilitation in an intensive 3-week interdisciplinary functional restoration program for neck pain and low back pain and found no major differences. It would thus seem reasonable to extrapolate that there are no major differences between persons with cervical pain and those with problems in the lower back. Given what is known about the psychosocial factors influencing these illnesses, this extrapolation seems logical.

PAIN MANAGEMENT

Many patients are too disabled to take part in a program that involves vigorous physical activity. The disability may be caused by either physical impairment or excessive emotional vulnerability. Usually, however, it is both, mind and body interacting in complex and ultimately poorly understood ways. Such patients have high levels of pain and are often taking a large number of pain-related medications. They have high levels of disability as measured with, for example, the Oswestry disability questionnaire (11). They are markedly disabled with limitations of function in most domains, such as work, self-care, and leisure. Frequently they are barely self-caring, relying on walking aids and other supports, such as collars and corsets or even wheelchairs. They have high levels of depression and anxiety as measured with interview and psychometric questionnaires.

Treatment of such persons involves helping them to manage their symptoms and optimize quality of life. For most persons with pain, the prospect of full rehabilitation is not realistic. Treatment is aimed at optimizing function within the constraints of the illness. Inevitably this means helping the person with pain come to terms with limitation of function. The treatment is delivered by an interdisciplinary team well versed in psychologic techniques in general and cognitive therapy in particular (26). Staff on such a program includes physicians, psychologists, physiotherapists, occupational therapists, and nurses.

The concept of pain management takes its validity from examination of persons who have chronic pain problems but who manage to function normally and enjoy a good quality of life. When scrutinized, such people seem to do the following:

• Understand the likely cause of pain and have overcome fears about it
• Take as few medications as possible
• Maintain physical fitness and keep as active as possible
• Pace activities and avoid overdoing or getting into overactivity or underactivity cycles
• Have methods for coping with flare-ups and setbacks
• Keep their mood positive and avoid catastrophizing
• Use a relaxation technique

The aims of a pain management program are to teach persons with pain the aforementioned skills and to help them improve physical performance with a stretching and exercise regimen. Treatment typically is delivered in a group with 8 to 10 patients receiving intensive treatment over a number of weeks. In the United Kingdom, this is either organized as an outpatient program of 6 to 8 weeks' duration or as a residential package of 3 or 4 weeks (27).

Outcome data from such programs indicate that substantial changes can be made in a number of domains that equate with better quality of life. There are few outcome data specific to pain from the cervical spine. In a recent metaanalysis, Morley et al. (22) reported that compared with control treatment conditions, cognitive behavioral interventions showed clear superiority in pain level, cognitive coping, and reduction in behavioral expression of pain.

REFERENCES

1. Abram SE. Pain mechanisms in lumbar radiculopathy. *Anesth Analg* 1988;67:1135–1137.
2. Barnsley L, Lord SM, Wallis BJ, et al. Lack of effect of intraarticular corticosteroid for chronic pain in the cervical zygoapophyseal joints. *N Engl J Med* 1994;330:1047–1050.
3. Boden S, McCowin P, Davis D, et al. Abnormal magnetic resonance scans of the cervical spine in asymptomatic subjects. *J Bone Joint Surg Am* 1990;72:1178–1184.
4. Bogduk N. The clinical anatomy of the cervical dorsal rami. *Spine* 1982;7:319–330.
5. Bovim G, Berg R, Dale LG. Cervicogenic headache: anaesthetic blockade of the cervical nerves and facet joint. *Pain* 1992;49:315–320.
6. Bovim G, Schrader H, Sand T. Neck pain in the general population. *Spine* 1994;19:1307–1309.
7. Burton AK, Tillotson M, Main CJ, et al. Psychosocial predictors of outcome in acute and subchronic low back trouble. *Spine* 1995;20:722–728.
8. Bush K, Hillier S. Outcome of cervical radiculopathy treated with periradicular/epidural corticosteroid injections: a prospective study with independent clinical review. *Eur Spine J* 1996;5:319–325.
9. Cousins MJ, Bridenbaugh PO. *Neutral blockade in clinical anesthesia and pain management,* 2nd ed. Philadelphia: JB Lippincott, 1988.
10. Dwyer A, Aproll C, Bogduk N. Cervical zygoapohphyseal joint pain patterns, I: a study in normal volunteers. *Spine* 1990;15:453–457.
11. Fairbank JCT, Couper J, Davies JB, et al. The Oswestry Low Back Pain Disability Questionnaire. *Physiotherapy* 1980;66:2781–273.
12. Grenier B, Castagnera L, Maurette P, et al. Neuralgie cervico-brachiale chronique traitee par injection peridurale cervicale de corticoides: resultats a long terme. *Ann Fr Anesth Reanim* 1995;14:484–488.
13. Hodges SD Castleberg RL, Miller T, et al. Cervical epidural steroid injection with intrinsic spinal cord damage: two case reports. *Spine* 1998;23:2137–2142.
14. Jackson RP. The facet syndrome: myth or reality? *Clin Orthop* 1992;279:1110–1121.
15. Kendall M, Main CJ, Linton SJ, et al. Letter. *Pain* 1998;78:223–225.
16. Kendall NA. Psychosocial approaches to the prevention of chronic pain: the low back paradigm. *Baillieres Best Pract Res Clin Rheumatol* 1999;13:545–554.
17. Koes BW, Scholten RJ, Mens JM, et al. Efficacy of epidural steroid injections for low-back pain and sciatica: a systematic review of randomized clinical trials. *Pain* 1995;63:279–288.
18. Lord SM, Barnsley L, Wallis BJ, et al. Percutaneous radiofrequency neurotomy for chronic cervical zygoapophyseal joint pain. *N Engl J Med* 1996;335:1721–1726.
19. Lord SM, Barnsley L, Walis BJ, et al. Chronic cervical zygoapophyseal joint pain after whiplash: a placebo controlled prevalence study. *Spine* 1996;21:1737–1744.
20. Manchikanti L. Cervical epidural steroid injection with intrinsic spinal cord damage. *Spine* 1999;24:1170–1172.
21. Mayer TG, Gatchel H, Mayer H, et al. A prospective two year study of functional restoration in industrial low back injury: an objective assessment procedure. *JAMA* 1987;258:1763–1767.
22. Morley S, Eccleston C, Williams A. A systematic review and meta-analysis of randomized controlled trials of cognitive behavioral therapy and behavior therapy for chronic pain in adults excluding headache. *Pain* 1999;80:1–13.
23. Niv D, Devor M. Transition from acute to chronic pain. In Aronoff G, ed. *Evaluation and treatment of chronic pain,* 3rd ed. Baltimore: Williams & Wilkins, 1998.
24. Roy DF, Fleury J, Fontiane SB, et al. Clinical evaluation of cervical facet joint infiltration. *Can Assoc Radiol J* 1988;39:118–120.
25. Stav A, Ovadia L, Sternberg A, et al. Cervical epidural injection of cervicobrachialgia. *Acta Anaesthesiol Scand* 1993;37:562–566.
26. Turk DC, Meichenbaum D, Genest M. *Pain and behavioral medicine: a cognitive behavioral perspective.* New York: Guildford Press, 1983.
27. Turner JA. Efficacy of cognitive therapy for low back pain. *Pain* 1993;52:169–177.
28. van Suijlekom, Weber WEJ, van Kleef M. Treatment of spinal pain by means of radiofrequency procedures, II: thoracic and cervical areas. *Pain Rev* 1999;6:175–191
29. Vervest A, Stolker R. The treatment of cervical pain syndromes with radiofrequency procedures. *Pain Clin* 1991;4:103–112..

30. Vervest A, Stolker R, van Kleef M, et al. Effects and side effects of a percutaneous thermal lesion of the dorsal root ganglion in patients with cervical pain syndrome. *Pain* 1993;52:49–53.
31. Waddell G. *The back pain revolution.* Edinburgh: Churchill Livingstone, 1998:119–134.
32. Wallis BJ, Lord SM, Bogduk N. Resolution of psychological distress of whiplash patients following treatment by radiofrequency neurotomy: a randomized, double blind placebo-controlled trial. *Pain* 1997;73:15–22.
33. Watts RW, Silagy CA. A meta-anaysis on the efficacy of epidural corticosteroids in the treatment of sciatica. *Anaesth Intensive Care* 1995;23:564–569.
34. Williams A. Measures of function and psychology. In: Wall PD, Melzack R, eds. *Textbook of Pain,* 4th ed. Edinburgh: Churchill Livingstone, 1999;427–444.
35. Wright A, Mayer TG, Gatchel RJ. Outcomes of disabling cervical spine disorders in lumbar spinal disorders. *Spine* 1999;24:178–183.

Surgical Treatment Modalities

The Degenerative Cervical Spine,
edited by Marek Szpalski and Robert Gunzburg
Lippincott Williams & Wilkins, Philadelphia © 2001.

17

Anterior Cervical Decompression and Fusion Without Instrumentation

Henry Vernon Crock

Spinal Disorders Unit, Cromwell Hospital, Cromwell Road, London SW5 OTU, United Kingdom

PREPARATIONS FOR ANTERIOR CERVICAL FUSION OPERATIONS
ANESTHESIA
SKIN INCISION
DISSECTION
DOWEL CUTTING
REMOVAL OF DISC REMNANTS
GRAFT HARVESTING
GRAFT IMPACTION
RESULTS
POSTOPERATIVE CARE

Techniques of anterior cervical spinal fusion were introduced in 1955 by Robinson and Smith (4) and in 1958 by Cloward (2). In the early 1960s, modified instrumentation was developed by Crock (3). By the end of the twentieth century this procedure had become the most commonly performed operation for the management of a wide variety of lesions affecting the cervical spine. At the beginning of twenty-first century, profound changes in attitudes toward spinal surgery in general and to cervical spinal surgery in particular are gathering pace. In the United States, Wall Street investors have continued to support the rapid growth in the development of surgical implants and instruments for use in spinal surgery. Set-up costs and purchase prices for individual items such as plates, screws, and cages are high.

Education in the use of much of this new equipment has been taken over largely by the manufacturers. Surgeons are enticed to attend workshops staged during congress meetings or held as isolated events of short duration, designed to launch new products. A new phrase, "the learning curve," has crept into use in surgical education. For example, when a young orthopedic surgeon was questioned about his use of that phrase in relation to the operation of synchronous combined anterior and posterior fusion of the lumbar spine with internal fixation, he replied, "We lost two patients on the operating table." In another incident, a middle-aged patient who had come to medical attention with brachial neuralgia awoke from anterior cervical fusion with internal fixation, performed by a young neurosurgeon, with complete paralysis of both arms. After urgent revision surgery, the patient died. Clearly the steeper the learning curve, the more hazardous is the outcome, for both the patient and the surgeon.

Complications of anterior instrumented arthrodesis of the cervical spine were presented by Casamitjana et al. (1) in a lecture at the Annual Meeting of the Spine Society of Europe held in Munich in September 1999. Six hundred seventy-four of these operations had been performed between 1991 and 1998. The authors reported 2 deep hematomas; 1 tracheal rupture; 2 esophageal fistulas; 3 severe cases of dysphagia; 10 mild cases of dysphagia; 1 esophageal pseudocyst; 10 peripheral neurologic complications, including 2 hypoglossal nerve palsies and 5 facial mandibular branch nerve injuries; 5 pseudoarthroses; and 4 complications of graft donor sites. The review raises many questions about the advisability of routine use of internal fixation devices in anterior cervical fusion.

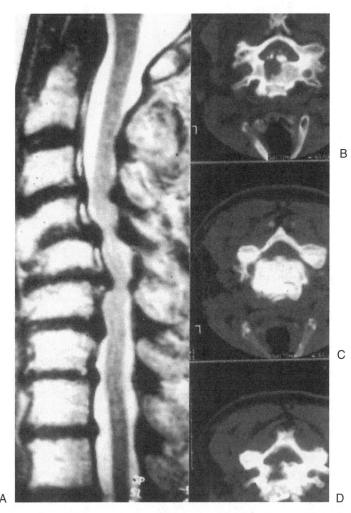

FIG. 17.1. Images of an 80-year-old man with myelopathy who has used a wheelchair for 1 year. He is unable to lie prone because of cardiac surgery. **A:** Midsagittal magnetic resonance image of cervical spine shows severe canal stenosis at C4-5 and C5-6. **B, C:** *Top right,* postoperative computed tomographic images. Ossicles remain attached to the dural sac anteriorly. **D:** *Lower right,* less than 3 months after canal decompression and interbody fusion, the patient could walk with two canes, and improvement has been maintained at one year.

The purpose of this chapter is to present a detailed account of a technique that I have practiced regularly for 35 years in nearly 1,000 operations using a dowel grafting method without the addition of internal fixation devices. The instruments needed are inexpensive but reliable. They are suitable for use by surgeons working in hospitals where funds are not available for purchasing the expensive imaging equipment and consumable items needed for internal fixation of the spine (Fig. 17.2).

PREPARATIONS FOR ANTERIOR CERVICAL FUSION OPERATIONS

Anterior cervical spinal fusion operations are rated as high-risk surgery. The patient's informed consent should be obtained personally by the surgeon. In discussing potential

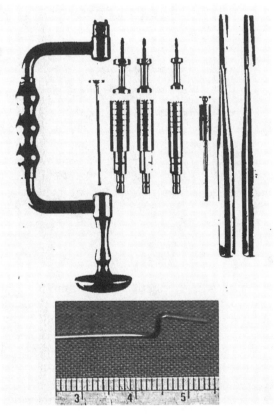

FIG. 17.2. Top: Photograph shows the Crock instruments used for dowel cutting in anterior cervical interbody fusion. *Left,* Hudson brace. Cutters of three sizes are shown. The starter center pieces have been removed from each of these. To the left of the cutters is a pusher, which fits inside the cutters and can be used to eject the starter center pieces or graft bone. To the right of the cutters is a pusher with a tubular segment of metal measuring 12.5 mm in depth. When this "dummy" is slotted into the cutter it acts as a guard to prevent the cutter from penetrating deeper than 12.5 mm into the cervical vertebral bodies. Dummies are provided in three sizes, 10 mm, 12.5 mm, and 15 mm, for use according to the vertebral dimensions in individual cases. *Right,* two tooled gouges, which fit into the cuts made into adjacent vertebral bodies (see Fig. 17.3. The cutters have circular rings marking the outer surfaces at intervals of 5 mm. **Bottom:** Photograph shows 23-gauge hypodermic needle bent in a *Z* shape to prevent penetration of the spinal canal when used as a marker in the disc space. (From Crock, HV. *A short practice of spinal surgery.* New York: Springer-Verlag, 1993, with permission.)

complications, the minor inconveniences of graft donor site pain, transient sore throat. and difficulty with swallowing should be addressed first. The risks of major complications, such as serious wound infection and injuries to the cervical spinal cord or nerve roots, should be dealt with in detail, especially if a patient has myelopathy, for which multilevel fusions or strut grafts are to be used after decompression of the dural sac (Fig. 17.1).

ANESTHESIA

The surgeon must warn the anesthetist to avoid hyperextension of the neck during intubation in operations on patients with cervical canal stenosis or in the presence of large disc prolapses. In some of these operations, transnasal intubation with endoscopy may be needed. The patient's eyes should be protected with thick padding, and the endotracheal tube fixed in the midline of the forehead. On the operating table, a small pillow should be placed under the shoulders and a rolled towel in the hollow of the neck with the occiput resting on a ring-shaped support.

SKIN INCISION

Before the operative area is sterilized and surgical drapes applied, the siting of the skin incision should be planned. Approaches through the right side of the neck can be used routinely with safety. In operations on patients with degenerative disc disease at one or two levels, anteriorly projecting osteophytes can be palpated with the surgeon's index finger, and the level of the skin incision outlined with a marking pen. In operations on patients with very long necks in which the vertebral bodies from C2 to T1 are visible on the lateral radiograph and in other patients with very short, fat necks in which only the upper four cervical vertebrae may be visible on a lateral radiograph, it is wise to use a metal marker on the neck on a preliminary lateral radiograph to plan the skin incision.

DISSECTION

Surgical drapes should be attached over the lower margins of the mandible, at the level of the manubrium sterni inferiorly and laterally on each side behind the sternocleidomastoid muscle attachments. The anterior half of the right iliac crest should be exposed for harvesting of bone grafts. Short, oblique incisions may be made at the desired level extending from the anterior border of the sternocleidomastoid toward the midline. The platysma muscle is exposed by means of dissection of the subcutaneous tissue from its outer surface upward and downward. During this stage of dissection, it may be necessary to isolate one of the large anterior cervical veins, although it is rarely necessary to ligate and divide it.

The fibers of the platysma muscle are split longitudinally in the gap between the anterior margin of the sternocleidomastoid muscle and the larynx and trachea. The encircling layer of deep cervical fascia is split longitudinally with a fine, blunt-nosed scissors. In the process, the upper or lower margins of the superior belly of the omohyoid muscle are defined, depending on the level of the vertebral column to be exposed. During this stage of dissection it is rarely necessary to ligate and divide any of the major branches of regional arteries and veins unless the thyroid gland is enlarged, in which case, the superior thyroid artery or a middle thyroid vein may have to be isolated, ligated, and divided. After this careful blunt dissection, a gap is opened between the midline structures of esophagus, larynx, and trachea and the laterally placed carotid sheath.

The surgeon should insert the tip of the index finger to palpate the front of the vertebral column, sweeping the digit easily upward and downward to separate the soft tissues and prepare for insertion of retractors. In some patients, all subcutaneous tissue is extremely fibrous, rendering exposure tedious. In most patients, however, the soft tissues in the prevertebral space are supple and separate easily. A blunt-ended retractor is placed under the esophagus, and the midline structures are retracted toward the left side. A second retractor is inserted to the level of the anterior surface of the cervical spine, and the carotid sheath retracted laterally until the medial border of the longus colli muscle can be seen. The thin, transparent prevertebral fascia should be split in the midline and dissected with a scissors upward and downward until the anterior surface of the disc and adjacent vertebral bodies is exposed. This fascia normally strips off the anterior longitudinal ligament easily until the medial borders of both the right and left longus colli muscles are clearly seen. With a suction device in the left hand and a bayonet-shaped forceps in the right, the surgeon coagulates the vessels along the medial border of the right-sided longus colli muscles and separates the muscle laterally so that the right-sided retractor can be placed beneath it, thereby avoiding constriction of the vessels in the carotid sheath. Exposure of the anterior surface of the vertebral column and of the intervertebral disc is then complete.

DOWEL CUTTING

A 23-gauge needle, the end of which is bent in a *Z* shape (Fig. 17.2), is inserted into the disc space, and a control radiograph is obtained taken to confirm the vertebral level and to provide an accurate guide to the actual depth of the disc space between the anterior and posterior margins. Once the correct level has been identified, the needle is removed and the dowel-cutting instrument inserted. The centering pin is pushed into the center of the disc so that when the instrument is oscillated in a semicircle, ellipses of bone of equal dimension cut into the adjacent vertebral bodies on either side of the disc space.

The instrument is withdrawn and the centering pin removed. A safety device of predetermined length is set in the dowel cutter. Meanwhile with a fine probe, the margins of the cut surfaces of the vertebral bodies are checked to ensure that the path of the dowel cavity to be cut between the vertebral bodies is correct.

The dowel-cutting instrument is reinserted and oscillated until the instrument reaches the desired depth (Figs. 17.2 and 17.3). As the cutter is oscillated in semicircular motions, the surgeon is aware of a grinding sensation transmitted through the Hudson brace. When the cutter has reached the desired depth, this sensation changes to one of smooth gliding. The cutter is removed and the specially designed gouge slotted carefully first into one vertebral body. The ellipse of bone is levered out, and the device is slotted into the other vertebral body and the second ellipse levered out. The cylinder of tissue consisting of adjacent vertebral body margins and intervening disc tissue is lifted out directly with a pituitary rongeur of appropriate size.

Where the disc space is narrow, owing to advanced disc resorption, the vertebral end plates are very close together, and it is usually necessary to remove remnants of disc tissue and end-plate cartilages before the gouge can be used to lever out the ellipses of bone. In operations on some elderly patients, brisk venous hemorrhage may occur from the vertebral bodies during preparation of the dowel cavity. The bone plugs should be removed quickly and the hemorrhage readily controlled by means of applying bone wax to the cut surface of the vertebral body.

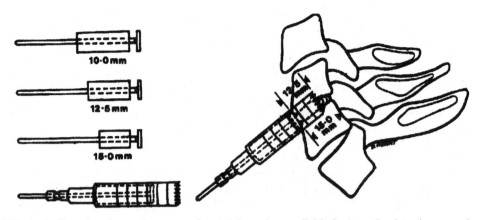

FIG. 17.3. Drawing shows the range of metal dummies available for insertion into the zero-size cutter to allow preparation of dowel cavities of predetermined depth depending on the depth of the disc space in individual patients. The depth of the space is checked with a control radiograph with the use of the bent needle as in Fig. 17.2. *Bottom,* dummy assembled inside the cutter. Drawing of the cutter in use (*right*) shows the mechanism of safety protection provided by the 12-mm dummy, which is inserted after removal of the starter centerpiece. The surgeon can count the rings on the outer side of the cutter to doublecheck safety. (From Crock, HV. *A short practice of spinal surgery.* New York: Springer-Verlag, 1993, with permission.)

REMOVAL OF DISC REMNANTS

Attention is focused on removal of disc remnants from the base and sides of the dowel cavity. This is done with fine, straight, and angled curettes in rotatory motions so that the remnants of vertebral end-plate cartilage can be separated from the vertebral end plates themselves. In the process the remaining disc remnants are removed with fine, straight pituitary rongeurs. Care must be taken not to penetrate the posterior longitudinal ligament or to damage the vertebral arteries on either side of the disc space as the disc remnants are curetted away.

When it is necessary to remove posterior osteophytes or ossific masses in the posterior longitudinal ligament, the use of a diamond-tipped, high-speed burr is essential. This instrument must be introduced into the depths of the dowel cavity before it is activated to avoid damage to the soft-tissue structures of the neck. Suction and irrigation and good lighting are essential for the safe use of these drills. An operating microscope is not essential, although use of a microscope is desirable if one is available.

The safe removal of any obstructing tissue from the cervical spinal canal demands rigid attention to detail. Fine 1- and 2-mm cup-sized curettes should be available. Straight and curved strong, fine spatula-shaped probes are useful in separating the dural sac from the tissues encroaching on it. Removal of osteophytic bars at one or two levels often is time consuming even if vertebrectomy is performed. Release of self-retaining retractors or removal of handheld retractors at regular intervals during these prolonged procedures is essential so that circulation in the retracted soft tissues can be reestablished intermittently to prevent postoperative complications such as severe dysphagia or recurrent laryngeal nerve palsy.

In some cases it may prove impossible to remove calcified or ossified tissues from the dural surface. If the dural sac has expanded in the course of the dissection and the ossified or calcified fragments are seen to move freely with the dural tissue, attempts to remove these fragments should be abandoned (Fig. 17.1).

At the completion of decompression at one or two levels, an intact bony ledge should be retained in the base of the dowel cavity to prevent posterior migration of the interbody graft when it is inserted. When preparation of the dowel cavity has been completed, a piece of gelatin foam sponge and a patty should be inserted and retractors withdrawn from the wound until the autogenous bone grafts have been harvested from the iliac crest.

GRAFT HARVESTING

An incision is made in the line of the anterior third of the right iliac crest. The musculo-tendinous attachments to the top of the crest should be divided along the top of the crest a few millimeters lateral to its inner margin. The muscles covering the inner table of the iliac crest can be separated from the crest to a depth sufficient to allow insertion of the tubular cutter, which passes from the inner to the outer table of the iliac crest, the grafts being withdrawn with the instrument after it has penetrated the outer cortex of the iliac crest. As the instrument is withdrawn, muscle fibers attached to the outer table of the graft bone are divided close to it with a fine scalpel. The graft is ejected from the tubular cutter. It should be handled with a gauze swab while remnants of soft tissue are removed from the inner and outer surfaces. The shape of the graft can be trimmed to appropriate size until ideally it is of tubular shape with parallel inner and outer surfaces. After removal of the graft plug from the iliac crest, the donor site should be packed with gelatin foam sponge while the graft is being finally prepared for impaction into the dowel cavity in the neck.

GRAFT IMPACTION

Retractors are replaced in the neck to expose the dowel cavities. The neck wound is re-exposed. The depth of each cavity should be measured and checked against the length of the dowel graft. Immediately before impaction of the graft, the neck should be gently elongated. This can usually be done by the anesthetist with fingers under the angles of the jaw and gentle traction exerted on the neck. The graft can be tapped into position. When the graft is almost completely seated, a plain-ended impactor is placed half-way across the graft and half-way across the adjacent vertebral body. Final seating of the graft occurs as the plain-ended impactor is tapped gently into place without any danger of penetrating the spinal canal.

Before wound closure, the operative field should be carefully inspected to make sure that there are no bleeding vessels at the grafted site. Sutures are placed in the platysma muscle, and subcuticular skin sutures are inserted. Wound drainage is not needed unless a large strut graft has been inserted. Routine closure of the wound over the right iliac crest is performed after checking that hemorrhage control at the donor site is satisfactory. If two or three grafts have been removed from the iliac crest, the wound should be drained.

RESULTS

The Crock instruments have been used in Australia for more than 30 years, in Singapore for 20 years, and in the United Kingdom for the past 15 years. There have been no reported cases of spinal cord injury after their use or of graft prolapse necessitating re-operation. Donor site pain has not been a problem when the harvesting method described herein is used. Meralgia paraesthetica has been reported in a few cases, usually in operations on obese patients during which exposure of the inner table of the iliac crest has been difficult. Nonunion of the grafts has been rare (Fig. 17.4).

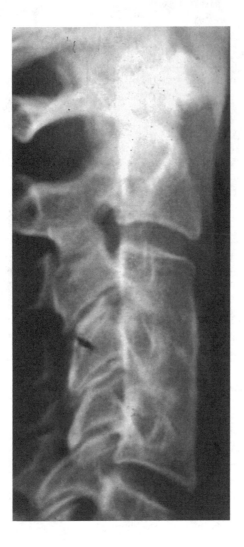

FIG. 17.4. Lateral radiograph of the cervical spine obtained 10 years after C3-4, C4-5 interbody fusion with autogenous dowel grafts.

POSTOPERATIVE CARE

A soft cervical collar is fitted in the operating theater. A firmer plastic collar is used once the patient is fully mobile. In special cases in which multiple dowel grafts or strut grafts have been inserted, halo-thoracic support may be needed. The hospital stay averages 5 to 6 days. Use of some form of neck support is recommended when traveling for 3 months after the operation.

REFERENCES

1. Casamitjana JA, Guerra E, Martinez I, et al. Complications of anterior instrumented arthrodesis of the cervical spine. *Eur Spine J* 1999;8:55(abstract).
2. Cloward RB. The anterior approach for ruptured cervical disc. *J Neurosurg* 1958;15:602–617.
3. Crock HV. *A short practice of spinal surgery.* New York: Springer-Verlag, 1993:238,246.
4. Robinson RA, Smith GW. Anterolateral cervical disc removal and interbody fusion for cervical disc syndrome. *Bull Johns Hopkins Hospital* 1955;96:223–224.

The Degenerative Cervical Spine,
edited by Marek Szpalski and Robert Gunzburg
Lippincott Williams & Wilkins, Philadelphia © 2001.

18

Laminoplasty of the Cervical Spine

Dan M. Spengler

*Department of Orthopaedics and Rehabilitation, Vanderbilt University Medical Center,
Nashville, Tennessee 37232*

INDICATIONS AND CONTRAINDICATIONS
TECHNIQUES
RESULTS
CASE EXAMPLE

Patients who with symptoms and signs of cervical myeloradiculopathy present a challenge to the surgeon. Because cervical myelopathy often can be present to an advanced degree without comparable pain, the diagnosis of this condition can be overlooked. Patients often have a history of mild imbalance while walking. Patients also may have weakness of the arms, legs, or both. Some patients may have more lower extremity weakness than upper extremity symptoms. Because many of these elderly patients also have evidence of lumbar stenosis, the lumbar spinal disorder may be managed initially and the cervical myelopathy overlooked. Patients with cervical myelopathy also may relate a history of clumsiness associated with the use of the upper extremities (1–5). These patients typically have difficulty buttoning their shirts or blouses. Patients also may report bilateral palmar paresthesia. This paresthesia often is misinterpreted as carpal tunnel syndrome.

The key point of this discussion is to emphasize that many patients, if not most, do not report pain relevant to the upper extremities or neck. The differential diagnosis of cervical myeloradiculopathy includes central disc herniation, tumor, multiple sclerosis, anterolateral sclerosis, subacute combined degeneration, and syrinx (5).

The evaluation of patients with cervical myelopathy can be quantified with the Japanese Orthopaedic Association/Revised Version 2 scoring system (see Appendixes 1 and 2). Once a patient has been interviewed and examined, appropriate confirmatory imaging studies are needed to confirm the presence of cervical compression consistent with myelopathy. High-resolution magnetic resonance imaging or computed tomographic (CT) myelography can be used to confirm the diagnosis. I use the CT myelography with 3-mm sections to clearly define the pathologic anatomic features. After the diagnosis is established and surgical treatment is chosen, several options can be considered. Patients with myelopathy can be treated with laminoplasty, laminectomy, laminectomy with fusion, or anterior corpectomy and fusion. This chapter focuses on cervical laminoplasty. The other options for surgical management are discussed in Chapters 17 through 29.

INDICATIONS AND CONTRAINDICATIONS

The classic indication for cervical laminoplasty is the presence of spinal cord compression associated with cervical myelopathy at three or more levels (1,2,4). In Asia, most patients considered for cervical laminoplasty have ossification of the posterior longitudinal ligament (OPLL) (5). Although this condition occurs in the United States, U.S. patients are more likely to have multilevel cervical stenosis or multilevel degenerative disc disease (3,5). For patients with one or two levels of cervical stenosis, anterior cervical decompression and fusion may represent a more appropriate procedure.

The main contraindication to cervical laminoplasty is the presence of considerable cervical kyphosis (1,2). Posterior decompression would be unlikely to afford much decompression of the cervical cord when kyphotic deformity is present. Patients with multilevel cervical compression and cervical kyphosis should undergo anterior decompression and fusion.

Age has also been mentioned as a relative contraindication to cervical laminoplasty (2). An elderly patient who is not in the best of health who has limited outcome expectations represents the type of patients to consider laminectomy. If laminectomy is performed at multiple levels, associated fusion may be warranted to minimize the development of subsequent cervical kyphosis.

TECHNIQUES

Although many types of cervical laminoplasty have been described, three main techniques predominate. These include Z-shaped laminoplasty, unilateral enlargement laminoplasty, and midline enlargement laminoplasty (Figs. 18.1, 18.2, 18.3). The experience at Vanderbilt has been exclusively with the unilateral enlargement technique of Hirabayashi (Figs. 18.3, 18.4). In this unilateral enlargement technique, a hinge is made

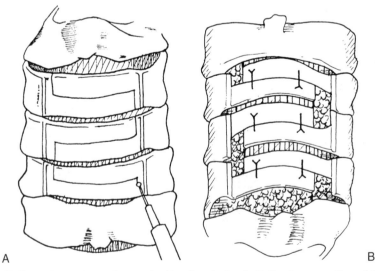

A   B

FIG. 18.1. Z-shaped osteotomy for cervical laminoplasty. **A:** Following resection of the cervical spinous processes, a small burr (3mm) is used to create the Z cuts in the cervical laminae. **B:** After Z cuts and expansion, sutures are used in each lamina to maintain expansion. (From Kawai S. Indications and techniques for cervical laminoplasty. In: Birdwell K, DeWald R, eds. *The textbook of spinal surgery,* 2nd ed. Philadelphia, Lippincott Williams & Wilkins, 1997:1421–1426, with permission.)

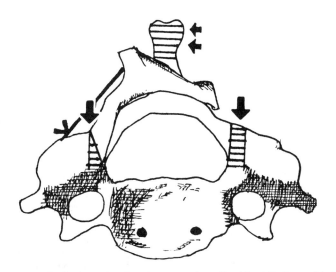

FIG. 18.2. Unilateral enlargement laminoplasty as described by Hirabayashi. (From Kawai S. Indications and techniques for cervical laminoplasty. In: Birdwell K, DeWald R, eds. *The textbook of spinal surgery,* 2nd ed. Philadelphia, Lippincott Williams & Wilkins, 1997:1421–1426, with permission.)

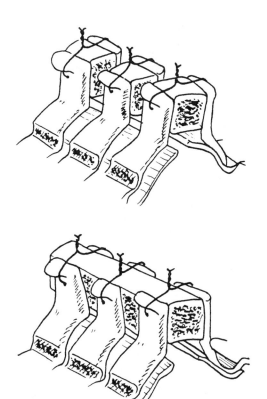

FIG. 18.3. Midline enlargement laminoplasty as originally described by Kurokawa. (From Kawai S. Indications and techniques for cervical laminoplasty. In: Birdwell K, DeWald R, eds. *The textbook of spinal surgery,* 2nd ed. Philadelphia, Lippincott Williams & Wilkins, 1997:1421–1426, with permission.)

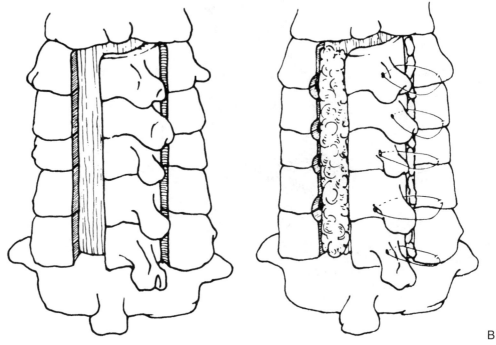

A   B

FIG. 18.4. The hinge and trough for the unilateral enlargement laminoplasty described by K. Hirabayashi. **A:** Open trough following unilateral enlargement laminoplasty (*left*). Hinge can be seen on right. **B:** Enlargement is maintained by suturing spinous processes to lateral masses. Mitek bone anchors work quite well. (From Watkins, *Posterior cervical spine surgery.* Philadelphia: Lippincott Williams & Wilkins 1981, with permission.)

at the junction of the facets with the lamina on the less symptomatic side. A similar trough is made on the open side but taken through both cortices with division of the ligamentum flavum. At this critical juncture, gentle pressure is placed on the cervical spinous process to encourage opening of the laminoplasty. This portion of the procedure should not be rushed, because rapid opening of the laminoplasty can cause a catastrophic neurodeficit. Once the opening is made, the separation nearly always remains greater than 1 cm. At this point, the opening of the laminoplasty is ensured by placing Mitek bone anchoring sutures in the lateral masses and tethering the spinous processes to maintain the opening. Regional bone or allograft can be used to encourage fusion in the region of the hinged trough. Postoperatively the patient wears a cervical collar.

RESULTS

Results of the open hinge laminoplasty of Hirabayashi have been reported by Lee et al. (4). Twenty-one of 24 patients (84%) had gait improvement. Hand tingling was alleviated for 87% of the patients, and bladder function improved for 77%. The 4 patients who had cervical radiculopathy in addition to myelopathy experienced resolution of the radicular symptoms. These results are graphically depicted in Fig. 18.5. Cervical laminoplasty does have complications. Although a precise incidence has not been reported, marked neurologic deterioration to the point of quadriparesis can occur. If the laminoplasty trough is placed too medially or laterally, facet fractures or lamina displacement can oc-

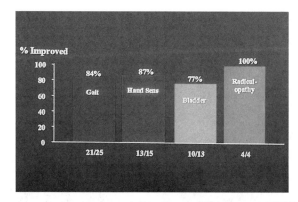

FIG. 18.5. Results of cervical laminoplasty. (From Lee TT, Orias JM, Andrews HL, et al. Progressive postraumatic myelomalacic myelopathy: treatment with untethering and expansive laminoplasty. *J Neurosurg* 1997;86:624–628, with permission.)

cur and cause root entrapment and radiculopathy. Traction injuries can occur in the C5-6 nerve root distribution. Traction injuries also have been reported among patients who undergo operations with an anterior approach. Restriction of range of motion of the cervical spine has occurred after cervical laminoplasty.

CASE EXAMPLE

A 68-year-old man came to the spine center with long-standing progressive cervical myelopathy. The main symptoms were gait imbalance, dysesthesia in the palms, and clumsiness of function of the upper extremities. Imaging studies (Figs. 18.6 through 18.8) depicted multilevel cervical compression due to OPLL and cervical stenosis. The patient had no evidence of cervical kyphosis. Because of the multilevel nature of the

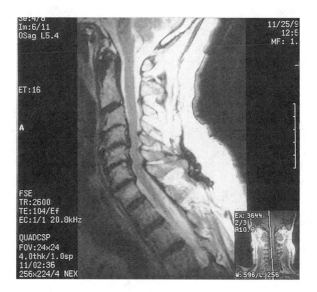

FIG. 18.6. Sagittal magnetic resonance image shows multilevel cervical stenosis.

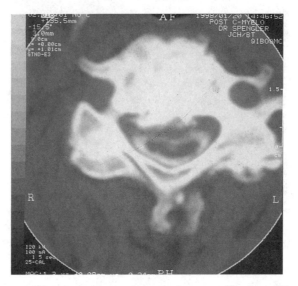

FIG. 18.7. Axial computed tomographic myelogram shows ossification of the posterior longitudinal ligament with central canal encroachment.

problem, cervical laminoplasty was offered and accepted. Figs. 18.9 through 18.11 are postoperative images that show marked improvement in the volume of spinal canal available for the cervical canal. The clinical outcome was good. The patient noticed marked improvement in gait and a decrease in dysesthesia in the palms. He continued to have mild dysfunction of dexterity.

In summary, cervical laminoplasty is a valuable procedure for patients with multilevel myeloradiculopathy from spinal cord compression who do not have cervical kyphosis.

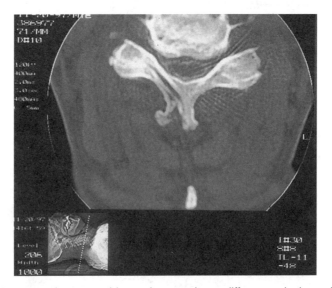

FIG. 18.8. Axial computed tomographic myelogram shows diffuse cervical canal stenosis without ossification of the posterior longitudinal ligament.

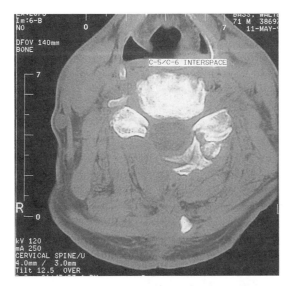

FIG. 18.9. Axial computed tomographic scan obtained after unilateral enlargement laminoplasty shows a marked increase in the volume available for the cervical cord.

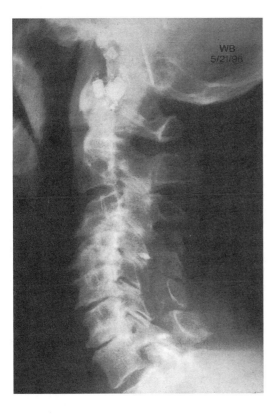

FIG. 18.10. Sagittal radiograph of the cervical spine obtained after cervical laminoplasty shows evidence of posterior enlargement. Mitek sutures are visible within the lateral masses.

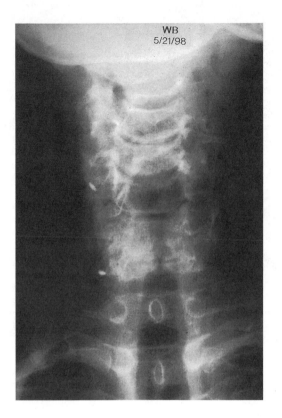

FIG. 18.11. Anteroposterior radiograph of the cervical spine obtained after unilateral enlargement laminoplasty. The spine is well aligned. The Mitek sutures are visible in the lateral masses. These sutures hold the laminoplasty open during healing.

Prospective studies with more patients would be quite helpful for critical evaluation of the various treatment options.

REFERENCES

1. Daftari T, Herkowitz H. Open door laminoplasty in posterior cervical spine surgery. In: Dillin W, Simeone F. *Posterior Cervical Spine Surgery*. Philadelphia: Lippincott-Raven, 1998;161–170.
2. Kawai S. Indications and techniques for cervical laminoplasty. In: Birdwell K, DeWald R, eds. *The Textbook of Spinal Surgery,* 2nd ed. Philadelphia: Lippincott-Raven, 1997;1421–1426.
3. Lee TT, Green B, Gromelski E. Safety and stability of open-door cervical expansive laminoplasty. J Spinal Disord 1998;11:12–15.
4. Lee TT, Orias JM, Andrews HL, et al. Progressive postraumatic myelomalacic myelopathy: treatment with untethering and expansive laminoplasty. *J Neurosurg* 1997;86:624–628.
5. Yonenobu K, Sakou T, Ono K. *OPPL*. Tokyo: Springer-Verlag, 1997.

The Degenerative Cervical Spine,
edited by Marek Szpalski and Robert Gunzburg
Lippincott Williams & Wilkins, Philadelphia © 2001.

19

A Comparison of Cervical Percutaneous Laser Disc Decompression with Holmium:YAG and KTP532 Wavelengths: Prospective Research in Progress

Martin T.N. Knight, Anukul Kumar Deb Goswami, Janos Patko

The Spinal Foundation, The Arbury Centre, Rochdale 0L11 4LZ, United Kingdom

---

BACKGROUND
METHODS
  Inclusion Criteria • Exclusion Criteria • Protocol • Operative Procedure • Data Collection
RESULTS
  History of Onset • Paresis • Neck Pain • Sensory Deficits • Radicular Pain • Headache • Complications • Postoperative Course • Postoperative Drug Consumption
DISCUSSION

BACKGROUND

Choy et al. (3–7) found that 1,000 J of neodymium:yttrium-aluminum-garnet (Nd:YAG) energy inserted in to the center of a lumbar disc reduces the internal pressure by 50% or more. From this finding, they extrapolated that phenomenon could effect decompression of lumbar compressive radiculopathy (1,2). However, 1,064-nm Nd:YAG laser is not well absorbed by disc material, and internal scatter may penetrate 5 to 10 mm. Well known for its ability to coagulate and vaporize tissue through flexible fibers, potassium titanyl potassium:YAG (KTP532 frequency-doubled 1,064 neodymium) is somewhat better absorbed by disc tissue and well absorbed by vascular tissues containing ferritin. Penetration in disc material is estimated to be 3 to 4.5 mm. The specific uptake in vascular tissues would be expected to result in absorption of energy in areas of anular neovascularization and in coagulation of these newly formed vessels. These areas also are concurrently found to be sites of neoneuralization (10), and laser application may effect concomitant denaturation of the anular neoneuralization and amelioration of pain. The 2,100-nm holmium:YAG wavelength energy is better absorbed by water and produces more discrete disc tissue ablation, with tissue penetration limited to 0.2 to 0.5 mm, and less tissue heating at equivalent distances from the probe (17–21) than Nd:YAG or KTP532 laser energy (11).

Efficacious clinical outcomes with all wavelengths have been reported after lumbar laser disc decompression. The greater depth of penetration and the forward-firing configuration of the Nd:YAG system caused us concern. The Holmium:YAG and KTP532 systems had side-firing probes with directional guides, and the wavelengths were more discretely absorbed and directed away from end plates and bone marrow. Accordingly, our study was confined to these two wavelengths. The energy penetration differential preserved by using the Nd:YAG and KTP532 wavelengths raised the possibility of defining whether the mechanism of action of laser disc decompression arose from a central intradiscal mass ablation effect or from the effect of heating the posterior wall of the anulus.

Hellinger (16) in 1990 started effecting cervical laser disc decompression with the Nd:YAG laser. He claimed satisfactory outcome in the management of monosegmental noncompressive radiculopathy. We began using KTP532 cervical laser disc decompression in 1991 in the care of patients with broad-based soft disc protrusions in noncompressive radiculopathy. The therapy was successful, and in 1991 we extended the indications for the technique to include patients with multilevel compressive and noncompressive radiculopathy with symptoms that persisted despite extensive conservative therapy for more than 3 months. We began holmium cervical laser disc decompression in 1992. The randomized clinical trial began in 1992.

METHODS

Inclusion Criteria

Patients with broad-based soft disc protrusions with neck pain and compressive or noncompressive radiculopathy of at least 6 months' duration were included in the study. Patients with leaking discs or zones of high intensity at the index level also were included.

Exclusion Criteria

Patients with extruded or sequestrated disc protrusion, tumor, pregnancy, dorsal vertebral or foraminal osteophytosis and retrolisthesis or olisthesis of 3 mm or more, previous surgery at the same level, cord compression, or fracture were excluded.

Protocol

Patients filled in a questionnaire consisting of the Vernon-Mior functionality scale, visual analog pain scale, pain manikin, and the Zung index and Dram score. Patients with signs of myelopathy or compressive radiculopathy underwent electromyography. All patients underwent radiography with images obtained in the frontal plane and in the lateral plane in full flexion and extension. Those fulfilling the entrance criteria underwent magnetic resonance imaging and were entered in to a physiotherapy gateway for 3 months during which self-help kinetic muscle balance physiotherapy was performed. Patients not responding to this therapy were prescribed laser disc decompression and randomly allocated to a wavelength by means of a randomizing computer program related blindly to their hospital number.

Operative Procedure

At the outset of the procedure 1.5 g of Cefuroxime was administered intravenously. No intravenous steroids were administered. The patient was placed on an arched table with his or her neck extended and a transverse pillow placed under the shoulder blades with the occiput in the well of the arched, radiolucent table. No skull traction was necessary. Two assistants provided traction on the arms to display C5 and below for patients with a short neck or marked settling.

Neuroleptic (aware state) analgesia was provided with a 0.03 mg/kg bolus of midazolam (Hypnoval) at the beginning of the operation, 2 to 5 µg/kg fentanyl, and 30 to 70 µg/kg droperidol. Patient feedback is essential in these operations, in which the presence of anular leakage often is unexpected and causes intense irritation of the adjacent neural structures. Draping was the same as for thyroid surgery. The skin and subcutaneous tissue were infiltrated with local anesthetic—0.75 to 1.5 mg/kg 0.25% lidocaine (Xylocaine) with 1:200,000 epinephrine.

A lead strip was laid on the neck to identify the vertebral levels and to ascertain direct alignment of the approach in the lateral projection. The skin corresponding to the disc space was marked along the lower border of the strip after radiographic localization of the index disc space to be studied. The area between the carotid sheath and the esophagotracheal complex was palpated. The needle entry point over this area and in line with the lateral projection defined by the metal marker was infiltrated with local anesthetic and incised with a 2-mm incision.

The disc was approached on the side of the more severe symptoms. The cannula used had a diameter of 1.6 mm and had a separate long needle linked to the local anesthetic container with a flexible plastic extension tube. The local anesthetic was injected as the needle and cannula were advanced under radiographic control in two planes. The local anesthetic was massaged in to the tissues until the anterior border of the disc and vertebra was clearly felt. The anterior surface of the cervical spine was palpated, the trachea and esophagus were displaced medially, and the common carotid artery and sternocleidomastoid muscle were displaced laterally. After contact was made with the vertebra or the disc, the deep tissues and the longissimus cervicis muscles were probed to determine the distribution of the evoked pain and thereafter infiltrated with local anesthetic.

The correct point of entry was established when the tip of the cannula rested on the anterior surface of the disc in the lateral projection. In the anteroposterior projection the tip of the needle was made to lie medially to a line drawn between the lateral borders of the vertebrae at their narrowest points. This position ensured that the needle did not pass along the lateral margin of the disc in patients with vertebrae and discs that tapered dorsally. The needle was advanced through the anulus until it reached the dorsal third of the disc diameter and pointed toward the middle of the disc in the anteroposterior projection.

Discography was performed to establish the geographic features of the degeneration as it was distributed throughout the disc (Fig. 19.1). The presence, position, and dispersal of leaks was documented, as were the distribution, severity of evoked pain, and whether these symptoms reproduced the initial symptoms. The needle was clipped and used as a guidewire. A trephine was passed along the guidewire within the cannula and used to open the anulus under radiographic control. The laser probe was checked for beam focus and replaced the trephine and guidewire. The direction of the side-firing laser beam was constantly controlled with a lug on the handpiece away from the end plate and bone marrow. Digital photodocumentation of the needle and probe position was obtained at each stage of the procedure.

The energy was applied with either a Laserscope Surgical Laser System KTP532 generator and a side-firing Laserscope Disckit with continuous suction or a Trimedyne Omnipulse 1210 holmium laser generator and a 30-cm side-firing Omni-tip CE0197 probe with continuous suction. The KTP532 setting was 12 W and 0.2-second duration with a

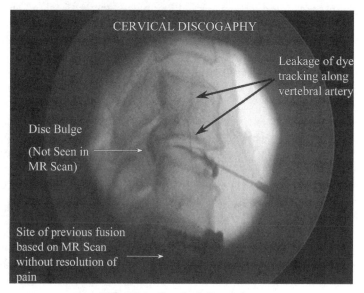

FIG. 19.1. Cervical discogram.

0.5-second interval, which corresponds to 2.4 J per pulse. The holmium:YAG setting was 12 W, 12 pulses per second with a maximum duration of 6 seconds before a pause. This corresponds to 0.5 J per pulse. Whenever pain occurred, application of laser energy was halted until discomfort ceased. After 600 to 800 J was reached, the procedure was completed and the disc was washed with 10 mL saline solution. Eighty milligrams depomedrone was instilled into the disc space at the end of each procedure.

When a leak was found, 2 mL of blood was sampled under sterile conditions after routine laser application was completed. The blood was injected into the disc in 1-mL aliquots and polymerized with 50 J of energy totaling an additional 100 J when polymerization with the fibrin sealant effect (9) and posterior wall annealing were sought (12–15).

Some patients had diffuse pain radiating to the neck, interscapular region, or shoulder region. This pain subsided a few moments after application laser energy was halted. After the procedure the patient was encouraged to perform self-help kinetic muscle balance physiotherapy rather than maintain malposture and muscle atrophy by wearing a collar. Physiotherapy supervision began within 5 days of surgery. Patients who could tolerate them were offered nonsteroidal anti-inflammatory drugs (NSAIDs) to avoid flares of symptoms which usually occurred approximately 5 days after the surgery.

Data Collection

All patients completed a questionnaire containing the Vernon-Mior scale and a visual analog pain (VAP) scale substratified for neck pain, shoulder and arm pain, a pain manikin, and Zung and Dram psychologic profiles. Patients completed the same questionnaire containing an additional satisfaction score 6 weeks and 3 months after the operation and once a year thereafter. When the patient was no being treated, the questionnaire was completed by mail. When there was a divergence in results between serial questionnaires, the patient was contacted by telephone and in the event of deterioration recalled for examination on clinical grounds. Data were entered in to an access database and analyzed with the Cognos software suite linked to the statistical SPSS package. This allowed comparison of preoperative scores with postoperative scores as an index and statistical analysis. Because this research is ongoing, the statistical results are omitted.

Percentage Change in Vernon-Mior Score: The Vernon-Mior Index

Vernon-Mior disability scores were substratified for neck, shoulder, and arm pain. The outcome was measured by means of observing the percentage change in Vernon-Mior score—the Vernon-Mior index (VMI) (22)—as shown in the following the formula:

$$\Delta DI = \frac{\text{Preoperative DI} - \text{Postoperative DI}}{\text{Preoperative DI}} \times 100$$

A VMI of 100% was deemed an excellent result, 50% deemed good, and 20% deemed improved. A VMI less than 20% was deemed poor, and negative values were deemed a worse result.

Percentage Change in Visual Analog Pain Scores

Preoperative and follow-up VAP levels (VAP index) were measured with a VAP scale with the following guidelines to patients: pain level 10, excruciating pain unbearable for any time; 9, horrible pain bearable for only a short time; 6, distressing pain bearable for some time; 3, mild pain; 0, no pain. These results were presented as the VAP index, calculated as follows:

$$\text{VAP Index} = \frac{\text{Preoperative score} - \text{Postoperative score}}{10} \times 100$$

These results were substratified for neck, shoulder, and limb pain.

Patient Satisfaction

Patient satisfaction was determined with a satisfaction rating questionnaire. Patients decided whether they were delighted, satisfied, did not get any benefit, or were not happy. Those delighted or satisfied were considered satisfied with the results.

RESULTS

Between January 1992 and January 1999, 122 patients underwent discography at 275 cervical levels. Percutaneous laser disc decompression was performed at 108 levels on 105 patients. All patients were contacted for evaluation since July 1999 for postoperative follow-up information. Of the 105 patients, 6 could not be contacted, and 2 patients had died. Sixty-four questionnaires were returned by patients and the data verified and entered into the database. Cohort integrity was only 61% when this report was written.

The follow-up period ranged from 6 months to a maximum of 7 years. The average follow-up period was 37 months. The patients were 36 men and 69 women ranging in age from 19 to 76 years with a mean of 41 years. Six patients had abnormalities (identifiable painful site reproducing all symptoms during probing and discography) at C2-4, 15 at

C4-5, 47 at C5-6, 23 at C6-7 and 6 at C7-T1. Three patients needed intervention at two levels. Fifty-four patients underwent holmium:YAG laser disc decompression, and 51 underwent KTP532 laser disc decompression. Forty-one patients (39%) underwent posterior wall supplementation with polymerized blood. The results of percutaneous laser disc decompression are given in Tables 19.1 through 19.4.

TABLE 19.1. *Results of PLDD with holmium-YAG laser*

Vernon and Mior index	Good to excellent ≥50	Fair, good, excellent ≥20	Fair 20–49	Poor 0–19	Worse <0
Neck	48	73	25	8	19
Shoulder	43	75	32	7	18
Arm	52	73	21	10	17

Values are percentages.
PLDD, percutaneous laser disc decompression; YAG, yttrium-aluminum-garnet.

TABLE 19.2. *Results of PLDD with KTP*

Vernon and Mior index	Good to excellent ≥50	Fair, good, excellent ≥20	Fair 20–49	Poor 0–19	Worse <0
Neck	53	73	20	17	10
Shoulder	33	70	37	20	10
Arm	53	82	29	6	12

Values are percentages.
PLDD, percutaneous laser disc decompression; KTP, potassium titanyl phosphate.

TABLE 19.3. *Results of PLDD with posterior wall reconstruction*

Vernon and Mior index	Good to excellent ≥50	Fair, good, excellent ≥20	Fair 20–49	Poor 0–19	Worse <0
Neck	55	75	20	15	10
Shoulder	41	70	29	17	13
Arm	55	72	17	17	11

Values are percentages.
PLDD, percutaneous laser disc decompression.

TABLE 19.4. *Results of PLDD without posterior wall reconstruction*

Vernon and Mior index	Good to excellent ≥50	Fair, good, excellent ≥20	Fair 20–49	Poor 0–19	Worse <0
Neck	53	74	31	13	13
Shoulder	40	79	39	10	11
Arm	51	78	27	11	11

Values are percentages.
PLDD, percutaneous laser disc decompression.

History of Onset

The mean duration of symptoms before referral was 3.4 years. The onset was spontaneous in 58% of cases, caused by a fall in 16%, caused by a road traffic accident in 13%, was sport related in 9%, and was vocational in 3% of cases.

Paresis

Thirty-three patients (31%) had paresis preoperatively, and this number decreased to 7 patients (6%) after the percutaneous laser disc decompression. In 2 of these patients the weakness was alleviated but not fully resolved. One of the 7 patients had considerable pain 5 days after surgery without signs of infection. Excessive ingestion of a NSAID had caused a thrush infection of the throat, which was found with gastrointestinal endoscopy. Preoperative paresis had been alleviated but recurred 5 days after the operation and progressed to become transiently partial quadriparesis with edema of the cord from the pons to T2. These symptoms resolved almost completely. This complication occurred despite the use of the less penetrating holmium:YAG wavelength and a total of 700 J with no intraoperative leakage.

Neck Pain

One hundred two patients reported persistent cervical pain before the procedure that was unresponsive to conservative treatment. During the follow-up period, 18 patients reported residual pain but for 11 of these, the symptoms were more than 50% alleviated.

Sensory Deficit

Fifty-seven of the patients (54%) had a sensory deficit before the operation. After the operation, 2 patients had residual deficit, and 9 (8%) described the symptoms a heaviness or leadenness of limb without sensory deficit.

Radicular Pain

Radicular pain was intrusive for more than 49 of the patients (46%) before the operation. During the follow-up period, 9 patients (8%) continued to have radicular symptoms, but for 4 the symptoms were more than 50% alleviated.

Headache

Headaches were reported by 67 patients (63%) before surgery. During the follow-up period, headaches had resolved for all but 21 patients. Among the the others the headache was ameliorated in 10.

Complications

No patient had postoperative infection, hematoma, or hoarseness. Two patients reported transient postoperative swallowing discomfort. One patient with marked preoperative settling needed autofusion.

Postoperative Course

Eighty-five percent of patients had improvement within the first 5 postoperative days. Thirty-seven (35%) had a transient recurrence of symptoms that lasted about 3 weeks. The resolution was such that 80% of patients reported clinical improvement at the 6-week review point. At 3 months, 75% of patients reported sustained clinical improvement.

Postoperative Drug Consumption

All of the patients used pain medication (analgesia or an NSAID) regularly before the operation. Four patients needed morphine sulfate before surgery. At follow-up evaluation, 18 needed medication on an occasional basis, and none needed morphine sulfate.

DISCUSSION

The cohort integrity of this study has reached only 61%, so this represents an outcome study still in progress. However the numbers of patients in both the holmium:YAG and KTP532 groups equate, and some guarded conclusions can be drawn. We differentiated between clinical improvement taken as 20% improvement in the VMI and meaningful clinical improvement taken as a 50% improvement in the VMI. Our results indicate that whichever wavelength was used, 50% of patients achieved clinically sustained significant improvement an average of 37 months after surgery. The results were evident early in the postoperative period. More than 75% reported clinical functional improvement. However, over the ensuing years approximately 10% of good or excellent results deteriorated to mere improvement. The total number of patients who benefited from the procedure remained approximately 75% throughout the period.

The sustained nature of the response rules out a placebo response, because a placebo response usually is short lived (8). Patients with a leaking disk appeared to have no benefit conferred by the use of a blood patch, but the number in this subgroup was small.

The finding that both wavelengths achieved comparable outcomes caused us to question the concept that the benefit is conferred primarily by reduction of intradiscal pressure. That two wavelengths with widely different tissue ablative and tissue penetrative effects achieve closely allied results suggests that efficacy is related to tissue heating, collagen annealing (12–15), coagulation of neovascularization and neoneuralization, and an effect on the release of painful irritants from within the disc that produce secondary external irritation in the epidural space and foramen.

Laser disc decompression is proving to be a valuable technique for obviating conventional open surgery in the care of 96% of patients with soft, broad-based disc protrusion. Selection has to be constrained. We recommend that this intervention be restricted to patients without serious stenosis of the lateral recess, retrolisthesis or olisthesis of 3 mm or more, marked dorsal or foraminal osteophytosis, extrusion, or sequestration. For patients with these features, endoscopic amplification of the technique may allow these pathologic limitations to be overcome and managed with minimally invasive surgery. Laser disc decompression offers a valuable minimally invasive technique for operations on elderly and infirm patients. It causes minimal trauma and allows the patient to avoid general anesthesia.

The one case of transient quadriparesis represents an inadequately explained complication despite careful application of the laser, and this event remains a source of concern. The use of side-firing suction probes has rendered this technique a simple atraumatic technique in which the laser energy can be directed discretely and precisely to the discal pain source and limits unwanted application of the laser to adjacent vertebral bone marrow and end plate. The technique can be use for outpatient or overnight-stay surgery.

Anterior probing has proved valuable in determining the segment causing the pain among patients with elusive noncompressive radiculopathy. In many cases of noncompressive radiculopathy, the causal segment showed a leaking disc, and the symptoms mimicked symptoms normally conceived to be arising at an adjacent level. The symptoms arising from a leak usually manifested periodicity and characteristics of global diffuse limb and interscapular involvement with disproportionate degradation of function and limited magnetic resonance findings.

Cervical laser disc decompression effected sustained and substantial clinical benefit among more than in 50% of patients observed for a mean period of 37 months. An additional 25% had functional benefit. Despite the longevity and cause of symptoms, neck pain, headaches, and radicular pain responded to discrete and targeted application of the laser. Paresis, sensory deficits, neck pain, brachialgia, and headache were alleviated considerably for most patients. Cervical laser disc decompression does not preclude subsequent conventional open surgery. In this study, only 2% of the patients needed additional surgery in the extended review period.

REFERENCES

1. Ascher PW. Status quo and new horizons of laser therapy in neurosurgery. *Lasers Surg Med* 1985;5:499–506.
2. Ascher PW, Holzer P, Sutter B, et al. Nucleus-pulposus-Denaturierung bei Bandscheibenprotrusionen. In: Siebert WE, Wirth CJ, eds. *Laser in der Orthopadie*. Stuttgart: Thieme, 1991:169–172.
3. Choy DSJ. Clinical experience and results with 389 PLDD procedures with Nd:YAG laser, 1986 to 1995. *J Clin Laser Med Surg* 1995;13:209–214.
4. Choy DSJ, Altmann P. Fall of intradiscal pressure with laser ablation. *J Clin Laser Med Surg* 1995;13:149–152.
5. Choy DSJ, Ascher PW, Ranu HS, et al. Percutaneous laser disc decompression: a new therapeutic modality. *Spine* 1992;7:949–956.
6. Choy DSJ, Case RB, Fielding W, et al. Percutaneous laser nucleolysis of lumbar discs. *N Engl J Med* 1987; 317:771–772.
7. Choy DSJ, Michelsen L, Getrajdman G, et al. Percutaneous laser disc decompression: an update. *J Clin Laser Med Surg* 1992;6:177–184.
8. Cleophas TJ. Clinical trials: specific problems associated with the use of a placebo-control group. *J Mol Med* 1995;73:421–424.
9. Dunn CJ, Goa KL. Fibrin sealant: a review of its use in surgery and endoscopy. *Drugs* 1999;58:863–886.
10. Freemont AJ, Peacock TE, Goupville P, et al. Nerve ingrowth into diseased intervertebral disc in chronic back pain. *Lancet* 1997;350:178–181.
11. Gamache FW, Morgello S. Histological effects of CO_2 versus KTP laser or brain and spinal cord: a canine model. *Neurosurgery* 1993;32:100–104.
12. Hayashi K, Markel MD, Thabit G 3rd, et al. The effect of nonablative laser energy on joint capsular properties: an in vitro mechanical study using a rabbit model. *Am J Sports Med* 1995;23:482–487.
13. Hayashi K, Nieckarz JA, Thabit G 3rd, et al. Effect of nonablative laser energy on the joint capsule: an in vivo rabbit study using a holmium:YAG laser. *Lasers Surg Med* 1997;20:164–171.
14. Hayashi K, Thabit G 3rd, Bogdanske JJ, et al. The effect of nonablative laser energy on the ultrastructure of joint capsular collagen. *Arthroscopy* 1996;12:474–481.
15. Hayashi K, Thabit G 3rd, Vailas AC, et al. The effect of nonablative laser energy on joint capsular properties: an in vitro histologic and biochemical study using a rabbit model. *Am J Sports Med* 1996;24:640–646.
16. Hellinger J. Technical aspects of the percutaneous cervical and lumbar laser-disc-decompression and nucleotomy. *Neurol Res* 1999;21(1):99–102.
17. Siebert WE. Nucleus pulposus vaporization experimental investigations on use of lasers on the intervertebral disc. In: Mayer HM, Brock M (eds). *Percutaneous nucleotomy*. Berlin: Springer-Verlag, 1989.
18. Siebert WE. Percutaneous laser disc decompression: the European experience. *Spine* 1993;7:103–133.
19. Siebert WE. Percutaneous laser disc decompression of cervical discs. *J Clin Laser Med Surg* 1995;13:205–209.
20. Siebert W. Percutaneous nucleotomy procedure in lumbar intervertebral disc displacement: Current status. *Orthopade* 1999;28:(7):598–608.
21. Siebert W. Use of lasers in orthopaedics. Proceedings of 3rd World Congress of International Musculoskeletal Research Society (IMLAS) November 7–10, 1996, Kassel. *Orthopade* 1997;26(4):394–398.
22. Vernon H, Mior S. The Northwick Park Neck Pain Questionnaire, devised to measure neck pain and disability. *Br J Rheumatol* 1994;33:1203–1204.

The Degenerative Cervical Spine,
edited by Marek Szpalski and Robert Gunzburg
Lippincott Williams & Wilkins, Philadelphia © 2001.

20

Laminoplasty versus Laminectomy and Fusion for the Management of Cervical Spondylotic Myelopathy: Surgical and Economic Considerations

Eric C. Chamberlin, Edward N. Hanley Jr.

Department of Orthopedic Surgery, Carolinas Medical Center, Charlotte, North Carolina 28203

ETIOLOGY
COURSE OF DISEASE
CLINICAL MANIFESTATIONS
IMAGING
NONOPERATIVE TREATMENT
OPERATIVE TREATMENT
   Indications • Anterior Approaches • Posterior Approaches) • Results
ECONOMIC CONSIDERATIONS
CONCLUSIONS

Cervical spondylotic myelopathy (CSM) is a protean disorder caused by extrinsic compression of the spinal cord with resultant clinical manifestations of myelopathy. Patients with CSM have characteristic symptoms and signs, including altered gait, coordination, strength, and sensation. Pain may or may not be a component of the disorder. Because signs and symptoms may be subtle, the diagnosis of CSM often is missed. However, CSM is a relatively common disorder among the elderly, and the diagnosis should be sought when a patient reports gait or fine motor disturbances.

ETIOLOGY

As the name suggests, CSM is caused by degenerative cervical processes that damage the spinal cord. Theories of the pathogenesis are mechanical and vascular in nature. Spondylosis progresses from disc degeneration to reactive hyperostosis of the uncovertebral joints and facet joints. These changes along with other possible processes, including invagination of the ligamentum flavum, ossification of the posterior longitudinal ligament (PLL), instability, or a congenitally narrow canal conspire to decrease the amount of space available for the spinal cord. Damage to the cord and the resultant clinical manifestations are a reflection of both direct compression and compression-induced neuroischemia (2,5).

Mechanical factors that contribute to CSM include a developmentally narrow canal and dynamic factors such as movement between adjacent cervical segments. Movement between adjacent levels can cause a pincer effect in which the posterior aspect of one vertebral body compresses the cord against the lamina of an adjacent vertebra. This motion decreases the relative space for the spinal cord. The relative space for the cord can be measured as an absolute distance from the posterior edge of the vertebral body to the spinolaminar line of 13 mm or less. In a study involving 63 patients, Edwards and LaRocca (8) found stenosis and myelopathy in patients with less than a 13-mm measurement. The healthy control group had a distance of 17 mm, and the average cord diameter was a relatively constant 10 mm throughout the cervical spine. An alternative is to measure the Pavlov-Torg ratio, which is the width of the vertebral body on a lateral radiograph divided by the distance from the posterior edge of the vertebral body to the spinolaminar line. A normal value is said to be greater than or equal to 0.8 (4,8,27).

Other causes of cervical myelopathy-like symptoms include congenital ossification of the PLL, syringomyelia, Chiari malformations, myopathy, neuropathy, tabes dorsalis, hydrocephalus, rheumatoid disease, tumor, multiple sclerosis, and arteriovenous malformation. These other causes of myelopathy must be ruled out because treatment recommendations are different (4).

COURSE OF DISEASE

The variable nature of CSM predicts the contradicting opinions in the literature. Clarke and Robinson (7) in 1956 believed that most patients exhibited persistent motor deficits without regression but with most patients having several episodes of new signs and symptoms with continuous deterioration. In their study of 120 patients, they found CSM progresses in three general patterns: stepwise degeneration in 75%, relentless progression in 20%, and stable in 5%. Lees and Turner (18) advocated nonoperative treatment because of slow progression of the disease with the existence of long plateaus. Symon and Lavender (25) in 1967 concluded that approximately one third of patients improved or stayed in stable condition whereas the conditions of two thirds of patients deteriorated. In summary, for any given patient, it is impossible to predict which course the disease will take. LaRocca (17) in 1988 concluded that there is not enough information for precise operative indications because the range of outcomes is from gradual and mild progression to rapid and catastrophic.

CLINICAL MANIFESTATIONS

Patients with CSM have characteristic symptoms, including gait disturbance (wide-based and stooped), balance problems (unsteady on feet), loss of manual dexterity, upper extremity greater than lower extremity weakness, numbness and paresthesia, and bowel and bladder dysfunction, which is uncommon. Sensory findings may range from radiculopathy and neck pain to paresthesia. The most characteristic symptom, gait disturbance, is the basis of the Nurick (21) classification of myelopathy:

Grade 0. Root signs and symptoms, no evidence of cord involvement
Grade 1. Signs of cord involvement, normal gait
Grade 2. Mild gait involvement, employable
Grade 3. Gait abnormality limiting employment
Grade 4. Ambulate with assistance only

Grade 5. Chair bound or bedridden

Signs of CSM often may be elicited during a physical examination before the patient realizes there is a problem. Signs include typically lower motor neuron signs at the level of the lesion (cell body, lower-tract involvement) and upper motor neuron signs below the level of the lesion. Lower motor neuron signs include weakness and hyporeflexia. Upper motor neuron signs include spasticity, hyperreflexia, clonus, and Babinski sign, which is a late finding. Subtle signs of upper motor neuron dysfunction are the Hoffman sign, the inverted radial reflex and recruitment. These signs may occur early and bring the condition to the attention of the examiner. The Lhermitte sign is an electric shock sensation down the spine with neck flexion and is another sign of myelopathy (6).

IMAGING

The first imaging test for patients with suspected cervical abnormality is plain radiographs (1). From these views the absolute diameter of the canal and the Pavlov-Torg ratio is calculated. Flexion and extension views are used to assess the stability of the vertebral column and may show the pincer effect. Axial imaging whether computed tomography (CT) or magnetic resonance imaging (MRI) is essential for confirmation of decreased canal diameter and for preoperative planning. Penning et al. (23) showed that myelopathy occurred when there was a 30% decrease in cross-sectional area at CT. MRI has the added advantage of soft-tissue definition, which allows visualization of changes in the cord. Myelomalacia is visible on MR images and may help with the decision to operate. Wade et al. (26) compared MRI with CT myelography and found the only important prognostic factors to be the transverse area of the cord on CT myelograms, the duration of symptoms, and the number of blocks on the myelogram. MRI or CT myelography remains the choice of the investigator. We favor MRI.

NONOPERATIVE TREATMENT

Nonoperative treatment may be helpful in the early period of CSM. CSM often is insidious in presentation and varies considerably in course. Therefore operative indications are for the most part relative. For this reason, early treatment often is nonoperative and suggested for patients with symptoms that are not functionally disabling and for patients who are poor operative candidates regardless of the severity of disease. Immobilization in a cervicothoracic collar may alleviate symptoms for 50% of patients. Other interventions include intermittent bed rest; use of nonsteroidal antiinflammatory drugs (NSAIDs), oral steroids, muscle relaxants, epidural steroids, physical therapy modalities, and cervical traction (4).

OPERATIVE TREATMENT

Indications

Because the course of CSM is not entirely known, the mere presence of myelopathy is not an absolute indication for surgery. The primary indication for operative management of CSM is progressive neurologic deterioration. In general, the best results are obtained by patients with milder disease (Nurick grades 1 through 3) and by patients with short duration of symptoms. Bernard and Whitecloud (3) suggested that patients operated on within 1 year of onset of symptoms and whose condition was Nurick grades 1, 2, or 3, had the greatest success with surgery. That said, the difficulty lies in the unpredictable course of the disease and in determining which patients will benefit from surgery. Because patients do better when operated on early in the course of the disease, diligent observation for the often subtle signs of progression of the disease is the best way to decide on the timing of surgery.

Relatively poor surgical candidates include the very elderly, the very ill, and those with severe neurologic compromise. These patients have a relatively poor chance of recovery, though surgery may be considered to halt progression of disease. The choice of operative procedure depends on the cause of stenosis and the patient's cervical alignment.

Anterior Approaches

In general, anterior approaches are recommended for patients with normal to kyphotic cervical alignment. For patients with kyphotic alignment, laminectomy alone has been shown to destabilize the spine and lead to further kyphosis. Decompressing a kyphotic spine posteriorly leaves the cord compressed anteriorly by the posterior aspect of the vertebral bodies and the discs. Another potential advantage of the anterior approach is that in patients with any instability or subluxation visible on flexion and extension radiographs, fusion is indicated which can be achieved by means of anterior iliac crest or strut grafting.

Anterior decompression and fusion consists of removal of the compressive, degenerative structures followed by fusion of the segments adjacent to the decompression. Preoperative imaging studies depict the sites of compression and from them, the extent and location of the operation is planned from removal of one disc and surrounding osteophytes to removal of several discs, partial vertebrectomy, and strut graft fusion.

The operative procedure consists of careful positioning of the patient's head to avoid hyperflexion or hyperextension. A shoulder roll is placed to extend the neck. A doughnut is used for discectomy and fusion, while corpectomy and strut grafting generally are performed with Gardner-Wells tongs with about 10 lb (4.5 kg) of traction. Most authors suggest somatosensory evoked potential monitoring during the operation.

For one- or two-level surgery, a transverse incision is made that corresponds to the level of the lesion with the hyoid at C3, the thyroid cartilage at C4-5, and the cricoid cartilage corresponding to C6. The carotid artery is retracted laterally while the esophagus and trachea are taken toward the midline. The prevertebral fascia is located beneath the pretracheal fascia. The prevertebral fascia is incised at this point in the midline to expose the anterior longitudinal ligament and the longus colli muscles bilaterally. With the disc and vertebral body thus exposed, discectomy or corpectomy is performed. For discectomy, disc material is removed down to the PLL posteriorly and to the uncovertebral joints laterally. A high-speed burr is used to remove the bony end plates down to bleeding subchondral bone. A tricortical iliac crest graft is formed into a horseshoe shape and placed into the disc space.

Longer lengths of decompression and fusion commonly are obtained through multilevel discectomy and fusion and, more frequently, corpectomy and strut grafting. Corpectomy and strut grafting is accomplished by means of continuing bone removal through the vertebral body to the level of the PLL. If the patient has ossification of the PLL, the PLL is removed to expose the dura. Laterally the corpectomy is continued to the level of the uncovertebral joint. At this point the strut graft, either tricortical iliac crest graft (two levels or fewer) or fibula (three levels or more), is recessed into the vertebral body above and below to prevent graft extrusion. An anterior cervical plate sometimes is placed to allow earlier mobilization and potentially to increase fusion rates. The indications for the use of instrumentation are debated and are evolving (9). The benefit of an anterior approach is that the site of compression is addressed directly. Disc, osteophytes from uncovertebral and facet joints, and in some cases the PLL, can be directly removed (10).

Posterior Approaches

Laminectomy, laminectomy with fusion with or without instrumentation, and laminoplasty are the posterior approaches used for decompression of the cervical spine. Common to all of these approaches is the concept that with removal of or opening of the lamina, the diameter of the spinal canal will be increased, decreasing the potential for stenotic compression of the cord. Direct decompression of the nerve roots by means of foraminotomy is possible in cases of concomitant radiculopathy. The posterior approaches are indicated in operations on patients with lordotic or neutral alignment of the cervical spine with multiple levels of compression and those with congenital stenosis. Laminectomy and laminoplasty usually involve levels C3 through C6 or C7.

Laminectomy

Cervical laminectomy, the historical surgical standard, is performed through a midline posterior incision. Care must be taken in preoperative positioning with the neck in neutral position. In hyperextension, the anteroposterior diameter of the canal is lessened and in hyperflexion, and the cord is under tension. Prone positioning avoids the potential complication of air embolism, which may occur when the patient is in the seated position. Another potential complication is hypoperfusion of the the cord, which is prevented by having the anesthesiologist avoid hypotensive anesthesia. Most authors recommend somatosensory evoked potential monitoring during the operation.

A standard approach to the lamina is performed. Decompression is performed by means of either en bloc removal of the laminae or piecemeal lamina excision with Kerrison rongeurs. For en bloc laminectomy, a 3-mm burr is used to make two troughs in the lamina just lateral to the dura, where the lamina begins to widen into the facet joint. Levels to be included in the decompression include one above and one below the level of compression. As the ligamentum flavum begins to be exposed, the surgeon changes to a 1 mm Kerrison rongeur to cut the remaining lamina and protect the underlying dura, nerve roots, and cord. Once through the most caudal level to be decompressed, a towel clip is applied to the spinous process, and the process is lifted upward. The ligament is then sharply incised and the laminae are lifted and removed en bloc. Meticulous closure is performed with a drain and the patient is placed in a soft collar.

Laminectomy can be followed by posterior fusion with instrumentation to further increase the stability of the cervical spine and restore and maintain lordosis. This approach is gaining popularity, the indications being multilevel involvement, a neutral or lordotic sine, spondylolisthesis, and iatrogenic instability (with previous laminectomy). Fusion is accomplished by means of facet fusion, plate or rod fixation, lateral mass 14- to 16-mm screws, and bone graft.

Complications encountered with laminectomy for CSM include paralysis, perfusion injury and hematoma, C5 root problems, dural injury, air embolism, and most frequently, postlaminectomy kyphosis and neck pain (25%) (11,12,19).

Laminoplasty

Laminoplasty is a procedure developed originally in Japan. It is used to increase the diameter of the cervical spinal canal while maintaining most of the structural integrity, protecting the spinal cord, and preserving motion. Several methods have been described, all of which involve cutting the laminae and hinging them open. Indications for laminoplasty include congenital stenosis, CSM that is multisegmental, and continuous or mixed-type ossification of the PLL. Some authors recommend laminoplasty for radiculopathy or one- or two-level spondylosis associated with congenital stenosis. The only absolute contraindication to laminoplasty is kyphotic cervical alignment.

The expansive open-door laminoplasty described by Hirabayashi et al. (15) is discussed herein. There are several other described techniques, including the original Z-plasty of Hattori, the en bloc laminoplasty of Itoh and Tsuji (31), and French-door laminoplasty. All are basically variations on a theme. Open-door laminoplasty is begun much as laminectomy is, but instead of a complete cut through both sides of the laminae from C3 to C7, only one side is completely cut and the other side is used as a hinge. The open side should ideally correspond to the more symptomatic side. Sutures are placed from the facet capsules into the corresponding laminae or spinous processes to keep the door open. An alternative is to use bone graft from the iliac crest or allograft to prop open and fuse the door.

Disadvantages of laminoplasty include neck stiffness (30% to 70%), pain (50%), and loss of lordosis (25%). Potential complications include those of laminectomy, such as wound problems, C5 palsy (5%), and axial pain as well as risk of door closure (30).

RESULTS

Anterior Approach

The operative results of anterior decompression and fusion are in general very good and are the main reason that anterior techniques may be considered the standard in the management of CSM. Most studies have shown major improvement of symptoms among most patients. Bernard and Whitecloud (3) found in a study of 21 patients treated with anterior decompression and fibular strut grafting that 16 of 21 patients improved by at least one Nurick grade. Of those not improving, beneficial arrest of neurologic deterioration was believed to have been achieved. These authors believe and other authors have suggested (28) that the best results are achieved in operations on patients who have had symptoms for less than 1 year and for those who have Nurick grade 1, 2, or 3 disease. Emery et al. (10) also found the best predictor of recovery to be preoperative severity of myelopathy. In their study of the care of 108 patients, they found 71 of 82 patients had improved gait and 80 of 87 patients had resolution or partial resolution of the neurologic deficit. Okada et al. (22) found at least one Nurick grade improvement among 36 of 37 patients treated with various anterior decompression and fusion techniques.

The most common cause of return of symptoms or deterioration of initially good results after anterior decompression and fusion for CSM is new spondylosis at a level adjacent to the fusion (10,22). The risk of major neurologic complication during anterior decompression and fusion is quite rare. Flynn (13) found the incidence of major neurologic complication in anterior cervical discectomy and fusion to be 0.01% in a questionnaire sent to 1,358 neurosurgeons in 1974. Other common complications of anterior surgery for CSM include hoarseness, graft displacement, hematoma, cerebrospinal fluid leak, esophageal perforation, infection, and donor site morbidity.

Posterior Approaches

In the proper patient population, laminectomy and laminoplasty have very good results. Among patients with stable cervical spines and lordotic alignment, 70% to 80% of patients can expect satisfactory results with laminectomy (18). Hirabayashi et al. (15) found good results among 66% of 40 patients undergoing laminoplasty for CSM as determined by the Japanese Orthopaedic Association scale. In this series there were 29 cases of ossification of the PLL, 11 cases of spondylosis, and 9 combined cases. Satomi et al. (24) in a long-term follow up study of laminoplasty for CSM found the recovery rate, again based on Japanese Orthopaedic Association scores, to be approximately 60%.

Several studies have compared directly the results of laminectomy and laminoplasty and both posterior operations for CSM with anterior decompression and fusion. Hukuda et al. (16), compared French-door laminoplasty with laminectomy in terms of Japanese Orthopaedic Society functional grade. No significant difference was found between the two groups. Both laminoplasty and laminectomy had a 30% incidence of postoperative kyphosis and instability. Mikawa (20) found change in alignment of the cervical spine among 36% of patients undergoing laminectomy for CSM, ossification of the PLL, or tumor. Instability was found among 14% of patients in this study, which spanned 24 years. Herkowitz (14) compared anterior cervical fusion, cervical laminectomy, and cervical laminoplasty and found the success rate (percentage of excellent and good results) to be 92% for anterior cervical fusion, 66% for cervical laminectomy, and 86% for laminoplasty in the management of multiple-level spondylotic radiculopathy. He found laminoplasty to most limit cervical range of motion. Other complications in this series were clinically insignificant pseudarthrosis in 22 of 58 (37%) levels fused in patients undergoing anterior cervical fusion, kyphosis in 3 of 12 patients undergoing laminectomy, and door closure in 2 of 15 undergoing laminoplasty. In a study involving 854 patients, Yonenobu (29) found improvement after surgery among 38% of those undergoing laminectomy alone, 50% of those undergoing laminoplasty, 55% of those undergoing anterior cervical diskectomy and fusion, and 45% of those undergoing anterior cervical fusion.

ECONOMIC CONSIDERATIONS

At our institution, the average length of stay, surgical costs, and length of operation were determined for each of four procedures—laminectomy, laminoplasty, laminectomy with fusion, and anterior corpectomy and fusion. Length of stay is one of the most important figures in terms of hospital costs. Length of stay for this group was 2 days for laminectomy, 2 days for laminoplasty, 3.5 days for laminectomy with fusion, and 4 days for anterior corpectomy and fusion. Hospital charges exclusive of surgeons' fees were similarly distributed. Laminectomy cost an average of $11,000 U.S., laminoplasty $11,500 U.S., laminectomy and fusion $15,300 U.S. Operating room time was 1.8 hours for laminectomy, 3.2 hours for laminoplasty, 3.2 hours for laminectomy and fusion, and 3.2 hours for corpectomy and fusion. Economic concerns suggest that in instances such as multiple-level stenosis of the neutral to lordotic spine, in which posterior or anterior procedures are equally appropriate, posterior approaches including laminoplasty may be favorable.

CONCLUSIONS

Although CSM is a protean disease without a well-defined course or a consensus on operative indications, general conclusions can be made. The surgeon must carefully take

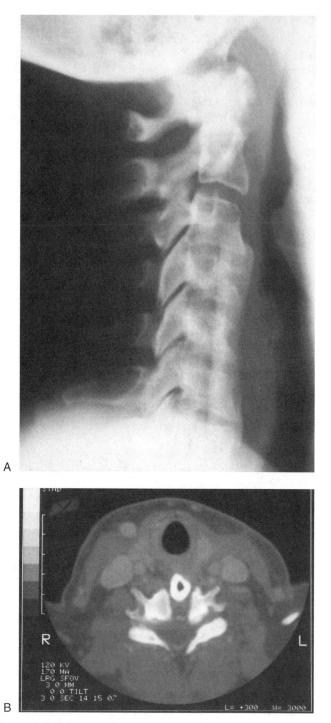

FIG. 20.1. A: Lateral radiograph shows cervical spine after anterior cervical decompression and fibular strut grafting. **B:** Computed tomographic scan shows position of fibular strut graft.

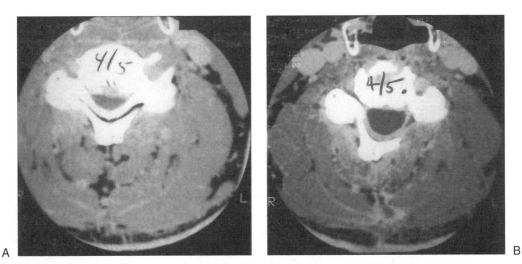

FIG. 20.2. A: Computed tomographic (CT) scan shows spondylosis and stenosis. **B:** CT scan of cervical spine after Hirabayashi open-door laminoplasty.

into account the cause of the particular patient's symptoms and consider the alignment of the cervical spine to choose the correct operative technique. With good preoperative planning and meticulous technique, complications can be minimized and improvement expected by most patients. Laminectomy is used least often, laminoplasty to treat selected patients, and an anterior operation for most patients. Laminectomy with instrumented fusion appears to be gaining popularity (Figs. 20.1, 20.2).

REFERENCES

1. Alker G. Neuroradiology of cervical spondylotic myelopathy. *Spine* 1988;13:850.
2. Benner BG. Etiology, pathogenesis, and natural history of discogenic neck pain, radiculopathy and myelopathy. In: *The cervical spine.* Philadelphia: Lippincott-Raven, 1998:735–740.
3. Bernard TN, Whitecloud TS. Cervical spondylotic myelopathy and myeloradiculopathy: anterior decompression and stabilization with autogenous fibula strut graft. *Clin Orthop* 1987;221:149–160.
4. Bernhardt M, Hynes RA, Blume HW, et al. Current concepts review: cervical spondylotic myelopathy. *J Bone Joint Surg Am* 1993;75:119–128.
5. Bohlman HH, Emery SE. The pathophysiology of cervical spondylosis and myelopathy. *Spine* 1988;13:843–846.
6. Clark CR. Cervical spondylotic myelopathy. History and physical findings. *Spine* 1988;13:847–849.
7. Clarke E, Robinson PK. Cervical myelopathy: a complication of cervical spondylosis. *Brain* 1956;79:483–507.
8. Edwards WC, LaRocca H. The developmental segmental sagittal diameter of the cervical spinal canal in patients with cervical spondylosis. *Spine* 1983;8:20–27.
9. Emery SE. Anterior approach for cervical myelopathy. In: *The Cervical spine.* Philadelphia: Lippincott-Raven, 1998:825–837.
10. Emery SE, Bohlman HH, Bolesta MJ, et al. Anterior cervical decompression and arthrodesis for the treatment of cervical spondylotic myelopathy. *J Bone Joint Surg Am* 1998;80:941–951.
11. Epstein JA. The surgical management of cervical spinal stenosis, spondylosis and myeloradiculopathy by means of the posterior approach. *Spine* 1988;13:864–869.
12. Epstein NE, Epstein JA. Operative management if cervical spondylotic myelopathy. In: *The cervical spine.* Philadelphia: Lippincott-Raven, 1998:839–848.
13. Flynn TB. Neurologic complications of anterior cervical interbody fusion. *Spine* 1982;7:536–539.
14. Herkowitz H. A comparison of anterior cervical fusion, cervical laminectomy and cervical laminoplasty for the surgical management of multiple level spondylotic radiculopathy. *Spine* 1988;13:774–780.
15. Hirabayashi K, Watanabe K, Wakano K, et al. Expansive open-door laminoplasty for cervical spinal stenotic myelopathy. *Spine* 1983;8:693–699.
16. Hukuda S, Ogata M, Mochizuki T, et al. Laminectomy versus laminoplasty for cervical myelopathy: brief report. *J Bone Joint Surg Br* 1988;70:325–326.

17. LaRocca H. Cervical spondylotic myelopathy: natural history. *Spine* 1988;13:854–855.
18. Lees F, Turner J. Natural history and prognosis of cervical spondylosis. *Br J Med* 1963;2:1607–1610.
19. Malone DG, Benzel EC. Laminotomy and laminectomy for spinal stenosis causing radiculopathy or myelopathy. In: *The cervical spine*. Philadelphia: Lippincott-Raven, 1998:817–823.
20. Mikawa Y, Shikata J, Yamamuro T. Spinal deformity and instability after multilevel cervical laminectomy. *Spine* 1987;12:6–11.
21. Nurick S. The natural history and the results of surgical treatment of the spinal cord disorder associated with cervical spondylosis. *Brain* 1972;95:101–108.
22. Okada K, Shirasaki N, Hayashi H, et al. Treatment if cervical spondylotic myelopathy by enlargement of the spinal canal anteriorly followed by arthrodesis. *J Bone Joint Surg Am* 1991;73:352–364.
23. Penning L, Wilmink JT, van Woerden HH, et al. CT myelographic findings in degenerative disorders of the cervical spine: clinical significance. *AJNR Am J Neuroradiol* 1986;146:793–801.
24. Satomi K, Nishu Y, Kohno T, et al. Long-term follow-up studies of open-door expansive laminoplasty for cervical stenotic myelopathy. Spine 1994;19:507–510.
25. Symon L, Lavender P. The surgical treatment of cervical spondylotic myelopathy. *Neurology* 1967;17:117–127.
26. Wada E, Yonenobu K, Suzuki S, et al. Can intramedullary signal change on magnetic resonance imaging predict surgical outcome in cervical spondylotic myelopathy? Spine 1999;24:455–462.
27. White AA, Panjabi MM. Biomechanical considerations in the surgical management of cervical spondylotic myelopathy. Spine 1988;13:856–860.
28. Yang KC, Lu XS, Cai QL, et al. Cervical spondylotic myelopathy treated by anterior multilevel decompression and fusion: follow-up report of 214 cases. *Clin Orthop* 1987;221:161–164.
29. Yonenobu K, Hosono N, Iwasaki M, et al. Neurologic complications of surgery for cervical compression myelopathy. Spine 1991;16:1277–1282.
30. Yonenobu K, Yamamoto T, Ono K. Laminoplasty for myelopathy. Indications, results, outcome, and complications. In: *The cervical* spine. Philadelphia: Lippincott-Raven, 1998:849–864.
31. Itoh T, Tsui H. Technical improvements and results of laminplasty for compression myelopathy in the cervical spine. *Spine* 1985;10:729–736.

The Degenerative Cervical Spine,
edited by Marek Szpalski and Robert Gunzburg
Lippincott Williams & Wilkins, Philadelphia © 2001.

21

Occipitocervical Fusion

Bernard Jeanneret

Department of Orthopaedic Surgery, University of Basel, CH-4012 Basel, Switzerland

SURGICAL TECHNIQUE OF OCCIPITOCERVICAL STABILIZATION WITH THE CERVIFIX
  Screw Insertion in the Occiput • Transarticular Screw Insertion C1-2 • Screw Insertion in the Lower Cervical Spine (C3-7) • Screw Insertion in the Upper Thoracic Spine • Bone Grafting
POSTOPERATIVE CARE
CONCLUSION

Occipitocervical fusion may be indicated in the presence of posttraumatic changes in the upper cervical spine (unstable Jefferson fracture, dislocated fracture of the lateral masses of the atlas, dislocated fracture of the occipital condyles, atlantooccipital dislocation), developmental abnormalities (atlantoaxial instability in the presence of atlas assimilation, cephalic instability of the cervical spine in the presence of a complex anomaly at the occipitocervical junction, basilar impression), aseptic inflammation with occipitocervical

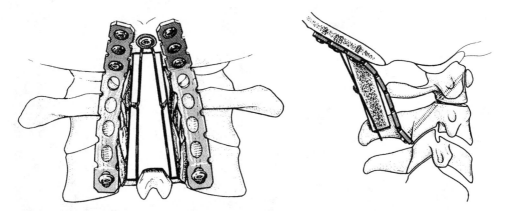

FIG. 21.1. Principle of occipitocervical fixation. A plate or a rod is fixed to the occiput with two or three screws and to C1 and C2 with a transarticular screw. If needed, the construct can be extended to the lower cervical spine as far as desired. In the lower cervical spine, articular mass screws are used. In the upper thoracic spine, transpedicular screws are used. Bone grafting always is performed with autologous bone graft, except in the presence of metastatic disease. In such cases, bone cement can be used (Fig. 21.2).

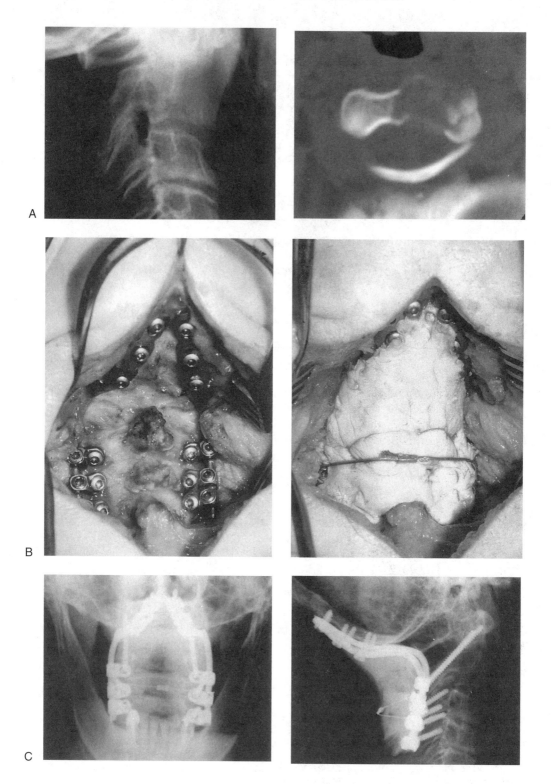

instability (rheumatoid arthritis), and tumor or infection with destruction of the occipital condyles of C1 or C2. There are three operative techniques of posterior occipitocervical fusion: (a) onlay bone grafting without metal implants, (b) bone grafting with internal fixation with wires, rods, Luque rectangles, plates and screws, or other implants, (c) stabilization with methyl methacrylate.

For many years, my colleagues and I have preferred a plate and screw technique (Fig. 21.1) transarticular screw fixation of C1-2 in which a plate is fixed to the occiput with screws (1,6). This technique provides a stable construct that can, if needed, be extended over one or more additional segments of the lower cervical spine and even be extended to the thoracic spine. This may be necessary for some patients with neuromuscular disorders or high quadriparesis, such as after atlantooccipital dislocation. We have developed a rod and screw system, CerviFix (3), which is versatile and does not have the disadvantages of plate fixation, such as varied distances between the screw holes and limited angulation of the screws. We use this implant system whenever it is indicated (Fig. 21.2). The surgical technique described is based on this implant system. However, a 3.5-mm AU reconstruction plate fixed with screws may be used as well.

SURGICAL TECHNIQUE OF OCCIPITOCERVICAL STABILIZATION WITH THE CERVIFIX

The patient is placed in a prone position. In unstable situations, reduction of C1 on C2 is checked with fluoroscopy immediately after positioning of the patient. If necessary, closed reduction is performed by means of positioning the head in the optimal position. A posterior midline incision is made. The occiput, posterior ring of the atlas, the posterior elements of C2, spinous processes, vertebral arches, and articular masses of the lower cervical vertebrae to be included in the fusion are exposed subperiosteally. For transarticular screw fixation of C1-2, the isthmus of C2 is exposed on both sides.

A template is bent in such a way that the cranial end, adjacent to the midline, is situated just caudad to the external occipital protuberance and that the rod passes over the lateral rims of the articular processes of C2, C3, and so on. The occipital rod is cut and bent according to the template. If necessary, residual C1-2 dislocation is reduced under image intensification. First, the holes for the C1-2 transarticular screws are drilled as described later (2,4). To provisionally stabilize C1-2, the drill bit is left in place on one side while instrumentation is performed on the other side.

Fig. 21.2. Clinical example. A 63-year-old woman had massive neck pain as a consequence of a pathologic dens fracture with instability of C1-2 due to destruction of C2 by metastasis from breast cancer. The patient had been bedridden for several weeks. Posterior stabilization of C0-4 was performed. The rod was fixed to the occiput with screws inserted through the plate-shaped end of the CerviFix device. On both sides, a C1-2 transarticular screw was inserted through the corresponding clamp. To allow secure fixation in the metastatic and osteoporotic bone, fixation was carried to C4 with the clamps designed for the lower cervical spine. Because autologous bone grafting was not indicated, bone cement was used for additional stabilization. The bone cement was fixed with a wire inserted around the rods. The patient could be mobilized the second day after the operation without any difficulty with a soft collar. **A:** Preoperative radiographs and computed tomographic scan show pathologic dens fracture. **B:** Postoperative radiographs. **C:** Intraoperative view shows occipitocervical stabilization before and after addition of bone cement.

The most caudal screw hole in the vertebrae to be stabilized is now drilled into the lateral mass according to the technique described later (5). All planned clamps are provisionally mounted and loosely fastened on the rod, which is now positioned over the vertebrae. The C1-2 transarticular screw is inserted first through its corresponding clamp. The occipital screw holes are drilled through the plate, and the screws are inserted (care must be taken to place the cranial end of the plate as close as possible to the midline of the skull to have the best possible purchase). The most caudal screw of the assembly is inserted. Through the corresponding intermediate clamps, the intermediate screw holes are drilled as desired, and the screws inserted. The other side is instrumented accordingly.

Screw Insertion in the Occiput

The thickest bone is found at or close to the midline. Therefore the screws should be placed as close as possible to the midline. The most cranial screw is placed immediately below and as close as possible to the external occipital protuberance. Three screws usually are used on each side.

Transarticular Screw Insertion at C1-2

The entering point for the screw is found on a straight sagittal line passing though the medial aspect of the isthmus and is located at the lower edge of the lamina of C2, about 2 mm cranially and laterally to the medial border of the caudal articular process of C2. The screw aims sagitally, straight forward, toward the medial aspect of the isthmus of C2 and toward the posterior part of the atlantoaxial joint, crosses the atlantoaxial joint, and enters the lateral mass of the atlas, from which it exits anteriorly immediately underneath the base of the skull.

Screw Insertion in the Lower Cervical Spine (C3-7)

The screw enters the vertebra 1 to 2 mm medially and cranially to the center of the articular mass. It is inserted parallel to the adjacent facet joint and is directed 20 to 30 degrees laterally, aiming toward the anterolateral corner of the upper articular process. This screw location minimizes the risk of injury to the vertebral artery and to the nerve root and provides maximal strew length and therefore optimal purchase for the screw.

Screw Insertion in the Upper Thoracic Spine

Transpedicular screw insertion has been shown effective. In selected cases, good fixation also can be obtained by means of inserting the screw into the transverse processes.

Bone Grafting

Between the occiput and the spinous process of C2 a corticocancellous bone graft shaped like a clothespin is inserted to act as a buttress. Bone graft chips are added and placed over the posterior elements of the vertebrae of the lower cervical spine to be fused. In operations on patients with metastatic disease and limited life expectancy or patients with tumor in the posterior elements, no autologous bone graft is used, because the bone material can be destroyed quickly by residual tumor cells. In these cases, we use methyl methacrylate to supplement the rod and screw construct.

POSTOPERATIVE CARE

The patients are allowed to get up the first or second day after surgery, and they use a four-poster orthosis for 3 months. In cases of pronounced osteoporosis or if the patient is unreliable, a Minerva cast can be used. If methyl methacrylate has been used, the patient wears a Philadelphia collar for life. In all other cases, the fusion usually is solid after 3 months and allows walking without an orthosis.

CONCLUSION

The problem of achieving stable occipitocervical fusion in a reduced position has been solved for almost all conditions. The technique described allows solid fixation and early mobilization even in extreme conditions in which other techniques fail or necessitate prolonged immobilization in bed or in a halo brace.

REFERENCES

1. Jeanneret B. Posterior fusion of the cervical spine. In: Grob D, ed. *Spine: state of the art reviews.* Philadelphia: Hanley & Belfus, 1992.
2. Jeanneret B. Posterior transarticular screw fixation of C1-C2. *Tech Orthop* 1994;9:49–59.
3. Jeanneret B. Posterior rod system of the cervical spine: a new implant allowing optimal screw insertion. *Eur Spine J* 1996;5:350–356.
4. Jeanneret E, Magerl P. Primary posterior fusion C1-2 in odontoid fractures: indications, technique and results of transarticular screw fixation. *J Spinal Disord* 1992;5:464–475.
5. Jeanneret P, Magerl F, Halter Ward E, et al. Posterior stabilization of the cervical spine with hook plates. *Spine* 1991;[Suppl 216]:56–63.
6. Sasso RC, Jeanneret B, Fischer K, et al. Occipitocervical fusion with posterior plate axed screw instrumentation: a long-term follow-up study. *Spine* 1994;19:2364–2368.

The Degenerative Cervical Spine,
edited by Marek Szpalski and Robert Gunzburg
Lippincott Williams & Wilkins, Philadelphia © 2001.

22

Cervical Plating in Degenerative Disease by Means of a New Semiconstrained System: The Aline Experience

Peter M. Klara, Maurice D. Gosby

Department of Neurosurgery, Eastern Virginia Medical School, Norfolk, Virginia 23507

It has been 20 years since Bohler and Gaudermak (2) reported using plates and screws as an adjunct to anterior cervical surgery. Caspar (3) designed plates and screws specifically for use in anterior cervical surgery. He also described retractors and a new vertebral body distractor to facilitate the procedure. Despite initial favorable reports by U.S. surgeons (12), widespread acceptance of cervical plating was slow in coming. The technique was most readily accepted to manage traumatic injuries and gross instability (4). The use of plating to manage degenerative disease remains controversial. The routine use of plating to manage single-level spondylosis and herniated disc certainly has been shown to be unnecessary (1,6). Multilevel discectomy and corpectomy have been accepted as relative indications for plating (8).

Results of early biomechanical studies suggested that plates were inadequate to reestablish stability (5). Animal and human cadaveric models showed deficiencies, possibly because they failed to allow for the stabilizing effect of cervical musculature. Later studies with interbody grafts, not used in earlier work, documented the stabilization provided by cervical plating (13). Numerous clinical studies of both unconstrained and fully constrained systems documented the relative safety and efficacy of cervical plating

TABLE 22.1. *Patient statistics*

Variable	Value
Total no. of patients	181
Men	97
Women	84
Age range (yr)	19–74
Average age (yr)	46
No. with myelopathy	37
No. with radiculopathy	144
No. of smokers	64
No. employed	117
No. receiving workers compensation	13
Level fused (no. of patients)	
1	57
2	72
3	39
4	11
corpectomy (no. of patients)	
Level 1	15
Level 2	17
Level 3	10
Level 4	1
Level 5	1

(4,7,8,10,12). Unconstrained systems relied on bicortical screw fixation, and constrained systems involved unicortical purchase. The advantages and disadvantages of both systems and a review of their development can be found in previous publications (9). A discussion of the development of semiconstrained systems is contained herein. Current design trends seem to favor the semiconstrained form. At least three new semiconstrained systems are available. This chapter describes one surgeon's initial 5 years of experience with the Aline anterior cervical plating system in the management of degenerative disease.

PATIENT SELECTION

All patients had degenerative disease of the cervical spine, including spondylosis, herniated disc disease, postsurgical kyphosis, and pseudoarthrosis. All patients had had symptoms for a minimum of 8 weeks. The symptoms were refractory to a full course of conservative therapy that consisted of limitation of activity, medication with antiinflammatory, analgesic and antispasmodic agents, and physical therapy (Table 22.1).

SURGERY

Anterior cervical surgery was performed in a manner previously described (9). Allograft bone and a modified Smith-Robinson technique were used. Some corpectomy procedures were performed with a Harms interbody cage with morselized locally harvested bone augmented with allograft.

SURGICAL FOLLOW-UP

Patients were observed for as long as 5 years after the operation; mean follow-up period was longer than 2 years. The patients were evaluated with a modified Prolo scale, an analog pain scale, and a physical examination by two physicians, one of whom was not the operating surgeon. All patients were asked whether they were satisfied with the results of the operation, whether they would undergo the procedure again if needed, and whether they recommend the procedure to a friend.

Radiographic evaluation was performed immediately after the operation 1 month, 3 months, 6 months, 1 year after the operation, and annually thereafter. The radiographs were evaluated by two physicians at least one of whom was not the operating surgeon. Dynamic flexion and extension radiographs were obtained 3 months after the operation and yearly thereafter. Criteria for fusion included no hardware failure, no motion on dynamic radiographs, and patient satisfaction greater than 85%.

RESULTS

More than 94% of patients related more than 85% satisfaction with the procedure. All of these patients said they would undergo the procedure again if necessary and would recommend the procedure to a friend. Fusion was deemed to occur on the basis of the criteria stated earlier in 91% of cases. Analog pain scale score improved from an average of 6 before surgery to a level of 2 at 6 months after surgery. Prolo scale increased from an average of 4 before surgery to 9 at 6 months after surgery. Of the 117 patients employed before surgery, 91 returned to their jobs. All 13 of the workers compensation patients returned to work.

The most dramatic finding was the total absence of hardware breakage among this cohort. In the early development of the Aline system, screws broke during the operation. This was the result of poor design of the screwdriver and screw angulation in excess of the recommended 15 degrees. This problem has been alleviated by alterations in product design. The drill guide inhibits excessive angulation, and the fit of the screwdriver has been improved. Nevertheless, screw or plate breakage after implantation does not seem to occur.

EXPLANATION

In an attempt to explain the dramatic decrease in hardware breakage, we considered the various factors involved:

Subsidence
Fatigue (fracture)
Material
Modulus of elasticity
Etch sensitivity
System design
Patient factors
Surgeon factors

Although the titanium alloy used in the Aline Ti has material advantages, it is unlikely that use of this material is solely responsible for the absence of breakage. In their review of hardware breakage, Lowery and McDonough (10) related a high occurrence of breakage of stainless steel and titanium plates, both unconstrained and constrained and manufactured by various sources. The authors suggested that a semiconstrained system may show less breakage. If it is assumed that most of the factors listed are constants, it would seem that the semiconstrained system design is responsible for the decreased rate of breakage.

HEIGHT CHANGES

Disc height was measured 1 and 2 years postoperatively (Table 22.2, Fig. 22.1).

TABLE 22.2. *Height changes*

No. of levels	No. of patients	1 yr	2 yr	3 yr
1	4	↑1.14	—	—
2	10	↓2.69	↓3.90	↓9.7
3	4	↑0.97	—	—
4	2	↓1.07	—	—

Values are percentages. ↑, increased; ↓, decreased.

One Level

Twelve months after the operation, the height of the vertebral bodies of 4 patients who underwent one-level operations had increased an average of 1.14% of the immediately postoperative height. No measurements were obtained from patients who underwent a one-level operation and follow-up evaluation for 2 years.

Two Levels

The vertebrae of 10 patients who underwent two-level operations were measured 1 year postoperatively. Six of these patients' vertebrae were measured 2 years after the operation. The height of the vertebral bodies after 1 year showed an average decrease of 2.69% of the immediately postoperative height. Measurements obtained 2 years after the operation showed a decrease in height of 3.90% of immediately postoperative height. Measurements were obtained from 2 patients 3 years after the operation. Vertebral height had decreased 9.7% and 3.6%.

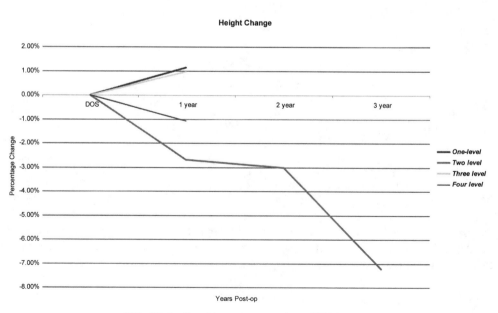

FIG. 22.1. Graphic representation of Table 22.2.

Three Levels

The vertebrae of 4 patients who underwent three-level procedures were measured 1 year after the operation. The average change was an increase in height of 0.97% of immediately postoperative height.

Four Levels

The vertebrae of 2 patients who underwent four-level procedures were measured 1 year after the operation. The two patients had a decreased height of 0.15% and 2.00%, and average of 1.07%.

CHANGES IN THE DISTANCE BETWEEN SCREWS

Changes in the distance between the screws are shown in Table 22.3 and Fig. 22.2.

One Level

The distance between the screws immediately and 1 year after the operations was measured for 3 patients. The average change was a 1.33% decrease from the immediately postoperative distance.

Two Levels

Twelve patients who underwent two-level operations had measurements obtained 1 year afterward. The average change was a 5.92% decrease from the immediately postoperative distance between the screws. Five of these patients had measurements obtained 2 years after the operation and had an average decrease of 3.02% of the immediately postoperative distance. Three of the 12 patients had measurements obtained 3 years after the operation. The average change was 7.23% of the immediately postoperative distance. In 11 patients the distance decreased after 1 year. In 1 of these patients the distance seemed to have increased at the 2-year measurement. In 1 patient the distance had increased after 1 year but seemed to have decreased at the 2-year measurement.

Three Levels

Four patients who underwent three-level operations had measurements obtained 1 year after the operation. The average change was a 0.877% decrease from immediately postoperative distance. One of the patients had measurements obtained 2 and 3 years after the operation, but the distance between the screws did not change.

TABLE 22.3. *Change in distance between screws*

No. of levels	No. of patients	1 yr	2 yr	3 yr
1	3	↓1.33	—	—
2	12	↓5.92	↓3.02	↓7.23
3	4	↓0.87	—	—
4	3	↓2.53	—	—

Values are percentages.
↓, decreased.

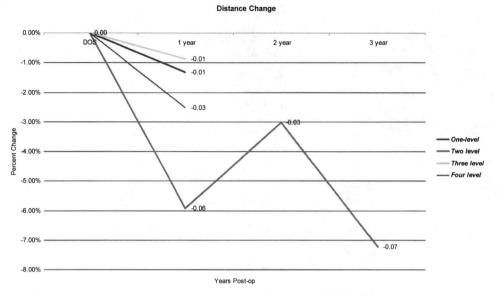

FIG. 22.2. Graphic representation of Table 22.3.

Four Levels

Three patients who underwent four-level cases operations had measurements obtained 1 year after the operation. The average change was a 2.53% decrease from the immediately postoperative distance between the screws.

CHANGES IN SCREW ANGLE

Changes in screw angle are summarized in Table 22.4 and Fig. 22.3.

One Level

The angles of the screws in 3 patients who underwent one-level operations were recorded immediately and 1 year after the operation. On average, the angles increased 1.6 degrees. The greatest change was a 2.8-degree increase; the smallest change was a 1.5-degree.

Two Levels

Screw angles in 12 patients who underwent two-level operations were measured immediately and 1 year after the operation. On average, the angles increased 4.48 degrees.

TABLE 22.4. *Change in screw angles*

No. of levels	No. of patients	1 yr	2 yr	3 yr
1	3	↑1.6	—	—
2	12	↑4.48	↑4.71	—
3	4	↑5.27	—	—
4	3	↑8.26	—	—

Values are degrees. ↑, increased.

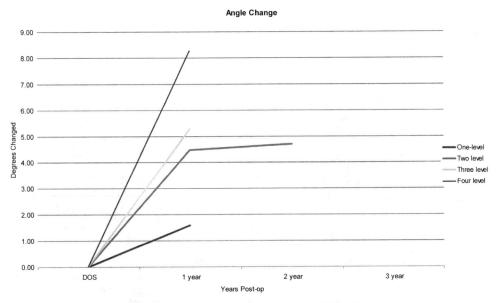

FIG. 22.3. Graphic representation of Table 22.4.

The greatest increase was 18.9 degrees; the greatest decrease was 8.4 degrees. In 9 patients the angles had increased 1 year after the operation; in 3 patients the angle had decreased. Six of the 12 patients had measurements obtained 2 years after the operation. The average change was a 4.71-degree increase. At the 2-year measurement, the angle increased in 5 patients. The greatest increase 2 years after the operation was 9.2 degrees. In 1 patient the angle had decreased 3.2 degrees.

Three Levels

Screw angles in 4 patients who underwent three-level operations were measured immediately and 1 year after the operation. The average change was a 5.27-degree increase. The greatest increase was 14.1 degrees; 1 patient had a decrease of 2.7 degrees. One of the 4 patients had measurements obtained 2 years postoperatively. The angle had not changed.

Four Levels

Screw angles were measured in 3 patients who underwent four-level operations. The average change was an 8.26-degree increase. None of the angles decreased.

CREEP

"A viscoelastic material deforms with time when it is subjected to a constant, suddenly applied load. The deformation curve approaches a steady state value asymptotically" (15). In an attempt to determine whether creep occurred during anterior cervical discectomy, cases were selected at random. Each patient's immediately postoperative appearance was compared with the appearance 1 and 2 years after the operation. Subsidence and

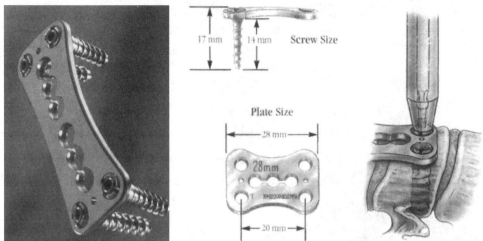

A,B   C

FIG. 22.4. A: The Aline implants and instruments are designed to provide the surgeon with variability of screw placement, the capability to place three screws into the vertebral body (superior or inferior), and a locking mechanism to help prevent screw back-out. The system consists of three implant components—bone screw, lock screw, and plate. The components are constructed of Ti13-13 to improve postoperative imaging. This proprietary titanium alloy undergoes a diffusion hardening and finishing process that minimizes the potential for wear debris generation. Aline is a trademark product produced by Surgical Dynamics, a subsidiary of United States Surgical Corporation. **B:** Diagram shows the Aline device. **C:** Locking screw expands the screw head, securing the screw to the plate. The system appears to allow creep, and this minimizes hardware breakage.

changes in screw angulation were measured as described in the next section. The results of the study suggested that as subsidence occurs, creep changes the relation (angle of the screw) between the screw and the plate. The ability of the screw and plate to creep prevents hardware breakage. Creep occurs with high rates of fusion and patient satisfaction (Fig. 22.4).

MEASUREMENT PROCEDURE

The results of this preliminary study showed decreased screw distance and increased screw angles. An unexpected finding was inconsistent change in height measurements. Because subsidence is known to occur, vertebral height should decrease, and this change should increase with multilevel surgery. A possible explanation for this inconsistency is a small sample size and measurement error. Ongoing study should provide clarification.

SUMMARY

Anterior cervical plating has evolved in a relatively short time. Problems such as the risk associated with bicortical screw penetration and screw and plate separation have been addressed with improved designs. High rates of fusion and good patient satisfaction can be obtained with no hardware breakage. The improved hardware, however, is not a substitute for careful and precise surgical technique. Furthermore, there is no substitute for careful patient selection. The results reported are one surgeon's experience, but they should provide the basis for ongoing study of the utility of anterior cervical plating.

For the Aline study, plain radiographs were measured with the X-Caliper device (Figs. 22.5) in the following manner

- Radiographs obtained immediately and 1 and 2 years after the operation are accumulated for patients who have Aline hardware.
- The width of the middle screw is measured with the X-Caliper device as a reference for magnification. Given a 4-mm screw width, one can accurately determine the distance between two points on the same radiograph. This minimizes variability caused by magnification.
- Points are determined as follows to record the distance between the screws at various intervals in the patient's history.
- Red lines are drawn down the middle of the two most visible screws at each end of the plate.
- The plain radiograph is marked with a grease pencil at the points where the middle of the screws end (the same screws in each picture).
- The distance between points A and D represents the distance between the vertebral bodies at a given point in time.
- The distance between points B and C represents the distance between the screws at a given point in time. By comparing the measurements with measurements obtained on different dates, one can determine whether and by how much the screws are moving closer together or farther apart.
- The angle of the screws is recorded. The acute angle is always the one used.

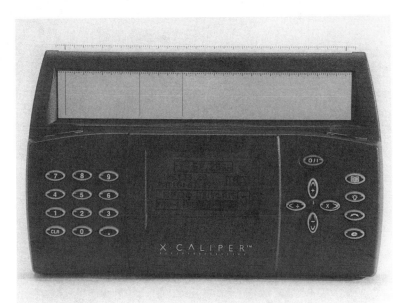

FIG. 22.5. The X-Caliper device is a product designed and distributed by Eisenlohr Technologies, Inc.

REFERENCES

1. Abraham D, Herkowitz H. Indications and trends in use in cervical spine fusion. *Orthop Clin North Am* 1998;29:731–744.
2. Bohler J, Gaudermak T. Anterior plate stabilization for fracture dislocations of the lower cervical spine. *J Trauma* 1980;20:203–205.
3. Caspar W. Die ventrale interkor porole stabilisierung mit der HWS-Trapez-Osteosyntheseplatte: Indication, Technik, Ergebnisse. *Orthopade* 1981;119:809–810.
4. Caspar W, Barbier D, Klara P. Anterior cervical fusion and Caspar plate stabilization for cervical trauma. *Neurosurgery* 1989;25:491–502.
5. Coe J, Warden K, Sutterlin CI, et al. Biomechanical evaluation of cervical spinal stabilization for unstable cervical spine fractures and/or dislocations. *Spine* 1989;14:1122–1131.
6. Connolly PJ, Esses SI, Kostuik JP. Anterior cervical fusion: outcome analysis of patients fused with and without anterior cervical plates. *J Spinal Disord* 1999;9:202–206.
7. Goffin J, Plets C, Van den Bergh R. Anterior cervical fusion and osteosynthetic stabilization according to Caspar: a prospective study of 41 patients with fractures and/or dislocations of the cervical spine. *Neurosurgery* 1989;25:865–871.
8. Illgner A, Haas N, Tscherne H. Review of the therapeutic concepts and results of operative treatment in acute and chronic lesions of the cervical spine: the Hannover experience. *Neurosurgery* 1991;5:100–113.
9. Klara PM. Anterior cervical plating: a historical perspective and recent advances. In: *Whiplash injuries: current concepts in prevention, diagnosis, and treatment of the cervical whiplash syndrome.* Philadelphia: Lippincott-Raven, 1998.
10. Lowery GL, McDonough RF. The significance of hardware failure in anterior cervical plate fixation. *Spine* 1998;23:181–187.
11. Randle M, Wolf A, Levi L, et al. The use of anterior Caspar plate fixation in acute cervical spine injury. *Surg Neurol* 1991;36:181–189.
12. Sutterlin CI, McAfee P, Warden K, et al. A biomechanical evaluation of cervical spinal stabilization methods in a bovine model. *Spine* 1988;13:795–802.
13. Tippets RH, Apfelbaum RL. Anterior cervical fusion with the Caspar instrumentation system. *Neurosurgery.* 1988;22:1008–1013.
14. Traynelis V, Donaher P, Roach R, et al. Biomechanical comparison of anterior Caspar plate and three-level posterior fixation techniques in a human cadaveric model. *J Neurosurg* 1993;79(1):96–103.
15. White A and Punjabi M. Biomechanisms A to Z. In: *Clinical Biomechanisms of the Spine,* 2nd ed. Lippincott: Philadelphia, 1990:646.

The Degenerative Cervical Spine,
edited by Marek Szpalski and Robert Gunzburg
Lippincott Williams & Wilkins, Philadelphia © 2001.

23

Surgical Indications and Results with Subtotal Corpectomy and Instrumented Fusion

Dan M. Spengler

*Department of Orthopaedics and Rehabilitation, Vanderbilt University Medical Center,
Nashville, Tennessee 37232*

TECHNICAL ASPECTS
DISCUSSION
CASE EXAMPLES

Subtotal corpectomy with instrumented fusion is a commonly performed surgical procedure for a variety of patients with myelopathy or radiculopathy and who have undergone imaging studies that show anterior compression, instability, or both. Cervical corpectomy ideally is limited to one or two vertebral bodies. Involvement of three or more levels can usually be managed by means of posterior laminoplasty.

Multilevel corpectomy can be performed when a patient has considerable kyphotic deformity. This chapter focuses on the indications, complications, and anticipated outcomes for patients who undergo anterior subtotal corpectomy and instrumented fusion. Recent information suggests that subtotal corpectomy with instrumented fusion should be considered in the treatment of smokers who need an anterior decompression procedure (5). Patients with one- or two-level compression due to ossification of the posterior longitudinal ligament also are appropriate candidates for corpectomy and fusion. In the United States, the largest group of patients to be considered for anterior corpectomy and fusion is patients with cervical spondylotic myelopathy (6–9).

TECHNICAL ASPECTS

Although it is not my intent to discuss detailed techniques for anterior procedures, I do want to emphasize several aspects of the procedure. The anterior approach is generally performed through a left-sided transverse incision over the cervical vertebrae of interest (3). After radiographic localization, self-retaining retractors are placed to ensure adequate visualization. Disc spaces above and below the level of corpectomy are partially removed. The uncovertebral joints or "goal posts" are identified. These structures are important landmarks to prevent injury to the vertebral artery, which is just lateral to these structures. The actual corpectomy is begun with a rongeur so that a high-speed carbide drill can be safely placed and controlled within the vertebral body. As corpectomy proceeds posteriorly, additional disc tissue is removed above and below the vertebral body until the entire discs have been removed. As the dissection proceeds posteriorly through the vertebral body, the carbide drill can be replaced with a diamond bur. The diamond bur in addition to being safer, also helps with hemostasis of the vertebral body. As the posterior cortical wall is removed, small angled curettes are of great assistance in initiating development of the proper planes to complete the corpectomy.

The width of corpectomy must be adequate to facilitate decompression centrally. General guidelines can be provided for the width of corpectomy, but a more precise way to assure adequate decompression is to calculate the width from the preoperative computed tomographic (CT) scans. Twelve millimeters can be a useful guideline, but the measurement must be flexible depending on the size of the vertebral body. No portion of the vertebral body lateral to the uncovertebral joints is removed to ensure protection for the vertebral artery.

Once corpectomy has been completed, an appropriate iliac crest structural graft is harvested. The graft is locked into place with one of the many cervical plates available for this purpose. Essential design features include screws that are unlikely to back out into the region of the esophagus. The plate must be placed in the midline to avoid injury to the sympathetic chain and vertebral artery. The wound is closed over a mastoid drain, and the patient is placed in a cervical collar.

DISCUSSION

Results of cervical corpectomy and of anterior cervical discectomy and fusion are generally quite good. Results are better for one-level anterior cervical discectomy and fusion than for two-level discectomy and corpectomy (2,4,6,9). Bohlman et al. (2) reported successful fusion for 90% of patients who underwent cervical discectomy and fusion. In regard to cervical myelopathy, published failure rates range from 18% to 60% (1). Spinal cord injury or myelopathy caused by the procedure occurred among 0.35% to 1.8% of patients in a large series (1). Pseudarthrosis has been variably reported to occur at a rate of 4% to 20% (1). Graft extrusions are uncommon in one-level procedures, but before plate fixation, the graft extrusion rate can range from 1.5% to 20% for multilevel corpectomy.

The advantages of plate fixation of the cervical spine include increased stability, a decrease in the graft extrusion rate, an enhanced fusion rate, and a decreased need for prolonged postoperative immobilization devices such as a halo (4,6–8). Disadvantages of plate fixation include the amount of operating room time necessary to add the plate, the cost of the additional implant, and the theoretic increased opportunity for additional complications. Other complications that are theoretically possible include a higher rate of adjacent segment disease among patients who have undergone plate fixation. Complication rates also could be theoretically higher among patients who have undergone previous surgery, either an anterior or a posterior approach (8).

CASE EXAMPLES

Figures 23.1 through 23.3 show two complications associated with plate fixation of the cervical spine. In the first situation, a 55-year-old man continued to have chronic pain despite multiple attempts to stabilize the spine. This patient underwent a cage procedure and anterior plate fixation as well as posterior lateral mass plate reconstruction. This is an example of poor preoperative decision analysis because one can question the need for this

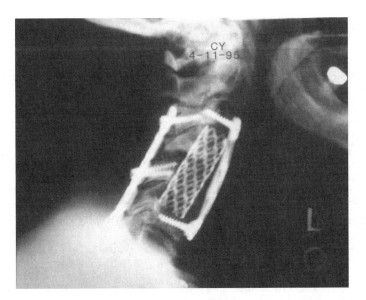

FIG. 23.1. Lateral radiograph shows anterior cervical cage reconstruction with anterior plating. The patient also underwent a posterior lateral cervical plating procedure. The patient continued to be incapacitated by severe chronic pain.

aggressive intervention in the care of someone with fairly minor degenerative changes (Fig. 23.1).

The case of the second patient (Figs. 23.2, 23.3) illustrates the problems associated with malposition of the plate. The plate has been placed too laterally. The CT scan shows the proximity of the screw to the vertebral artery. The artery was not injured, even though

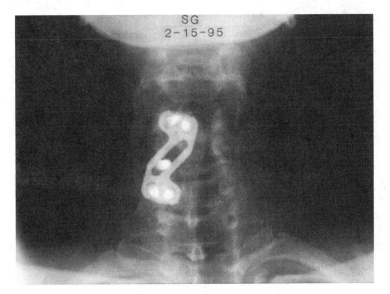

FIG. 23.2. Anteroposterior radiograph of the cervical spine shows malposition of plate.

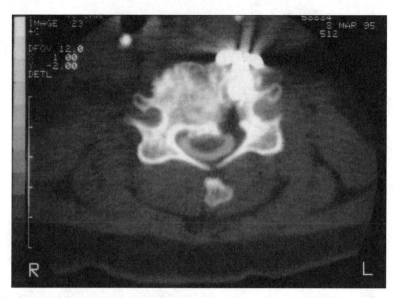

FIG. 23.3. Axial computed tomographic myelogram shows two points. First, lateral placement of the plate with the screw approaches but does not violate the vertebral artery. Second, the preoperative pathologic findings were not addressed in the initial procedure.

the patient did have irreversible Horner syndrome. Revision surgery was necessary to address the pathologic process not addressed during the initial operation. The final revision and the appropriate plate fixation are shown in Fig. 23.4.

The 55-year-old man who smoked had long-standing cervical radicular problems. He had minor neurologic deficits, and his quality of life was limited. He had not responded to nonoperative measures. Representative CT myelograms are shown in Fig. 23.5. Post-

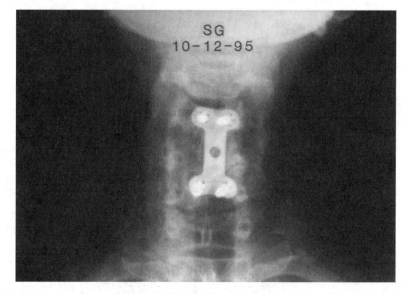

FIG. 23.4. Anteroposterior radiograph of the patient depicted in Figs. 23.2 and 23.3 after satisfactory decompression and proper plating.

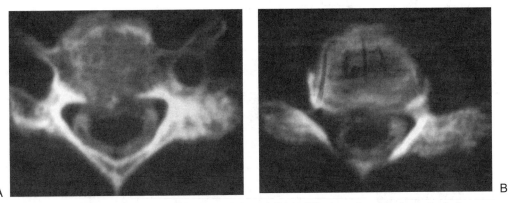

FIG. 23.5. Axial CT scans through C5-6 **(A)** and C6-7 **(B)** show two-level cervical disc encroachment on the subarachnoid space in the cervical spinal canal.

operative radiographs are shown in Fig. 23.6. The patient was a heavy smoker. His imaging studies showed two-level cervical disc herniation with minor osteophytes. In lieu of two-level cervical discectomy, I performed subtotal corpectomy and discectomy at both levels. A graft was placed in the corpectomy trough and fixed with an anterior plate. Postoperatively the patient did well and gained fusion. One other technical point is based on data (10) that suggest the left-sided approach to the cervical spine may be somewhat safer than the right-sided approach. In anatomic studies and clinical reviews, authors have suggested that risk of injury to the recurrent laryngeal nerve may be higher with the right-sided approach (10).

Perhaps the most important point concerns revision cervical spinal surgery. I believe that all patients who undergo revision surgery should undergo an evaluation of vocal cord function to ensure that the cords are intact. One would be reluctant to consider a left-

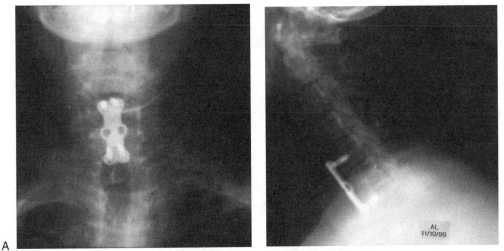

FIG. 23.6. Anteroposterior **(A)** and lateral **(B)** radiographs of the cervical spine of the patient depicted in Fig. 23.5 after subtotal corpectomy and instrumentation with a cervical plate.

sided approach for a patient who has undergone a right-sided approach if the right-sided vocal cord is inoperative. This puts the patient at too great a risk of injury to the intact vocal cord. In summary, I believe that subtotal corpectomy with fusion is a safe, predictable procedure. Precise surgical technique is an essential for optimal results.

REFERENCES

1. Balderston RA, An HS. *Complications in Spinal Surgery.* Philadelphia: WB Saunders. 1991.
2. Bohlman HH, Emery SE, Goodfellow DB, et al. Robinson anterior cervical discectomy and arthrodesis for cervical radiculopathy: long-term follow-up of one hundred and twenty-two patients. *J Bone Joint Surg Am* 1993;75:1298–1307.
3. Delamarter R. Cervical vertebrectomy. In: Bradford D, ed. *Master techniques in orthopaedic surgery: the spine.* Philadelphia: Lippincott-Raven, 1997;57–73.
4. Ebraheim N, DeTroze R, Rupp R, et al. Osteosynthesis of the cervical spine with an anterior plate. *Orthopaedics* 1995;18:141–147.
5. Kwiatkowski TC, Hanley EN Jr, Ramp WK. Cigarette smoking and its orthopaedic consequences. *Am J Orthop* 1996;25:590–597.
6. Lowery GL, Swank ML, McDonough RF. Surgical revision for failed anterior cervical fusions: articular pillar plating or anterior revision. *Spine* 1995;20:2436–2441.
7. Natio M, Kurose S, Oyama M, et al. Anterior cervical fusion with the Caspar instrumentation system. *Int Orthop* 1993;17(2):73–76.
8. Riew KD, Hilibrand AS, Palumbo MA, et al. Anterior cervical corpectomy in patients previously managed with a laminectomy: short-term complications., *J Bone Joint Surg Am* 1999;81:950–957.
9. Villas C, Martinez-Peric R, Preite R, et al. Union after multiple anterior cervical fusion: 21 cases followed for 1-6 years, *Acta Orthop Scand* 1994;65:620–622.
10. Weisberg N, Spengler D, Netterville J. Stretch-induced nerve injury as a cause of paralysis secondary to the anterior cervical approach. *Otolaryngol Head Neck Surg* 1997;116:317–326.

The Degenerative Cervical Spine,
edited by Marek Szpalski and Robert Gunzburg
Lippincott Williams & Wilkins, Philadelphia © 2001.

24

Anterior Decompression and Fusion with the BAK-C Cage in the Management of Cervical Spondylosis

Guy Matgé

Department of Neurosurgery, Centre Hospitalier, L-1210 Luxembourg, Luxembourg

---

METHODS AND PATIENTS
Operative Indications • Data Collection • Patient Population • Surgical Technique
RESULTS
Hospital Data • Clinical Results • Radiologic Results • Case Example • Complications and Reoperations
DISCUSSION
CONCLUSION

Anterior decompression with interbody fusion is the procedure of choice in the management of cervical spondylosis for patients with discogenic neck and radicular pain or myelopathy (13,28). Decompression alone may relieve radiculopathy or myelopathy, but because some patients continue to have neck pain and kyphotic deformity after the operation, routine interbody fusion at the same operation may be necessary (1,6,24). The conventional techniques pioneered 40 years ago by Cloward (10) and Smith and Robinson (23) yield good results, but a number of complications occur owing to graft collapse and expulsion, pseudarthrosis and harvest-site morbidity, mainly iliac pain (4,5,10,12, 14–24,26,27). Bone quality is not always good among the elderly population, and the cosmetic defect is not well accepted by young persons (22). Allografts suffer from irregular strength and weaker fusion than autologous bone (3,6,11). Additional anterior plating to enhance stabilization and fusion with allografts has new limitations due to material breakage and migration (14,25). These pitfalls together lead one to favor interbody cage fusion, as pioneered by Bagby (2).

The data presented are from an observational study representing 4 years of experience with the cervical BAK (BAK-C) device, a further development of the lumbar threaded titanium interbody fusion cage promoted by Kuslich et al. (16). The aim of the study was to determine whether it was possible to achieve equivalent or even better results with this implant than with traditional techniques without autograft or allograft complications and with a reduction in operative time and hospital stay.

METHODS AND PATIENTS

Operative Indications

Most patients had discogenic neck and radicular pain at one or two levels from C3 to C7-T1. A few had cervical myelopathy. Patients with persistent or recurrent pain with pseudarthrosis from previous failed discectomy or fusion were included in the series. Exclusion criteria were the presence of active infection, severe osteoporosis, vertebral tumor, or traumatic subluxation.

Data Collection

Patients completed a 10-point visual analog scale regarding neck and arm or shoulder pain. They also underwent a neurologic examination for radicular deficit or myelopathy. Imaging studies included dynamic radiography, computed tomographic (CT) myelography, or magnetic resonance imaging (MRI), or a combination of these modalities to detect disc herniation, degenerative discopathy, chronic instability such as kyphosis or listhesis, and the spinal cord lesions of myelopathy.

Patient Population

Starting in 1995, 146 patients underwent operations at 192 levels. Thirty-eight underwent operations at two levels and only one at three levels in the same session with the following distribution: C3-4, 3; C4-5, 18; C5-6, 94; C6-7, 74; C7-T1, 3. There were 80 men and 66 women 17 to 72 years of age (mean, 43 years); 136 had cervical radiculopathy, and 10 had myelopathy.

Surgical Technique

Slight neck extension under fluoroscopic control establishes or maintains lordosis. A standard anterior cervical approach is used with total discectomy and internal decompression as needed. An intervertebral spreader and microdrill are useful for posterior osteophyte resection. The posterior longitudinal ligament is resected if there are calcifications or free disc fragments; otherwise it is preserved as a tension band. Special instruments are provided to establish distraction and prepare the interbody space for the implant. These instruments include a bone-collecting reamer. With the BAK system, local bone graft is used as the osteoinductive material within the implant. The self-packing design of the cervical cage draws local bone into the implant on insertion. All instruments have positive stops on a safely seated drill tube of 10 or 12 mm diameter, depending on the cage size routinely used.

Correct distraction is import to achieve segmental stabilization by means of anular and posterior ligamental tension. Asymmetric drilling can cause end-plate weakening and must be avoided in operations on elderly patients with osteoporosis. Removing the anterior osteophytes and mainly the more protruding lip of the upper vertebra allows a better view and instrument alignment inside the interbody space. Another technical point to consider is sufficient reaming and tapping to prepare a bleeding bone bed. The recommended cage size is 2 to 4 mm larger than the distraction to allow good end-plate purchase. Adjusting the drill guide to 14 mm enables safe reaming and cage screwing about 2 mm behind the anterior vertebral border as cage depth is always 12 mm. Too short reaming risks cutting the bone threads (made by the tap) during cage insertion, a cause of implant migration, as is insufficient interbody distraction. Overdistraction can cause pain due to neural stretching and ligamental disruption. Lateral fluoroscopy is mandatory to control adapted distraction and final cage position.

RESULTS

Hospital Data

The operative time for one-level surgery was 45 to 60 minutes and for two-level procedures was 60 to 90 minutes. Blood loss was minimal (<100 mL) in 142 operations and acceptable (100 to 250 mL) in the other four. Hospital stay was 3 to 6 days (mean, 4 days). The mean stay for the Cloward procedure in our hospital was 6 days.

Clinical Results

The patient ratings of neck and radicular pain on the 10-point scale were as follows (the number in parentheses is the rating of radicular pain): 7.5 (7) before, 1.5 (1.0) 1 month after, 0.5 (0.0) 6 months after. Typical radicular arm pain was relieved completely for all patients, and very few had some neck discomfort 6 months after the operation. All radicular deficits also cleared. Resolution of neurologic symptoms was not as good among the 10 patients with myelopathy. Two recovered completely, and 6 had incomplete resolution, but 3 of these had an excellent result after further decompressive surgery. Two patients had unresolved neurologic symptoms.

Clinical outcome was good to excellent among 95% of patients with cervical radiculopathy and only 50% of those with myelopathy. A second staged decompressive operation relieved myelopathy among patients with a stenotic canal (30% in this group). All patients whose condition did not improve had spinal cord lesions with high signal intensity at preoperative MRI. Operation at this stage of disease may only prevent further deterioration.

Radiologic Results

Bone fusion was defined as no motion on lateral flexion-extension radiographs and no radiolucency around the device. According to these criteria, 90% of patients had fusion 6 months and 100% 12 months after the operation. Bridging bone around the cage was visible 12-months postoperatively, but bone inside the implant with similar density to vertebral body could be found only on CT bone scans. No segments fused in kyphosis greater than 10 degrees. One- to two-millimeter subsidence of the intervertebral spacer was regularly observed 1 year postoperatively, when bone union was complete. No pseudarthrosis was identified in this series.

Case Example

A 68-year-old woman had neck and C6 radicular pain that had lasted several months despite medical therapy. Neurologic examination revealed right weakness corresponding to signs of C6 nerve compression by hard disc herniation found at CT myelography and MRI. Degenerative discopathy was seen on flexion-extension radiographs without major instability. The operation was performed in a slight lordotic neck position by means of standard anterior discectomy and posterior decompression with a microdrill. The next

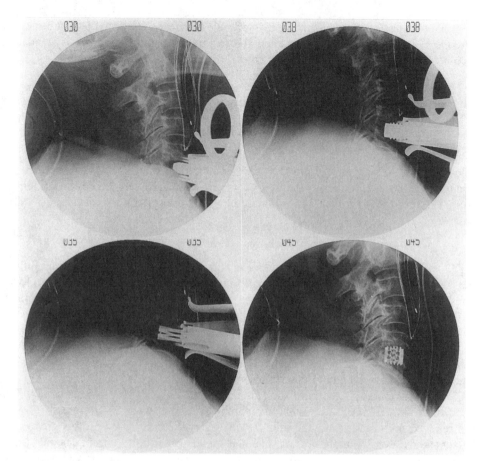

FIG. 24.1. Perioperative fluoroscopic image shows distraction, drilling, tapping, and implanted cage.

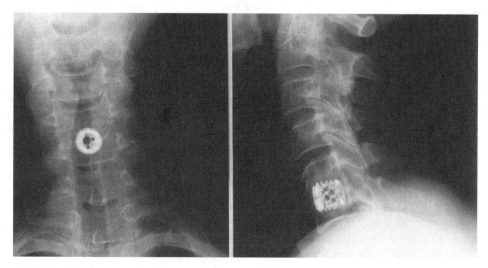

FIG. 24.2. Same patient as in Fig. 24.1. Excellent fusion is present 12 months after the operation.

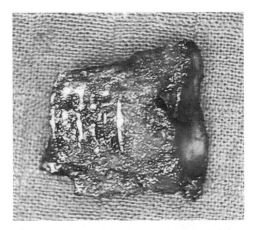

FIG. 24.3. Impressive fusion in a unique case of explantation of a cage during two-level corpectomy.

steps were 7-mm distraction, drilling, tapping, and screwing of a 10-mm cage (Fig. 24.1). The postoperative course was uneventful, and a 12-month evaluation showed excellent clinical results and fusion in this woman with slight osteoporosis (Fig. 24.2).

Complications and Reoperations

Neither hematoma nor infection occurred in this series. No patient had an implant- or instrument-related neurologic complication. One patient, a 70-year-old woman operated on at the C5-6 and C6-7 disc space, needed an early (first postoperative week) reoperation. She had symptomatic end-plate perforation and consecutive C6 vertebral body collapse. After anterior miniplate stabilization 1 week later the complications occurred, outcome was uneventful and bone fusion was good. Another patient had asymptomatic anterior migration, which was found at postoperative radiography. The supposed technical fault was too-short drilling and tearing of the bone thread during cage insertion. After deeper reaming of the interbody space and new tapping, the same cage was secured in the ideal position. This happened at the C6-7 space, where fluoroscopic control may be difficult in operations on heavy patients.

Late reoperations (6 months to 2 years) were performed to manage degenerative or stenotic conditions. Accelerated degeneration at an adjacent level occurred among 4 patients, who needed a cage at another level. Additional decompressive surgery was indicated in the care of 3 patients with myelopathy, insufficient neurologic recovery, and signs of residual stenosis at MRI. Four-level laminectomy was performed on 2 patients and anterior corpectomy on one with excellent outcome. The anterior column had fused, so there was no instability after laminectomy. In the third case, the cage was drilled out during C6-7 corpectomy to allow further anterior canal decompression and stabilization with a strut graft reinforced with a plate. Fusion was complete and impressive (Fig. 24.3) but not readily seen at radiographic and MRI evaluations.

DISCUSSION

Cervical spondylosis is a common disease facing spinal surgeons, who have to perform patient selection and choose an operative technique. A posterior approach may be indicated in the care of selected patients to manage soft disc herniation. There has been a trend to anterior surgery since the publications by Cloward and Smith and Robinson in 1958 (10,23). Painful posterior muscle splitting is avoided, and the more direct anterior approach allows better visualization and much better decompression of the spinal cord and nerve roots in the management of these mostly degenerative lesions (6). Decompression alone can relieve neurologic symptoms, but lasting postoperative neck pain with kyphotic deformity among some patients suggests the need for routine interbody fusion (1,4,6). Nowadays, anterior decompression and fusion in the same operation is the treatment of choice of patients with discogenic neck and radicular pain or myelopathy (1,4,6,10,24).

Conventional techniques pioneered 40 years ago yield good results, but there are a number of complications caused by graft collapse, graft expulsion, and pseudarthrosis at the cervical implantation site (4,6,13,26,28). Morbidity at the graft harvest site is even worse. The most frequent problem is iliac pain, the occurrence rate of which is greater than 10% in some publications (4,5,12,14–22,26,27). Less frequent complications are hematoma, infection, hernia, peritoneal perforation, fracture of the ilium, and nerve and arterial injury. Poor bone quality among the elderly and cosmetic deformity among younger patient are other concerns (22). Use of allografts may avoid these harvest problems and save operating time. I have found that allografts have irregular strength with time and weaker fusion than does autologous bone. The pseudarthrosis rate also is higher (3,6,11,18,19). Additional anterior plating to enhance stability and fusion with allografts has limitations caused by material breakage and migration (14,25). Newer dynamic ventral stabilization systems seem promising (8).

The pitfalls suggest that interbody cage fusion is a favorable option, as initiated by Bagby according to the principle of distraction-compression published in 1988 (2). In his initial work, Bagby performed fusion on horses with Wobbler disease, a form of cervical myelopathy, with impressive results. Later he worked with Kuslich, who in 1993 presented the first clinical results of use of a threaded lumbar titanium cage and local (autologous) bone graft—BAK-L (3,16). The cervical implant (BAK-C), in 1994, was a further development. I have used both devices since 1995 and with Leclercq submitted a paper on rationale of interbody fusion in 357 cervical and lumbar operations (20).

The BAK-C device is a cylindrical implant stabilized with tension forces of the anulus fibrosus and vertebral ligaments after adapted distraction (Bagby's distraction-compression principle) and precise preparation of the bleeding bone bed with a drill and tap into the vertebral end plates. Threads on the implant provide autostabilization better than that obtained with devices that are simply impacted (7,16). Local autologous graft is the osteoinductive material within the cage. It is obtained by means of decompression, use of a bone-collecting reamer, and self-packing during implant screwing.

Compared with a bone dowel, a titanium cage is noncompressible. The cage separates the mechanical and biologic properties of the interbody graft during healing to avoid collapse, expulsion, and pseudarthrosis. In vitro testing indicates better stability than is obtained with conventional grafting techniques. Histologic and radiologic analysis of use of the cage in operations on animals has shown good fusion (2,3). A biomechanical study by Butts et al. (7) confirmed segmental motion stabilization during implantation of rigid cylindrical spacer in a distracted disc space. The study also shows greater stiffness of the instrumented segment, suggesting accelerated degeneration at the adjacent level, as occurs with other fixation systems. Distraction with restoration of disc height in the degenerative spine increases foraminal volume and contributes to nerve root decompression (9).

The data presented are from an observational study representing my 4-year experience with the BAK-C device in 146 consecutive operations, 136 for cervical radiculopathy and 10 for cervical myelopathy. Indications for operation are discogenic neck and arm-shoulder pain with or without neurologic deficit at one or two levels between C3 and C7-T1. Persistent or recurrent pain after previously failed surgery or pseudarthrosis is also a good indication (20). Active infection, severe osteoporosis, considerable traumatic subluxation, and vertebral tumors are excluded.

The operative technique is similar to classic discectomy with decompression in a slightly lordotic neck position. Adapted distraction is the most important step in this operation. It allows restoration disc height with foraminal opening, segmental stabilization with correction of kyphosis and listhesis at the treated level (anulus tension) and the adjacent level (vertebral ligament tension). Distraction requires some feeling, and overdistraction can cause postoperative pain due to neural stretching and ligamental disruption. Insufficient distraction, however, suggests cage migration. Another consideration is to perform symmetric drilling to avoid end-plate weakening, mainly in operations on elderly women with osteoporosis, such as the patient in the series who needed early reoperation with plate fixation. Another technical fault is too-short reaming, which allows bone threads to be torn when the cage if inserted, as happened in the patient in this series who underwent reoperation because of anterior implant migration.

Operative time and hospital stay are shorter for the cage procedure than for the Cloward and Smith-Robinson procedures. Patients do not have iliac pain and do not need a cervical collar.

Clinical outcome is good to excellent after 95% of operations for cervical radiculopathy but only 50% of operation for myelopathy. Many patients with myelopathy have a stenotic canal (30% in this series), indicating the need for another decompressive operation such as laminectomy or corpectomy. This second operation, consisting of multilevel decompression, is offered to patients who have insufficient improvement after the most affected level is treated by means of interbody decompression and fusion. Persistent or recurrent stenosis found at follow-up MRI 6 months after the operation allows posterior decompression as the anterior column has fused. Unrelieved myelopathy already may have been associated with a spinal cord lesion (hyperintensity) at preoperative MRI. Operation at this stage can only prevent further neurologic deterioration.

Radiologic results are more difficult to analyze, especially at MRI, when a metallic implant is used than when a bone dowel or carbon cage is used. The degree of bone fusion as seen on dynamic lateral radiographs (no instability, no radiolucency around the device) is 90% at 6 months and 100% at 1 year, when bridging bone regularly appears around the cage. Bone inside the implant with similar density to the vertebral body can be seen only with CT bone scanning. Substantial kyphosis (greater than 10 degrees) and pseudarthrosis did not occur in this series, a finding different from results in the literature (1,5,14,27). I have found that 1- to 2-mm subsidence of the implant has occurred by the 1-year follow-up evaluation, when bone union is completed. Cage- or instrument-related complications did not occur in this study. The only device explanted during two-level corpectomy had impressive fusion that was not well detected with imaging.

CONCLUSION

Immediate stability with good clinical response, no graft-related morbidity, and decreased operative time and hospital stay are the advantages of use of the BAK-C implant compared with traditional fusion systems. This 4-year experience with BAK-C seems promising so far, but long-term follow-up in a multicenter study is needed.

REFERENCES

1. Baba H, Furusewa N, Imura S, et al. Late radiographic findings after anterior cervical fusion for spondylotic myelopathy. *Spine* 1993;18:2167–2173.
2. Bagby GW. Arthrodesis by the distraction-compression method using a stainless steel implant. *Orthopedics* 1988;11:931–944.
3. Bagby GW. Cages métalliques intersomatiques filetées pour arthrodèses rachidiennes. In: Duparc J, Schreiber A, Troisier O, eds. *Instabilités vertébrales lombaires.*Paris: Expansion Scientifique Française, 1995.
4. Bohlman HH, Esmont FJ. Surgical techniques of anterior decompression and fusion for spinal cord injuries. *Clin Orthop* 1981;154:57–67.
5. Boni M, Denaro V. Traitement chirurgical des cervicarthroses. Révision à distance (2–13 ans) chez les premiers cas opérés par voie antérieure. *Rev Chir Orthop* 1982;68:269–280..
6. Brunon J, Fuentes JM. Chirurgie antérieure et antéro-latérale du rachis cervical inférieur. *Neurochirurgie* 1996;42:105–122.
7. Butts MK, Kuslich SD, Bechold JE. Biomechanical analysis of a new method for spinal interbody fixation. In: Erdman A, ed. *Advances in Bioengineering*, Boston, 1987.
8. Cahill DW, Sonstein W. Anterior cervical instrumentation. *Tech Neurosurg* 1999;5:133–145.
9. Chen D, Fay LA, Lok J, et al. Increasing neuroforaminal volume by anterior interbody distraction in degenerative lumbar spine. *Spine* 1995;20:74–79.
10. Cloward RB. The anterior approach for removal of ruptured cervical disks. *J Neurosurg* 1958;15:602–617.
11. De Bowes RM, Grant BD, Bagby GW, et al. Cervical vertebral interbody fusion in the horse: a comparative study of bovine xenografts and autografts supported by stainless steel baskets. *Am J Vet Res* 1984;45:191–199.
12. Ducker TB, Zeidman SM. Cervical disk diseases, II: operative procedures. *Neurosurg Q* 1992;2:144–163.
13. Ebersold MJ, Pare MC, Lynn MQ. Surgical treatment for cervical spondylitic myelopathy. *J Neurosurg* 1995;82:745–751.
14. Fuentes JM. Les complications de la chirurgie par voie antérieure du rachis cervical. In: Saillant G, Laville C eds. *Echecs et complications de la chirurgie du rachis:* chirurgie de reprise. Sauramps Médical 1995:161–177.
15. Graham JJ. Complications of cervical spine surgery: a five-year report on a survey of the membership of the Cervical Spine Research Society by the Morbidity and Mortality Committee. *Spine* 1989;14:1046–1050.
16. Kuslich SD, Oxland TR, Jansen RC, et al. The BAK interbody fusion system: early clinical results of treatment for chronic low back pain. Presented at the North American Spine Society, San Diego, 1993.
17. Leclercq TA. Clinical results and rationale for lumbar interbody fusion with threaded titanium cages. *Spinal Surg* 1998;12:1–9.
18. Luitjes WF. Cervical interbody fusion with BAK-C cages. In: Gunzburg R, Szpalski M eds. *Whiplash injuries.* Philadelphia: Lippincott-Raven, 1998:259–269.
19. Matgé G. Anterior interbody fusion with BAK-cage in cervical spondylosis. *Acta Neurochir (Wien)* 1998; 140:1–8.
20. Matgé G, Leclercq TA. Rationale for interbody fusion with threaded titanium cages at cervical and lumbar levels: results on 357 cases. *Acta Neurochir (Wien)* 2000;142:425–434.
21. Mc Lellen, Tew J, Mayfield FH. Complications of surgery of the anterior spine. *Clin Neurosurg* 1976;23: 424–434.
22. Senter HJ, Kortyna R, Kemp WR. Anterior cervical discectomy with hydroxylapatite fusion. *Neurosurgery* 1989;25:39–43.
23. Smith GW, Robinson RA. The treatment of certain cervical spine disorders by anterior removal of the intervertebral disc and interbody fusion. *J Bone Joint Surg Am* 1958;40:607–623.
24. Teramoto T, Johmori K, Takatsu T, et al. Long-term results of the anterior cervical spondylodesis. *Neurosurgery* 1994;35:64–68.
25. Traynelis VC. Anterior and posterior stabilization of the cervical spine. *Neurosurgery Q* 1992;2:59–76.
26. Watters WC, Levinthal R. Anterior cervical discectomy with and without fusion. *Spine* 1994;19:2343–2347.
27. Whitehill R, Raynoff J, Ono K. Report of the Morbidity and the Mortality Committee. Presented at the 18th Annual Meeting of the Cervical Spine Research Society, San Antonio, November 28–December 1, 1990.
28. Zeidman SM, Ducker TB. Cervical disk diseases, I: treatment options and outcomes. *Neurosurgery Q* 1992;2: 116–143.

The Degenerative Cervical Spine,
edited by Marek Szpalski and Robert Gunzburg
Lippincott Williams & Wilkins, Philadelphia © 2001.

25

Evaluation of a New Monocortical Screw for Anterior Cervical Fusion and Plating by a Combined Biomechanical and Clinical Study

Tobias Pitzen, *Hans-Joachim Wilke, Wolfhard Caspar, *Lutz Claes, Wolf-Ingo Steudel

*Neurosurgical Department, University of Saarland, 66421 Homburg/Saar, *Department of Orthopaedic Research and Biomechanics, University of Ulm, 89081 Ulm, Germany*

MATERIAL AND METHODS
RESULTS
    Biomechanical Study • Clinical Study
DISCUSSION
CONCLUSION

After Cloward (6) and Smith and Robinson (14), Orozco and Llovet (10) in 1971 were the first to describe additional anterior cervical plating. Today anterior cervical fusion with plating has become a widely accepted technique in stabilization of the cervical spine for a variety of indications (1,2,12,15). The stabilization system, the special instruments, and the technical steps developed by Caspar (1) can be described as a classic cervical plating procedure. One of the main points in the development of this technique has been bicortical fixation of the plate. Stability is provided by means of anchoring the screws in the posterior cortex. This was shown in three studies (4,5,13) in which monocortical screw fixation with anterior cervical fusion and plating (ACFP) failed to achieve the stability of bicortical fixation. However, there is a risk of perforating the dura and damaging the spinal cord with bicortical screw fixation—even if intraoperative fluoroscopy is used (9,12).Therefore the most logical step for further evolution of ACFP had to be development of a monocortical screw that provides the same stability as fixation with the bicortical Caspar screw. The purpose of our biomechanical study was to evaluate the stability of such a screw for monocortical use.

MATERIAL AND METHODS

The classic Caspar plate for anterior osteosynthesis of the cervical spine is a trapezoidal, titanium plate that can be bent to the patient's lordosis (Fig. 25.1). Thus far it has been fixed onto the anterior aspect of the cervical spine with titanium, non–self-tapping

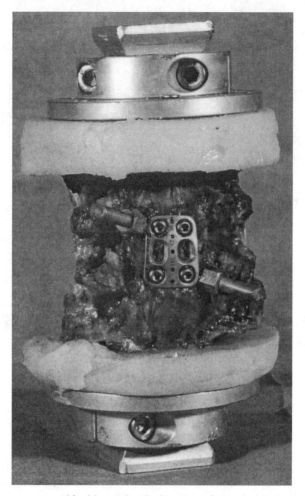

FIG. 25.1. Specimen prepared for biomechanical testing after anterior cervical fusion and plating. End plates of C4 and C7 fixed with polymethyl methacrylate. Modified Schanz screws are fixed in C5 and C6 for the motion analysis system.

screws also placed into the posterior cortex of the vertebral body. The new screw for monocortical fixation is a self-tapping, conical, screw 14, 15, 16, 17, or 19 mm long with an outer diameter of 4.0 mm and an inner diameter of 2.2 mm at the tip and increasing to 2.7 mm at the head (Fig. 25.2). The classic bicortical screw is not self-tapping, is available in 16 lengths from 10 to 28 mm with a constant outer diameter of 3.5 and an inner diameter of 2.2 mm. Both screws are made of titanium alloy with a corrundum-blasted surface over one third of the length at the tip.

Twelve fresh human cadaveric spinal segments (C4-7) were removed, frozen, and prepared for biomechanical testing. Great care was taken to avoid damaging any of the bony structures, the joint complexes, or the ligaments. The end plates of C4 and C7 were cleaned of fibrous material and three to five screws were drilled through the upper end plate of C4 and the lower end plate of C7. Lateral and anteroposterior radiographs were obtained to detect fractures, tumorous destruction, or spondylodiscitis. Bone mineral density (BMD) was determined to document bone quality (Stratec XCT-960A, Birken-

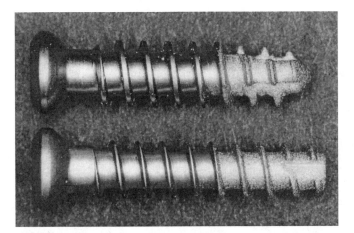

FIG. 25.2. The two types of screw. Monocortical (*top*) and and bicortical.w

feld, Germany). For matched-pair analysis (Table 25.1), specimens were selected according to the criteria for BMD, which was the main criterion influencing fixation of the screws (18). Mean BMD among patients who received monocortical screws was 216.2 mg/cm^3; among the patients who received bicortical screws mean BMD was 211.8 mg/cm^3. The mean ages of the two groups of patients were similar—55.5 years for the monocortical group and 56.2 years for the bicortical group. Overall mean BMD was 214 mg/cm^3, range 135 to 264 mg/cm^3.

The upper end plate of C4 and the lower end plate of C7 were anchored in polymethyl methacrylate (Fig. 25.1) to mount it in the spine tester (16). Testing of the specimen was performed without preload in flexion-extension, axial rotation (left, right), and lateral bending (left, right) in three cycles with pure moments of ±2.5 Nm (15,17). The range of motion (ROM) and neutral zone of the instrumented segment were documented with a motion analysis system (cmstrao V. 1.0; Zebris, Isny, Germany) fixed by screws in the anterior aspects of C5 and C6, and in C7 at the bottom of the spine tester (Fig. 25.3). The motion analysis system is ultrasound based. A single element of the system looks like a cross. The cross is fixed in the vertebral bodies of C5, C6, and C7. Each cross carries three ultrasound sources at its upper surface and three microphones at its lower surface. Thus, two crosses can communicate for measuring the distance between them. From these data a computer is used to calculate rotation and translation in each segment. The accuracy of the system is as high as 0.2 degrees without time-dependent drift.

TABLE 25.1. *Results of matched-pair analysis of two groups of C4-7 specimens*

	Monocortical instrumentation specimen		Bicortical instrumentation specimen	
Pair	Mineral bone density (mg/cm^3)	Age (yr)	Mineral bone density (mg/cm^3)	Age (yr)
1	261	35	211	67
2	243	63	264	39
3	208	86	232	65
4	241	54	230	49
5	209	35	161	66
6	135	60	173	51
Mean	216.2	55.5	211.8	56.2

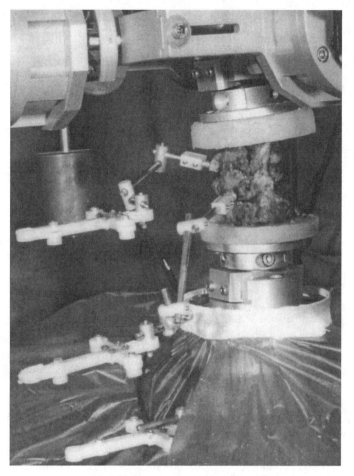

FIG. 25.3. Custom spine tester with specimen. The specimen has been fixed with polymethyl methacrylate plates and screws to the spine tester. Zebris system is fixed with screws in C5 and C6 and at the bottom of the spine tester.

The specimens were tested first intact then after complete discectomy with removal of the posterior longitudinal ligament and again after stabilization of this segment with bone graft and plating with either monocortical or bicortical screws. The bicortical screws were fixed in the posterior cortex, and the monocortical screws were chosen to be as long as possible without perforating the posterior cortex. All specimens were tested three times in each stage and each loading mode of the analysis but only the third cycle was evaluated. Statistical analyses were performed with the Mann-Whitney test with a P value less than .05 considered statistically significant.

The clinical study was performed as a prospective study involving 30 patients (15 men, 15 women, mean age 46 years, mean follow-up period 14.6 months) with cervical myelopathy (24 patients), radiculopathy (5 patients), or myeloradiculopathy (1 patient) caused by degenerative disease in one cervical motion segment (Table 25.2). None had severe instability. The surgical procedure was performed as discectomy and removal of the posterior longitudinal ligament, autologous bone graft fusion, and plating. Intraoper-

TABLE 25.2. *Clinical data on 30 patients*

Characteristic	Value
No. of men	15
No. of women	15
Mean age (yr)	46
Location (no. of patients)	
C4-5	4
C5-6	13
C6-7	12
C7-T1	1
No. of levels fused	
1	30
Disease (no. of patients)	
Radiculopathy	24
Myelopathy	5
Radiculomyelopathy	1

ative fluoroscopy was used to chose the optimal screw length. The screw should be as long as possible without penetrating the posterior cortical shell (Fig. 25.4).

A total of 120 screws were used; 118 screws were the new monocortical screws described earlier. Two screws were so-called oversize-rescue screws designed by Caspar. The rescue screws and eight monocortical screws, which had to be anchored with bone cement, had to be used, because sufficient screw torque of at least 40 Ncm could not be obtained in these cases. All patients wore a soft collar for 6 weeks after the operation. Clinical and radiologic (anteroposterior and lateral radiographs) examinations were performed immediately and 10 days, 3 weeks, 6 weeks, 3 months, 6 months, 12 months, and 18 months after the operation. Fusion was assessed with anteroposterior and lateral radiographs according to the criteria of bony bridging between the graft and the adjacent vertebral bodies and the absence of implant or graft dislocation. Lateral radiographs in flexion and extension were obtained when solid bony fusion was documented to show

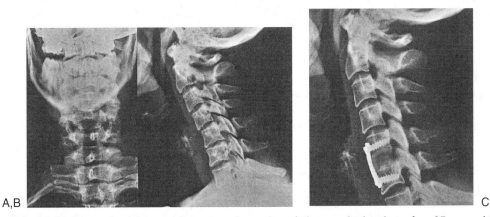

A,B   C

FIG. 25.4. Anteroposterior and lateral radiographs of the cervical spine of a 35-year-old woman who underwent anterior cervical autologous bone graft fusion and plating with monocortical screws at C5-6. **A,B:** Preoperative images. **C:** Images obtained 6 months after the operation. The screws are as long as possible but do not perforate the posterior cortical shell.

stability of the construct. Radiographic follow-up examinations were performed by an independent radiologist. The clinical follow-up examinations were performed by one of the authors (T.P.).

RESULTS

Biomechanical Study

Statistical analysis showed that ACFP provided the same stabilization for both groups of patients (Fig. 25.5). Mean ROM in the monocortical group was 9.8 ± 2.7 degrees for flexion-extension, 10.3 ± 4.0 degrees for rotation, and 8.1 ± 2.9 degrees for lateral bending. Mean ROM in the bicortical group was 10.6 ± 2.0 degrees for flexion-extension, 9.9 ± 3.5 degrees for rotation, and 10.6 ± 2.9) degrees for bending in the intact specimen. ROM increased after discectomy and resection of the posterior longitudinal ligament at C5-6. In the monocortical group the increase was 18.3 ± 4.3 degrees for flexion-extension, 12.9 ± 5.5 degrees for rotation, and 10 ± 4.1 degrees for bending. In the bicortical group the increase was 16.1 ± 4.3 degrees for flexion-extension, 12.4 ± 3.4 degrees for rotation, and 13.6 ± 4.2 degrees for bending. ACFP made the segment stiffer than it was in the intact specimen with slightly better results in the monocortical group of 1.2 ± 1.0 degrees for flexion-extension, 2.3 ± 1.2 degrees for rotation, and 1.4 ± 1.0 degrees for bending compared with 3.2 ± 3.8 degrees for flexion-extension, 3.6 ± 3.2 degrees for rotation, and 2.6 ± 2.7) degrees for bending in the bicortical group.

Clinical Study

Fusion had occurred in all patients at latest 12 months after the operation. No graft- or hardware-related complication such as graft height reduction, graft collapse, graft extrusion, graft compression fracture, screw breakage, or screw back-out occurred in any of the patients.

DISCUSSION

The results of this biomechanical matched-pair analysis and clinical study show that the new screw for monocortical fixation of Caspar plates provides the same stability as

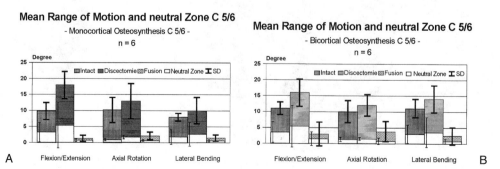

FIG. 25.5. Mean ROM and neutral zone with standard deviation. **A:** Monocortical screws. **B:** Bicortical screws. The values represent the sum of flexion plus extension, axial rotation left plus right, and lateral bending left plus right.

the classic bicortical screw but avoids the risks of bicortical fixation (dural perforation, spinal cord damage, epidural hematoma). The biomechanical test was performed on 12 cadaveric specimens of C4-7 human spine with a mean BMD of 214 mg/cm^3, range 135 to 264 mg/cm^3. Compared with results of another study (19), these findings are in the range of normal quality. The pure moments without preload and disregard of muscle forces in the study do not represent actual physiologic loading of the cervical spine. However, because this physiologic load is not known, the loading conditions used are widely accepted and even recommended for standardized testing (8,11,17). The clinical part of the study was performed after biomechanical results showed that there is no significant difference in the initial stability of both constructs.

Three earlier studies dealing with the evaluation of monocortical screw fixation in ACFP did not show stability comparable with that of bicortical screw fixation. Clausen et al. (5) compared the Caspar system with bicortical screws with the cervical spine locking plate system with monocortical locking screws. In that study of a model of complete C5-6 instability, the Caspar system with bicortical screws was superior to the system with the monocortical screws. Chen (4) compared the stability of ACFP using a porcine model with an H plate fixed monocortically and bicortically. The results showed comparable stability in both groups before cyclic loading; however, after cyclic loading bicortically fixed screws rendered additional stability. Ryken et al. (13) fixed a Caspar plate with monocortical and bicortical screws to compare stabilizing potentials. Monocortical screw placement gave inadequate stabilization in one half of the specimens.

The results of our study are in contrast to the results of Chen (4), Clausen et al. (5), and Ryken et al. (13). This difference may have occurred because different-shaped implants were used in the studies. The new implant we used has a special design—a self-threading screw with a conical inner diameter by which the cancellous bone is compressed when the screw is inserted. This may cause higher screw torque. We also chose to use the longest possible screw that would not perforate the posterior cortical shell to achieve maximal contact area between screw and bone. Finally, the designs of the studies with which our study is compared are different from our design. We did not use cyclic loading (4) for biomechanical testing of the implants. Repeated cyclic loading may be useful in biomechanical testing to simulate the "worst case." Cyclic loading, however, cannot simulate the biologic process of bony fusion in a segment, and the influence of an external orthosis is neglected completely. Whether cyclic loading is appropriate to mimic stress is not clear. Constant load is applied to the construct in conditions of cyclic loading, whereas a sudden increase in complex moments and forces causes failure of the construct in a stress situation. Thus clinical data seem to be more important for analyzing stress.

Because the results of the biomechanical part of the study showed no significant difference concerning the initial stability of both constructs, a prospective clinical study involving 30 patients was performed. At the latest follow-up evaluation, at which fusion was documented, no hardware- or graft-related complication had occurred. These clinical data underline the importance of initial stability in biomechanical testing. It seems to be a sufficient predictor of stability of osteosynthetic spinal constructs. Thus additional clinical data, as reported herein, seem to be needed to emphasize the results of the biomechanical part of the study.

Since its first description by Orozco and Llovet (10) and development by Caspar (1), ACFP has become a widely accepted technique in cervical spinal surgery for a variety of indications. Trauma, tumor, spondylodiscitis, and rheumatoid arthritis leading to segmental instability of the cervical spine all were thought to be indications for anterior decompression, fusion, and plating (1,2,12,15). But for degenerative pathologic changes, additional plating still is considered excessive treatment, although the rate of reoperation is markedly decreased with plating (3,7). There are arguments against the use of additional plating: longer operating time, need for intensive radiographic monitoring, and, when bicortical screws are used for plate fixation, the need for penetrating the posterior cortex and increased risk of dural perforation, epidural hematoma, and damage to the spinal cord (9,12). Three studies (3,4,13), however, have shown that the use of monocortical screws for ACFP leads to a drastic reduction in stability within the fused segment compared with ACFP with bicortical screws, so bicortical fixation should be favored in ACFP. The new device can be recommended for ACFP in the management of degenerative disease of the cervical spine. However, because of the design of the study, the results should be limited at this time to surgical therapy for monosegmental degenerative disc disease.

CONCLUSION

ACFP provides immediate stabilization, which leads to substantial reduction in graft-related complications, such as pseudarthrosis, graft collapse, and dislocation. Bicortical fixation has been favored in the past, because all former studies documented markedly better stabilization when bicortical screws were used for plate fixation. Use of bicortical screws, however, calls for penetration of the posterior cortex, which carries risk of dural perforation, epidural hematoma, and spinal cord damage. Although the use of intraoperative radiographic monitoring is recommended for monocortical screw fixation, the radiographs can be obtained more quickly. The results of this study showed that there is no statistically significant difference in stability within the fused segment when monocortical or bicortical Caspar screws are used for ACFP. Monocortical screw fixation with these special screws can therefore be recommended.

ACKNOWLEDGMENTS

The authors thank Mrs. Bettina Jungkunz for technical assistance. This study was supported by Aesculap AG, Tuttlingen, Germany.

REFERENCES

1. Caspar W. Die ventrale interkorporale Stabilisierung mit der HWS-Trapez-Osteosyntheseplatte: Indikationen, Technik, Ergebnisse. *Orthop Praxis* 1984;12:981–988.
2. Caspar W, Barbier D, Klara PM Anterior cervical fusion and Caspar plate stabilization for cervical trauma. *Neurosurgery* 1989;25:491–502.
3. Caspar W, Geisler FH, Pitzen T, et al. Anterior cervical plate stabilization in one- and two-level degenerative disease: overtreatment or benefit ? *J Spinal Disord* 1998;11:1–11.
4. Chen IH. Biomechanical evaluation of subcortical versus bicortical screw purchase in anterior cervical plating. *Acta Neurochir (Wien)* 1996;138:167–173.
5. Clausen JD, Ryken TC, Traynelis VC, et al. Biomechanical evaluation of Caspar and cervical spine locking plate systems in a cadaveric model. *J Neurosurg* 1996;84:1039–45.
6. Cloward RB. The anterior approach for removal of ruptured dics. *J Neurosurg* 1958;15:602–617.
7. Geisler FH, Caspar W, Pitzen T, et al. Reoperation in patients after anterior cervical plate stabilization in degenerative disease. *Spine* 1998;23:911–920.
8. Goel VK, Wilder DG, Pope MH, et al. Controversy: biomechanical testing of the spine—load-controlled versus displacement-controlled analysis. *Spine* 1988;20:2354–2357.
9. Karasick D. Anterior cervical spine fusion:Struts, plugs and plates. *Skeletal Radiol* 1993;22:85–94.
10. Orozco DR, Llovet TR. Osteosintesis en las lesiones traumaticas y degeneratives de la columna vertebral. *Rev Traumatol Chir Rehabil* 1971;1:45–52.
11. Panjabi MM. Biomechanical evaluation of spinal fixation devices, I: a conceptual framework. *Spine* 1988;13:1129–1134.
12. Papadopoulos MS. Anterior cervical instrumentation. *Clin Neurosurgery* 1993;40:273–285.

13. Ryken TC, Goel VK, Clausen JD, et al. Assessment of unicortical and bicortical fixation in a quasistatic cadaveric model: role of bone mineral density and screw torque. *Spine* 1995;20:1861–1867.
14. Smith GW, Robinson RA. The treatment of cervical spine disorders by anterior removal of the intervertebral disc and interbody fusion. *J Bone Joint Surg Am* 1958;40:607–624.
15. Tippits R, Apfelbaum R. Anterior cervical fusion with the Caspar instrumentation system. *Neurosurgery* 1989; 22:1008–1013.
16. Wilke HJ, Claes L, Schmitt H, et al. An universal spine tester for in vitro experiments with muscle force simulation. *Eur Spine J* 1994;3:91–97.
17. Wilke HJ, Wenger K, Claes L. Testing criteria for spinal implants: recommendations for the standardization of in vitro stability testing of spinal implants. *Eur Spine J* 1998;7:148–154.
18. Zink PM. Performance of ventral spondylodesis screws in cervical vertebrae of varying bone mineral density. *Spine* 1996;21:45–52.
19. Zink PM, Samii M, Luedemann, et al. Accuracy of single-energy quantitative computed tomography in the assessment of bone mineral density of cervical vertebrae. *Eur Radiol* 1997;7:1436–1440.

The Degenerative Cervical Spine,
edited by Marek Szpalski and Robert Gunzburg
Lippincott Williams & Wilkins, Philadelphia © 2001.

26

Upper Cervical Spine Fusion (C1-2)

Claes Olerud

Department of Orthopedics, Uppsala University Hospital, SE-75185 Uppsala, Sweden

---

PATIENTS AND METHODS
RESULTS
  Complications • Mortality • Follow-up
CASE PRESENTATION
CONCLUSIONS

Upper cervical fusion (C1-2 fusion) is most frequently indicated in the management of fractures and nonunion of the odontoid process and rheumatoid C1-2 subluxation. Other rarer indications are ligament laxity, such as Down or Marfan syndrome, or congenital deformity, such as os odontoideum.

The traditional wiring technique described by Gallie (3) is associated with an unacceptably high frequency of healing disturbances, mainly secondary displacement, graft resorption, and fibrous union (nonunion) (2). The principle of stability with the Gallie and other wiring techniques is that a cerclage wire under tension compresses the C1 and C2 arches against a solid block of bone (Fig. 26.1). Stability relies on the integrity of this bone block and its ability to withstand compressive forces. This is necessary for preservation of tension in the wire. In many patients with osteoporosis, bone quality does not allow optimal fixation with these techniques, so additional external fixation, such as a halo vest, frequently has to be added. In the Gallie technique, the wiring is merely posterior, which gives reasonably good stability against anterior or posterior rotational forces around a frontal axis, that is, flexion and extension. Translation along the frontal axis and translation and rotation around the sagittal and axial axes are poorly controlled.

The Brooks (1) technique consists of two sets of posterior wiring in different planes (Fig. 26.2). Thus a triangular configuration is constructed that makes this technique more stable than the Gallie fixation (4). However, the technique still relies on a structural bone graft, and passage of sublaminar wires under the C2 arch carries neurologic risk.

Various hook devices have been introduced, such as the Halifax clamp, but the stability and longevity of these systems have not proved ideal for C1-2 fixation (6). In these techniques a structural bone graft is used to produce the necessary counterforce to avoid nonphysiologic hyperextension of the motion segment, which would occur if the C1 and C2 arches were merely compressed against each other. Such hyperextension causes corresponding hyperflexion in the adjacent segments, which may increase the risk of degeneration or pain there. An other disadvantage of hook devices is that these techniques are strictly posterior and have the same inferior biomechanical properties as the wiring techniques.

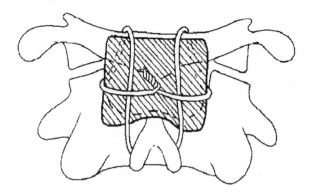

FIG. 26.1. The Gallie technique for posterior C1-2 fusion. The stability of the fixation relies on the tension of the wire, which depends on the integrity of the bone block. This is a problem because patients who need C1-2 fusion frequently have severe osteoporosis. The fixation is strictly posterior. It provides good stabilization against extension-flexion moment only.

When transarticular C1-2 screws are added to the Gallie wiring technique, the stability has been shown to increase. The frequency of solid union also increases, but a structural graft still is needed for tension on the the the wire (4,5). In an attempt to improve stabilization of the C1-2 articulation, a special instrument, the C1 claw device, has been developed (Fig. 26.3). The idea was to combine use of transarticular screws with posterior fixation of the C1 and C2 arches that did not require a structural bone graft. The transarticular screws give excellent stabilization against translational forces along all the three orthogonal axes and against rotation around the sagittal and axial axes. The posterior component stabilizes against rotation around the frontal axis. Thus forces in all six degrees of freedom are counteracted, which should result in superior biomechanical properties and a high frequency of solid union.

The implant consists of two counterpositioned hooks that form a claw designed to grasp the C1 arch. The shaft portion of the claw is built of two hemicircular profiles that together form a 3.5-mm rod. When the device is connected to a transarticular C1-2 screw,

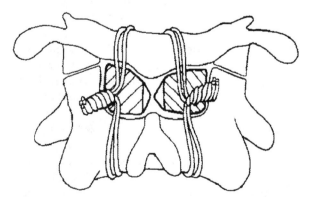

FIG. 26.2. The Brooks technique of posterior C1-2 fusion. The two posterior bone grafts are positioned at an angle to each other. The triangular configuration has better biomechanical properties than the Gallie technique, but the technique still necessitates use of a structural bone graft, and passage of sublaminar wires under C2 is risky.

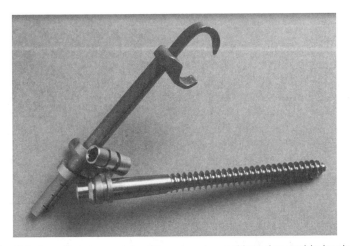

FIG. 26.3. The C1 claw device consists of two counterpositioned movable hooks designed to grip the C1 arch. The shaft of the claw device is connected to the bone screw with a screw link and a double-loop connector, which are the basic components of the Olerud cervical spine fixation system. When assembled, all parts of the device are mechanically locked to each other to form a rigid implant.

the claw is mechanically locked. The device is part of the Olerud cervical fixation system and combines anterior and posterior stabilization in the same fixation device.

The system has been subjected to biomechanical and clinical testing. The biomechanical studies were conducted in collaboration with Dr. Thomas Henriques, Uppsala, Sweden, and Dr. Brian Cunningham, Baltimore, Maryland. The results indicate that the device is superior to the Gallie technique with or without the addition of transarticular screws. The clinical studies were conducted in collaboration with Dr. Michael Cornefjord and Dr. Thomas Henriques, Uppsala, Sweden. A brief preliminary report of one clinical study is presented.

PATIENTS AND METHODS

The series consisted of 26 consecutively registered patients (14 women) with a mean age of 73 ± 14 years (range, 37 to 93 years) treated by means of posterior upper cervical fusion. The indications were odontoid fractures for 18 patients, rheumatoid C1-2 instability for 6, odontoid nonunion for 1, and os odontoideum with myelopathy for 1 patient. Two of the patients with a fracture also had concomitant spinal disease: 1 had rheumatoid arthritis, and the other had ankylosing spondylitis. The patient with nonunion also had rheumatoid arthritis. Five different surgeons performed the operations.

Follow-up evaluations were performed with clinical examinations and plain radiographs, and the follow-up period lasted an average of 13 ± 8 months. The radiographs were evaluated for signs of secondary displacement, instrument failure, and fusion healing. Bony union was evaluated according to the following three-point scale: Definitely healed—bone trabeculae bridging the fracture or fusion area; not healed but without signs of healing disturbances—bone trabeculae could not be seen bridging the fracture or fusion area. but no signs of mechanical failure of the fixation were present; established nonunion—fracture line still visible, radiolucent zone across the fusion mass, radiolucent zone around a screw, implant failure, or change in alignment or signs indicating nonunion.

RESULTS

Complications

There were no neurologic or vascular complications related to surgery, but three perioperative problems occurred. One patient was accidentally extubated during the operation after placement of the transarticular screws. She was rapidly turned around and reintubated, and the operation was continued. The episode did not result in any negative consequences to the patient. In two patients the transarticular screws cut out dorsolaterally in the isthmus of C2 during the operation, and there was insufficient purchase as a result. For one patient the situation could be solved by redirecting the insufficient screw. For the other the problem was resolved with pedicle screws in C3 as distal anchorage for the fixation. Minor postoperative complications occurred in three patients. One was successfully treated for urinary tract infection, one for oral fungal infection, and one for otitis media.

Mortality

Three patients died of unrelated causes 1 (intestinal obstruction), 4 (malignant tumor), and 8 (pneumonia) months postoperatively. At the time of death there were no signs of complications related to the neck surgery in any of these patients. No follow-up evaluation was conducted with the two patients with the shortest survival times. The patient who survived for 8 months was judged as not having healed but without signs of healing disturbances on the 6-month follow-up radiographs.

Follow-up Data

No secondary displacement have occurred, and no reoperation has been performed in the series. One patient could not be contacted for follow-up data collection. He died 25 months after the operation of myocardial infarction. According to his relatives, the patient had not had problems related to the cervical spine at the time of death. Two patients have undergone 3 but not 6 months of follow-up evaluation. Both have not healed but have no of healing disturbances. Nine patients have undergone 6 to 12 months of follow-up evaluation. All have radiographic signs of healing. Twelve patients have undergone 12 to 27 months of follow-up evaluation. All have radiographic signs of healing. In one of the patients with odontoid fracture, the fracture itself has healed, but the bone graft of the posterior fusion has resorbed. No dislocation has occurred, and the internal fixation device is in an unchanged position without signs of loosening. The clinical course of the patient has been uneventful.

CASE PRESENTATION

Radiographs obtained 1 year an operation on a 60-year-old woman with a displaced odontoid fracture sustained in a traffic accident are shown in Fig. 26.4. Treatment consisted of posterior fusion with the C1 claw device. The transarticular screws bridge the central portion of the C1-2 joints, and the C1 claws grasp the posterior arch of C1. Fusion was achieved with autologous bone chips from the iliac crest.

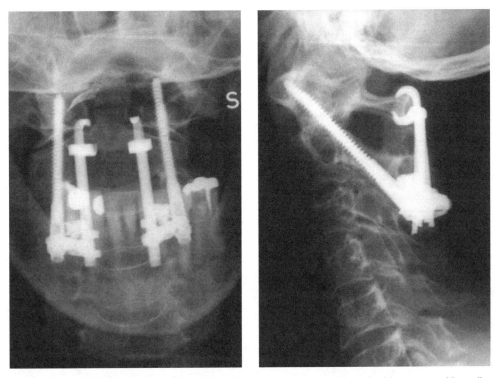

FIG. 26.4. Radiographs obtained 1 year after operation on a 60-year-old woman with a displaced odontoid fracture sustained in a traffic accident. Treatment consisted of posterior fusion with a C1 claw device. The transarticular screws bridge the central portion of the C1-2 joint, and the C1 claws grasp the posterior arch of C1. The fusion has been achieved with autologous bone chips from the iliac crest.

CONCLUSIONS

The early results of posterior C1-2 fusion with the C1 claw device of the Olerud cervical fixation system seem promising. No serious complications related to the use of the device have been encountered. Our experience is that this fixation device is quite easy to use. The stability of the implant obviates use of a solid bone block for graft and still results in a high frequency of fusion healing without secondary displacement.

REFERENCES

1. Brooks AL, Jenkins EB. Atlanto-axial arthrodesis by the wedge compression method. *J Bone Joint Surg Am* 1978;60:279–284.
2. Coyne TJ, Fehlings MG, Wallace MC, et al. C1-C2 posterior cervical fusion: long-term evaluation of results and efficacy. *Neurosurgery* 1995;37:688–692.
3. Gallie WE. Fractures and dislocations of the cervical spine. *Am J Surg* 1939;46:495–499.
4. Grob D, Crisco JJ 3d, Panjabi MM, et al. Biomechanical evaluation of four different posterior atlantoaxial fixation techniques. *Spine* 1992;17:480–490.
5. Jeanneret B, Magerl F. Primary posterior fusion C1/2 in odontoid fractures: indications, technique, and results of transarticular screw fixation. *J Spinal Disord* 1992;5:464–475.
6. Statham P, O'Sullivan M, Russell T. The Halifax Interlaminar clamp for posterior cervical fusion: initial experience in the United Kingdom. *Neurosurgery* 1993;32:396–398.

The Degenerative Cervical Spine,
edited by Marek Szpalski and Robert Gunzburg
Lippincott Williams & Wilkins, Philadelphia © 2001.

27

Anterior Cervical Discectomy and Vertebral Interbody Fusion Using a Carbon Fiber Cage with Allograft Bone versus an Iliac Crest Bone Graft

Valère Debois

Department of Neurosurgery, St. Maartens Ziekenhuis, B-2570 Duffel, Belgium

PATIENTS AND METHODS
SURGICAL TECHNIQUE
RESULTS
    Clinical Outcome and Radiologic Results • Complications
CONCLUSION

Cervical disc degeneration is multifactorial, resulting from anatomic, genetic, biomechanical, and electrophysiologic changes. It can lead to two different lesions—soft and hard herniation. Monosegmental cervical disc disease with radiculopathy necessitating operative intervention responds well to anterior disc excision and intervertebral fusion. As in the management of lumbar disc disease, the posterior approach was the main technique. The original descriptions of the anterior approach by Robinson and Smith (11), Cloward (1), and Dereymaeker and Mulier (2–4) in the 1950s recommended intervertebral fusion after removal of the disc. The compressive structures in the spinal canal were not removed. An iliac crest bone graft was used to stabilize the intervertebral space to preserve the height of the disc with secondary decompression of the nerve root. Stabilization by means of fusion would cause the regress compressing osteophytes to regress (5,11). The Cloward (1) technique also involved removal of compressive structures in the spinal canal. Other authors (6–9) emphasized removal of the compressive structures without fusion.

My colleagues and I prefer anterior discectomy and stabilization by means of fusion because we believe that it avoids kyphotic angulation, relieves overloading of the facet joints through restoration of the intervertebral space, reduces the risk of pseudarthrosis and growth of osteophytes, and restores the diameter of the intervertebral foramina.

We initially performed discectomy and fusion with autologous iliac bone graft from February 1989 until December 1995. Donor site morbidity (hematoma, infection, incapacitating pain) and complications at the fusion site (pseudarthrosis, graft dislocation) necessitated development of a new implant. A carbon fiber cage with allograft bone has been used in an attempt to avoid these complications.

TABLE 27.1. *Baseline data on 136 patients with soft cervical disc herniation*

Characteristic	Iliac crest bone graft group (n = 90)	Carbon fiber cage with allograft bone group (n = 46)
No. of men	46	19
No. of women	44	27
Mean age (yr)	43	44.2
Mean symptom duration (mo)	5.6	4.9
Mean follow-up period	2.6 yr	8 mo

PATIENTS AND METHODS

From February 1989 until September 1998, 136 patients with monosegmental soft cervical disc herniation underwent anterior discectomy with intervertebral fusion in our department. Patients with multisegmental or hard disc herniation and myelopathy were excluded. From February 1989 until December 1995, patients underwent discectomy and intervertebral fusion with iliac crest bone grafting. From January 1996 until September 1998 in operations on 46 patients, a carbon fiber cage with allograft bone was used for intervertebral fusion after discectomy. Demographically both groups were quite homogeneous (Table 27.1). As shown in Table 27.2, all patients had neck pain and brachialgia. Motor deficit or reflex changes or sensory deficit were present among 50% to 60% of the patients. Disc levels operated on are shown in Table 27.3. The neuroradiologic diagnosis of cervical root compression was made with computed tomography (CT) and CT after myelography (CTM). Magnetic resonance imaging (MRI) was more often as time went on.

SURGICAL TECHNIQUE

Standard anterior cervical discectomy was performed through a right-sided collar incision. Removal of the herniated disc, opening of the dorsal longitudinal ligament, and decompression of the nerve roots were performed with the aid of an operating microscope. Care was taken to achieve complete removal of the cartilaginous end plates and to prepare the fusion site to ensure maximum surface contact. Vertebral spreaders were used for distraction, and the carbon cage prosthesis with allograft bone was placed or tamped into the interspace with a detachable handle. Correct placement of the cage was confirmed with by intraoperative radioscopy. After meticulous hemostasis, the wound was closed in layers, preferably without leaving a prevertebral Redon drain.

The cage implant is made from long-fiber Hercules AS-4 carbon fibers in a polymer matrix of polyetherketone etherketone (Ultrapeek, DSM, ICI). The cage is square or rectangular and is available in a variety of sizes. The outer cage provides support and has a

TABLE 27.2. *Symptoms and signs*

Symptom or sign	Iliac crest bone graft group (n = 90)	Carbon fiber cage with allograft bone group (n = 46)
Neck pain	90 (100)	46 (100)
Brachialgia	90 (100)	46 (100)
Motor deficit	50 (55.5)	21 (45.6)
Reflex change	40 (44.4)	27 (58.6)
Sensory deficit	50 (55.5)	28 (60.8)

Values are numbers of patients with percentage in parentheses.

TABLE 27.3. *Operated disc level*

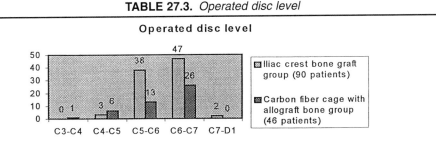

rough design to prevent slippage from the intervertebral space. The hollow inner space contains lyophilized allograft bone to assist bony fusion. The graft contains four titanium bars for radiologic visualization (Osteon).

RESULTS

Clinical Outcome and Radiologic Results

After the operation, all patients were evaluated clinically and radiologically at discharge, 6 weeks and 6 months postoperatively, and at annual examinations thereafter. The patients were evaluated according to the criteria of Odom et al. (10). *Excellent* means no reports of cervical neurologic symptoms, and the patient can continue with their daily occupation. *Good* means there is intermittent discomfort due to cervical abnormalities but it does not interfere with daily work. *Fair* means there is no improvement. *Poor* means symptoms are worse than before surgery. In the iliac crest bone graft group, excellent and good results were obtained by 96.6% of the patients. In the carbon fiber cage with allograft bone group, this percentage was 97.7% (Table 27.4).

Radiologic follow-up evaluation was conducted with plain anteroposterior and lateral cervical spinal radiographs in flexion and extension and in some cases with CT. In the iliac crest bone graft group, 86% of the patients had osseous fusion, and 14% had a pseudarthrosis. Slight kyphosis occurred among 11% of the patients. In the carbon fiber cage and allograft bone group, stable fusion was achieved by all patients. Slight kyphosis was present in 8.6% of the patients (Table 27.5). In many cases there was osseous bridging around the carbon fiber cage and allograft bone when the implant had a smaller diameter than the adjacent vertebral bodies. The appearance of the carbon fiber cage with allograft bone is shown in Figs. 27.1 through 27.3.

Complications

Cervical complications in the iliac crest bone graft group included one case of anterior dislocation of the graft. The patient needed a reoperation. One patient had a prevertebral

TABLE 27.4. *Clinical results (grading system of Odom)*

Result	Iliac crest bone graft group (n = 90)	Carbon fiber cage with allograft bone group (n = 46)
Excellent	73 (81.1)	35 (76.0)
Good	14 (15.5)	10 (21.7)
Fair	3 (3.3)	1 (2.1)
Poor	—	—

Values are numbers of patients with percentages in parentheses.

TABLE 27.5. *Radiologic results of surgery*

Result	Iliac crest bone graft group (n = 90)	Carbon fiber cage with allograft bone group (n = 46)
Osseous fusion	77 (86)	46 (100)
Pseudarthrosis	13 (14)	—
Slight kyphosis	10 (11)	4 (8.6)

Values are numbers of patients with percentages in parentheses.

hematoma, which was evacuated operatively. One patient had a recurrent nerve lesion, and two patients needed operations at a different level. Complications at the iliac crest donor site included 7 cases of infection. Seven other patients had prolonged disabling pain, and 1 patient had meralgia paresthetica. The only complication among the carbon cage allograft bone group was the need for one reoperation at a different level (Table 27.6).

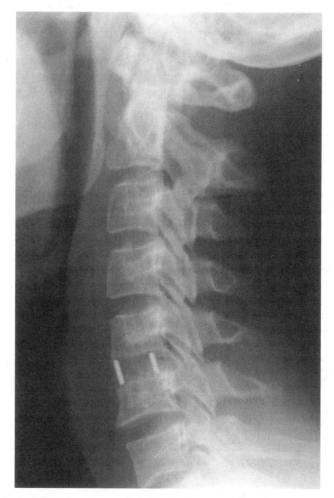

FIG. 27.1. Radiograph obtained immediately after the operation shows vertebral interbody fusion at C5-6 with a carbon fiber cage and allograft bone.

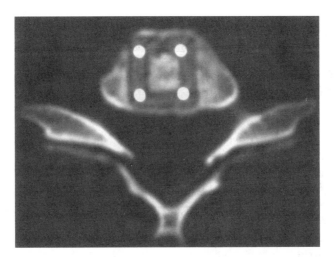

FIG. 27.2. Computed tomographic scan obtained 4 years after operation shows carbon fiber cage with allograft bone graft. Bony formation is present in and around the graft.

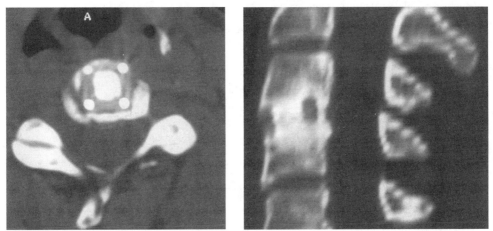

A   B

FIG. 27.3. Axial computed tomographic (CT) scan **(A)** and CT sagittal reconstruction **(B)** 3 years and 10 months after interbody fusion with a carbon fiber cage and allograft bone. Good bony fusion has been achieved.

TABLE 27.6. *Complications*

Complication	Iliac crest bone graft group (n = 90)	Carbon fiber cage with allograft bone group (n = 46)
Cervical spine		
Anterior dislocation of graft	1	—
Hematoma	1	—
Recurrent nerve lesion	1	—
Reoperation at different level	2	1
Iliac crest		
Infection	7	—
Prolonged pain	7	—
Meralgia paraesthetica	1	—

Values are numbers of patients.

CONCLUSION

Donor site morbidity and graft-related problems at the fusion site are frequent complications of cervical discectomy and intervertebral fusion with an iliac crest bone graft. In an attempt to eliminate donor-site problems and maintain acceptable fusion results, my colleagues and I replaced the iliac crest bone graft with a carbon fiber cage and allograft bone in the surgical treatment of patients with soft cervical disc herniation. The results showed that the clinical and neurologic outcomes were the same for both groups. All patients treated with a carbon fiber cage allograft implant had good fusion. It seemed that bone grows in the implant from the vertebral body. The graft appeared to be extremely stable after surgery, and no abnormal movement was seen on flexion and extension radiographs. The fusion rate was better than that among the iliac crest bone group and there were no complications related to the graft. It seems that with the use of a carbon fiber cage and allograft bone, complications related to an iliac crest bone graft can be avoided and the advantages of a fusion can be maintained. The results should be further investigated in a long-term follow-up study.

REFERENCES

1. Cloward RB. The anterior approach for removal of ruptured discs. *J Neurosurg* 1958;15:602–617.
2. Dereymaeker A. La fusion corporéale des vertébres cervicales en pathologie nerveuse. Presented at the Meeting of the Belgian Orthopedic Society, May 1, 1966, Brussels.
3. Dereymaeker A. Résultats à très long terme de la fusion intercorporéale dans la pathologie cervicale. *Acta Neurol Belg* 1987;87:57–65.
4. Dereymaeker A, Mulier J. La fusion vertébrale par voie ventrale dans la discopathie cervicale. *Rev Neurol (Paris)* 1958;99:99–103.
5. Gore DR, Gardner GM, Sepic SB, et al. Roentgenographic findings following anterior cervical fusion. *Skeletal Radiol* 1986;15:556–559.
6. Hankinson HL, Wilson CB. Use of the operating microscope in anterior cervical discectomy without fusion. *J Neurosurg* 1975;43:452–456.
7. Hirsch C, Wickbom I, Lidström A, et al. Cervical disc resection: a follow-up of myelographic and surgical procedure. *J Bone Joint Surg Am* 1964;46:1811–1821.
8. Lundsford LD, Bissonette DJ, Janetta PJ, et al. Anterior surgery for cervical disc disease, 1: treatment of lateral cervical disc herniation in 253 cases. *J Neurosurg* 1980;53:1–11.
9. Murphy MG, Gado M. Anterior cervical discectomy without interbody bone graft. *J Neurosurg* 1972;37:71–74.
10. Odom GL, Finney W, Woodhall B. Cervical disk lesions. *JAMA* 1958;166:23–28.
11. Robinson RA, Smith GW. Anterolateral cervical disc removal and interbody fusion for cervical disc syndrome. *Bull Johns Hopkins Hosp* 1955;96:223–224.

The Degenerative Cervical Spine,
edited by Marek Szpalski and Robert Gunzburg
Lippincott Williams & Wilkins, Philadelphia © 2001.

28

Cervical Fusion with Monocomponent PCB Plate

Jacques Benezech

Service de Neurochirurgie, Clinique Rech, 34000 Montpellier, France

MATERIALS AND METHODS
RESULTS

Despite a few contradictory publications, there is consensus about the changes in the cervical intervertebral disc space after discectomy. Interbody fusion occurs in about 90% of cases with a 70% incidence of cervical spinal deformity, mainly kyphosis. Careful analysis of this evolution leads to the following observations: global disturbance of spinal stability, a marked decrease in intervertebral disc height, segmental rigidity, facet joint dysfunction, and narrowing of the foramen in both the sagittal and the frontal axis (Figs. 28.1, 28.2).

To avoid such deformities and the related consequences, several authors have recommended use of bone grafts or, more recently, intervertebral cages. Whereas these systems address the orthopedic problem, they carry the inherent risk of anterior or posterior cage migration. To decrease the risk of migration, the graft or the cage has to be forcibly impacted in the disc space, which can exaggerate distraction of the intervertebral space or cause segmental hyperlordosis, which induces abnormal loads on the facet joints and causes pain.

The anatomic features of intervertebral disc space are a horizontal base, a convex roof, and slightly closed anterior and posterior ends (Fig 28.3). On a lateral radiograph the facet joint surfaces appear parallel (Fig 28.4). The ideal interbody cage should adapt exactly to that shape. From a biomechanical point of view, such a cage would have a neutralizing effect and absorb axial loads while maintaining parallel facet surfaces. This shape would make the system naturally stable with minimal risk of anterior or posterior migration. For increased security, the cage could be screwed to the adjacent vertebral bodies and increasing the rigidity of the construct. Following these anatomic and biomechanical considerations, my colleagues and I designed a monocomponent plate-cage system.

Shape and size are shown in Fig. 28.5. Figure 28.6 gives an overall view of the Plate Cage Benezech (PCB) implant. The anterior, superior, and inferior sides are widely fenestrated. Corticocancellous bone graft introduced through the anterior fenestration is used to fill the entire space with optimal contact with the end plates to achieve solid fusion. The closed posterior aspect of the cage prevents posterior extrusion of the graft. The

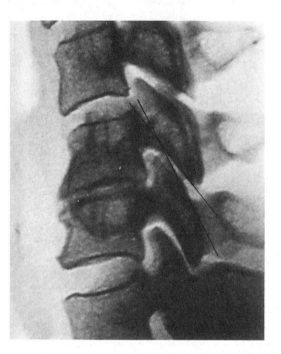

FIG. 28.1, 28.2. Spontaneous evolution of the intervertebral site after discectomy. Dysharmonic curvature, a loss of articular parallelism, and global narrowing of the foramen are present.

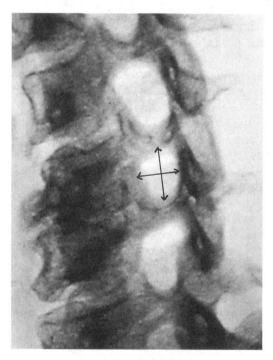

FIG. 28.2.

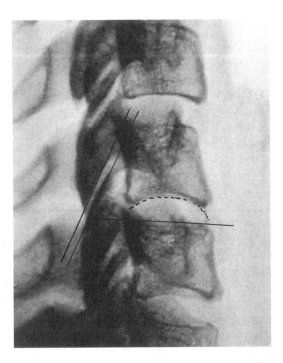

FIG. 28.3. Morphologic features aspect of the intervertebral space—horizontal base, convex roof.

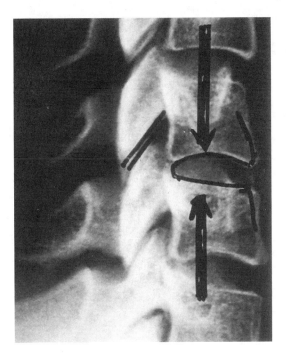

FIG. 28.4. Ideal theoretic cage.

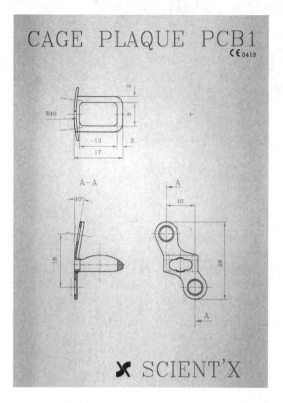

FIG. 28.5. Dimensions of the PCB cage.

upper fixation plate is slightly longer and more oblique than the inferior plate to allow a perfect fit on the upper vertebra. Most of the load is supported by the cage so that the plate fixation screws sustain minimal load and are therefore less subject to loosening. The triangulation of the construct gives it optimal mechanical properties. The lateral radiographic view in Fig. 28.7 shows an intact spinal curvature. The facet joint surfaces are parallel, and posterior osteophytes have been removed.

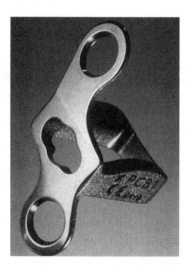

FIG. 28.6. View of PCB cage shows the widely fenestrated upper and lower aspects.

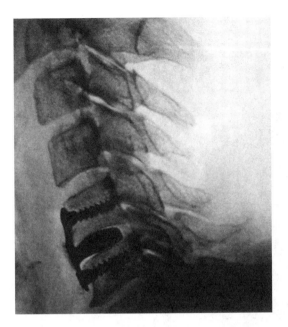

FIG. 28.7. Radiograph shows postoperative appearance. The parallelism of the facets is evident.

The diagonal orientation of the superior and inferior plates, easily seen on an anteroposterior radiograph, allows for fixation of two plates on the same vertebra and therefore treating several adjacent spaces (Figs. 28.8 through 28.10). The cage is wide enough as to enable a wide contact with the endplates for increased stability. A radio transparent model (polyetherketone) allows an easier follow-up assessment of the evolution of fusion (Fig. 28.11).

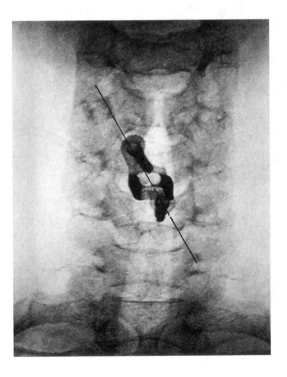

FIG. 28.8. Anteroposterior radiograph shows the diagonal orientation of the upper and lower plates.

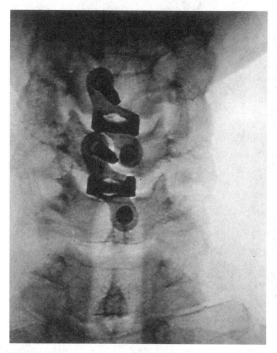

FIG. 28.9. Anteroposterior radiograph shows two-level fusion.

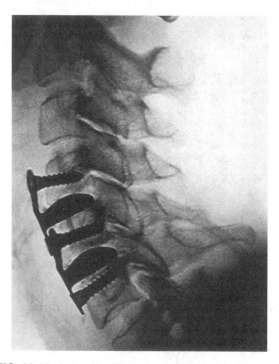

FIG. 28.10. Lateral radiograph shows two-level fusion.

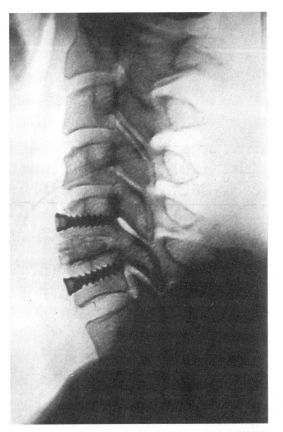

FIG. 28.11. Radiolucent polyetherketone cage allows follow-up evaluation of the fusion.

Different heights are available, but practically it appears that in more than 90% of cases, a single height of 5.5 mm suffices. Any remaining minor space is filled by the bone graft inserted with pressure. More than 1,000 PCB systems have been implanted worldwide. Herein are reported results of a retrospective study of 34 operations performed by one surgeon in 1995 and 1996. The follow-up period was at least 2 years. Clinical and radiologic assessments were conducted by an independent observer.

MATERIALS AND METHODS

Thirty-four patients participated in the study. Results were assessed according to the Prolo scale and Odom criteria (Tables 28.1 through 28.8). All patients had had severe cervicobrachial neuralgia not relieved with medical treatment and physical therapy. Two patients had a severe neurologic deficit due to degenerative myelopathy. Five patients underwent operations on two adjacent levels. The lesions most frequently encountered were soft herniation and degenerative osteophytes. The two patients with myelopathy also had spinal stenosis.

TABLE 28.1. *Demographics (N = 34)*

Characteristic	Value
No. of men	19
No. of women	15
Mean age (yr)	52
Age range (yr)	31–73

TABLE 28.2. *Clinical presentation*

Presentation	No. of patients (%)
Cervico brachial neuralgia	32 (94)
Complex neurologic deficit	2 (6)

TABLE 28.3. *Pathologic conditions (N = 39)*

Condition	No. of patients (%)
Herniated disc	19 (49)
Spondylosis	18 (47)
Spinal stenosis	2 (4)

TABLE 28.4. *Fused levels (N = 39)*

Level	No. of patients (%)
C6-7	22 (56)
C5-6	14 (36)
C4-5	3 (8)

TABLE 28.5. *Clinical results (N = 34)*

Result	No. of patients (%)
Cervical pain	
Absent	27 (80)
Permanent	3 (8)
Transient	4 (12)
Brachial pain	
Absent	30 (88)
Present	4 (12)

TABLE 28.6. *Rating of clinical results (N = 34)*

Rating	No. of patients (%)
Excellent	23 (68)
Satisfactory	9 (27)
Bad	2 (5)

TABLE 28.7. *Radiologic results (N = 34)*

Result	No. of patients (%)
Cervical spine	
Normal static view	28 (82)
Segmental difformity	6 (18)
Kyphosis	0
Upper and lower disc spaces	
Normal	25 (73)
Reduced height	5 (15)
Spondylosis	4 (12)

TABLE 28.8. *Complications (N = 34)*

Complication	No. of patients
Transient dysphagia	3
Transient dysphonia	2
Hematoma	1

RESULTS

The follow-up period was a minimum of 2 years. Seventy-seven percent of the patients did not have residual pain after surgery. Among those who continued to have pain, cervical pain was the most common. Cervicobrachial neuralgia had usually disappeared. Ninety-five percent of patients felt better, and 90% of those working before surgery returned to their professional activities. There was no secondary migration of the implant or loosening at the level of the screw. No patient had secondary angular kyphosis, and more than 80% had normal cervical stability. In more than 70% of cases, superior and inferior discs had no changed in height or other signs of degeneration. There were no instances of complications related to the implant itself. All the complications related to use of the anterior approach to the cervical spine spontaneously healed, but one retropharyngeal hematoma had to be surgically drained. The results show that this procedure is safe, effective, and reliable. It maintains cervical stability and can be offered as a simple method of interbody fusion.

The Degenerative Cervical Spine,
edited by Marek Szpalski and Robert Gunzburg
Lippincott Williams & Wilkins, Philadelphia © 2001.

29

Concept and Clinical Aspects of Computer-assisted Cervical Spinal Surgery

Dirk Vandevelde, *Heiko Visarius

*Department of Orthopaedic Surgery, University Hospital Antwerp, 2650 Edegem, Belgium;
Medivision Institute, 4436 Oberdorf, Switzerland

BACKGROUND
COMPONENTS
    Hardware • Software
METHODS
    Computed Tomographic Navigation • Fluoroscopy-based Navigation, or Virtual Fluoroscopy
DISCUSSION

The use of transpedicular screws in the cervical spine has been limited because of high risk of neurovascular complications. Although Roy-Camille et al. (18) and Smith et al. (20) described the applications of transpedicular screws without neurovascular complications, these procedures are still difficult for most surgeons who operate on the spine. Posterior instrumentation with screws in the cervical spine causes more complex problems than it does in other areas of the spine because of changes in pedicle shape, pedicle size, and body-pedicle angle (10). These changes in both angular and linear dimensions of the cervical vertebrae necessitate use of surgical techniques adapted for each vertebra, especially during blind maneuvers, such as placing screws in the cervical spine.

There also exists sufficient variation in the anatomic configuration of the cervical spine to conclude that transpedicular screw placement based on topographic landmarks is not safe and that additional anatomic data and technology are necessary to perform safe instrumentation of the cervical spine (21). Insufficient correlation exists between specific guidelines and the surgeon's assessment of surface landmarks to ensure safety during screw insertion in the cervical spine. Augmented accuracy and safety are needed so the surgeon can perform these operations without risk of damage to important neurovascular structures. Frameless stereotactic systems can help in these difficult operations to improve visual and tactile access to the cervical pedicle and enhance accuracy to improve the safety of transpedicular screw placement in the cervical spine.

Not only pedicle screw placement but also the placement of cervical lateral mass screws entails risks of injury to the vertebral arteries and cervical nerve roots as well as possible violation of the adjacent facet joints. Because here only the dorsal aspect of the vertebra is visible, the surgeon must use intuition to determine the location of this critical anatomic structure so that the intended screw trajectory avoids neurovascular and adjacent facet joints. Studies of cadavers and clinical experience have documented the limitations of the various surgical techniques described by Roy-Camille and Magerl (7). Clinical studies performed by Heller et al. (8) and Graham et al. (6) showed a rate of cervical nerve root injury of 5% to 14% and a high rate of subsequent surgical intervention for screw repositioning or removal. In a study of cadavers Foley et al. (3) used computer-assisted guidance to place lateral mass screws in 10 cervical spines from C3-7 bilaterally. Screw perfect was placement, no nerve roots were compromised, and all screws were placed bicortically as intended and planned. No violation of the vertebral artery, the transverse foramen or the facet joint occurred.

The management of cervical tumors such as osteoid osteoma and osteoblastoma, most commonly located in the lamina and other posterior elements, can be a challenge to surgeons. The most important determinant of successful operative removal of the tumor during therapy for osteoid osteoma and osteoblastoma is exact localization of the lesion (17). Management of these cervical tumors can be difficult because lesions can be located only with computed tomography (CT); radiographic findings are normal. It is likely that a lesion can be missed during open surgery. Accessibility of some lesions and the safety of the approach cannot be assessed perfectly under fluoroscopic guidance or without visualization. Perfect localization of the tumor can avoid unnecessary facet resection during removal of the tumor when the spine is unstable and a subsequent spinal stabilization procedure. It also avoids the multiple procedures necessary when the initial operation is performed on the wrong location. These procedures also can be performed better with under CT-based computer navigation (24).

Frameless stereotaxy has been described for procedures involving the anterior cervical spine to identify resection margins and the site to place anterior cervical screws (1). The potential benefit of using an image-guided Kerrison punch while performing foraminotomy during anterior cervical decompression on cadavers has been described (9). The use of a computer-assisted surgery (CAS) system for accurate placement of posterior or anterior surgical implants and for resection of tumor lesions within the cervical spine is explained.

BACKGROUND

The technology of CAS has emerged from the laboratory to find its way into the orthopedic operating theater. It is based on a combination of precise surgical navigation and tomographic image guidance. Clinical results of lumbar pedicle screw insertion have shown the benefit of CAS technology in operations on the spine (4,11,14–16,19). During acetabular cup placement and in periacetabular osteotomy reorientation this technology has proved its usefulness in hip surgery (12,22). Developments in the laboratory for other orthopedic applications, such as hip and knee endoprostheses and proximal femoral fracture fixation, are entering the clinical arena.

Image-guided surgery has its origins in neurosurgery, in which rigid fixation devices on the scull provide a fixed reference for fiducial registration between medical image and surgical navigation. Mechanical guides on this reference frame are used to locate anatomic structures with valuable image-generated data. The first complete description of the principles of and devices for stereotaxis was presented in 1906 in the classic paper by Clarke and Horsley (2). Evolution of this technology into the field of orthopedics was difficult because, unlike in the skull, bones are hidden deeply beneath soft tissue and must often undergo complex manipulations. To resolve these problems, orthopedic CAS systems take advantage of modern, mostly optical, tracking devices (Optotrak; Northern

Digital, Waterloo, Canada) and light weight references that allow real-time tracking of both tool and patient movement. The basic components of such a surgical system are (a) one surgical object, such as the vertebra, (b) the associated virtual object, such as the to-mographic image of the object, and (c) at least one surgical tool.

Correspondence between a preoperatively obtained medical image and the intraopera-tive tracking system is achieved through registration. Registration of the medical image with the navigation system allows exact visualization of tool position within the three-di-mensional anatomic structure. Considerable attention has been devoted to providing ad-vanced operator-machine interfaces that help the surgeon control the software au-tonomously while maintaining sterile conditions (23).

COMPONENTS

Hardware

The SurgiGATE system consists of an optoelectronic camera that can precisely (within 0.1 mm) locate light-emitting diodes in a large field of view (cube with 1.5-m side length). These diodes send out an infrared signal and are mounted on standard instru-ments for spinal surgery (STRATEC Medical; Medivision, Oberdorf, Switzerland), such as the Synthes USS Pedicle Awl and Probe. Further tools include a dynamic reference base to compensate for patient motion during the surgical procedure, a screw driver, a power drill, and a virtual keyboard, which in combination with a footswitch allows the surgeon to control the system directly without an on-site system engineer (23). The stan-dard tool set for spinal surgery is shown in Fig. 29.1. All tools have a cable attached that

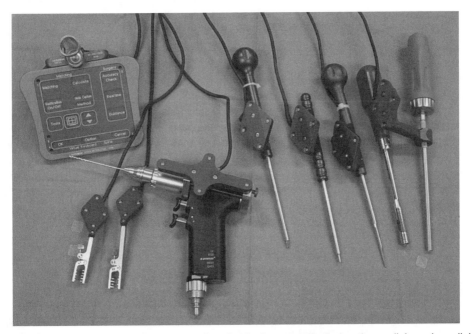

FIG. 29.1. The tool set for computer-assisted spinal surgery includes the pedicle awl, pedicle probe, dynamic reference base, virtual keyboard, space pointer, screw driver, and power drill.

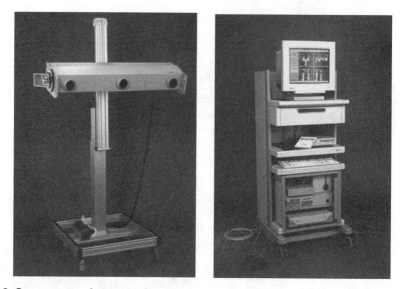

FIG. 29.2. Components of a system for computer-assisted surgery. The computer cart contains the electronic components. From here, connections are made to the camera and to the navigation instruments and fluoroscopic equipment.

is plugged into a distributor box. The plug contains a chip for self-identification of all instruments.

A separate planning computer system can be used with the same computer configuration as the operating room workstation computer. The electronics for the camera, the workstation computer, and the monitor for the surgeon are stored on a movable cart (Figs. 29.2). Integration of the fluoroscope necessitates adaptation with calibration of the fluoroscope and light-emitting diode attached to the C arm. A cable connection between the C arm and the computer unit is necessary to transfer C-arm images.

Software

The SurgiGATE software installed on the workstation provides modules for image data acquisition from various scanners, preoperative diagnosis, planning and simulation, tool check and calibration, skeletal registration (matching) based on paired points and surface, and two different modules for intraoperative support. The software is clearly structured with only six main buttons that guide the surgeon through the procedure. Inherent hierarchies help to control the program flow. For example, the matching modules cannot be accessed until a patient's information is loaded and tools are calibrated.

METHODS

Computed Tomographic Navigation

Preoperative planning is performed with the preoperative module of the planning station. Axial CT scans of all vertebrae to be operated on are obtained from the radiology department by means of hospital network, tape, or magnetooptical disc. The acquisition module reads image and header data and displays the patient. Using the mouse, the surgeon can select any view of the image data, including nonorthogonal cuts through the image volume. The surgeon can examine the vertebrae to be operated on. A three-dimensional model of the patient can be made in a semiautomatic manner within minutes.

Within the image, four to six anatomic landmarks are selected with a mouse click, labeled, and stored for intraoperative use during the matching procedure. As an alternative the surgeon can plan the procedure by defining an optimal axis (trajectory) for the pedicle screw or lateral mass screw by means of selection of an entrance and a target point in the image (Figs. 29.3 and 29.4). The chosen path can be displayed to simulate the operation and, if necessary, optimized further. This kind of preoperative planning is new to surgeons because they no longer have to depend on images radiologists provide on film.

During the usual preparation of the operating room, the computer cart and camera cart are positioned in the theater (Fig. 29.5). The positions of the cart and camera are arbitrary but should be chosen to ensure a good view of the screen for the surgeon and of the surgical site and tools for the camera. During standard posterior surgical exposure of the dorsal vertebral elements, the assistant prepares the navigation instruments. The plugs are dropped and connected to the distributor box, and the instruments are checked and calibrated by means of insertion into the calibration unit. This procedure should take no

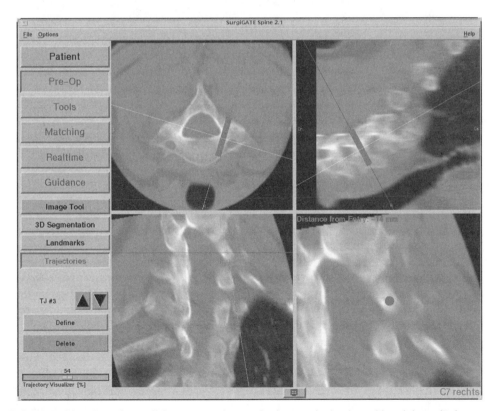

FIG. 29.3. Planning of a pedicle screw trajectory in the cervical spine with axial, sagittal, coronal, and pedicle views.

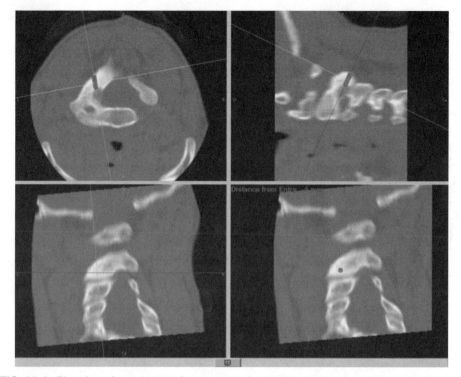

FIG. 29.4. Planning of a trajectory for removal of osteoid osteoma from the cervical spine.

longer than 5 minutes and does not delay the operation because it is performed in parallel with the surgical exposure.

The dynamic reference base (DRB) is mounted to a suitable anchor point, usually the spinous process, by the surgeon. Attaching the DRB to the patient compensates for any patient or camera motion during the procedure, because all instruments are tracked in the local, patient-fixed DRB coordinate system.

The next step, skeletal registration, is the most important. During this step the patient's anatomic features must be registered with the medical image. The simplest registration method involves identification of several anatomic landmarks, first preoperatively on the CT image of the anatomic features and then intraoperatively with respect to the surgical object in the navigation reference frame. Finding the transformation that maps these intraoperatively defined points to their corresponding CT coordinates is called *paired-point registration*. The preoperatively stored anatomic landmarks are shown on the screen one by one and located and digitized on the patient. For cervical spinal segments, four anatomic landmarks are typically selected. In most instances they are the tips of the bifid spinous process and the midpoint of each articular pillar at the inferior joint line. Because anatomic landmarks are difficult to precisely define on smooth anatomic structures, *surface registration* usually yields a better matching result. This involves intraoperative digitization of several points on the surface of the surgical object. The algorithm fits these points onto the surface by minimizing their distance to the CT-defined surface (5). A physical metaphor to this mathematical process is to fit a hat, defined by a cloud of points, onto a head. For cervical spinal surgery, a paired-point technique com-

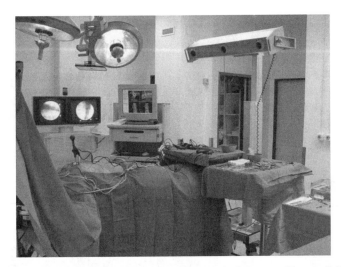

FIG. 29.5. Arrangement of CAS components in the surgical theater. The pedicle probe or drill is in the surgeon's hand. A marker carrier with light-emitting diode markers is attached to the standard tool. The dynamic reference base is visible on the patient.

bined with surface matching is used to find the transformation between the real world of the patient and the virtual world of the image.

After determination of the transformation, the overall accuracy of the system is verified. To do this, an instrument is placed at different places on the bony surface, such as the spinous process, and the surgeon confirms that the system indicates the identical position on the screen and that the instrument is exactly on the bony surface. The system is now ready for use. With the virtual keyboard, the surgeon can select a module for intraoperative guidance (see later).

The real-time trajectory mode (Fig. 29.6) provides the surgeon with a transverse and a sagittal cut through the tomographic volume at the location indicated by the tip of the tool. Seven image sections perpendicular to the current tool orientation are computed in different depths and indicate the future path of the tool. It can be described as the "What would happen, if I were to penetrate the bone in this direction?" view. The surgeon can see the position of the pedicle screw in the bone before any tissue is penetrated.

If preoperative planning data for a pedicle screw location or tumor localization were stored, they can be recalled intraoperatively and compared with the current tool position (Fig. 29.7). The guidance window also indicates the deviation of the tip and the orientation of the tool relative to the optimal path. The insertion depth is indicated in the upper left of that window.

Fluoroscopy-based Navigation, or Virtual Fluoroscopy

Mobile fluoroscopy devices are an integral part of the standard equipment used in orthopedic surgery to provide real-time feedback about bone and surgical tool positions. Mobile fluoroscopy has disadvantages such as only one single-plane view can be visualized at a time and the C arm has to be repositioned during the procedure when the surgeon needs multiplanar fluoroscopic visualization. The need for continued radiation exposure for visual control during spinal interventions is a risk for the surgeon.

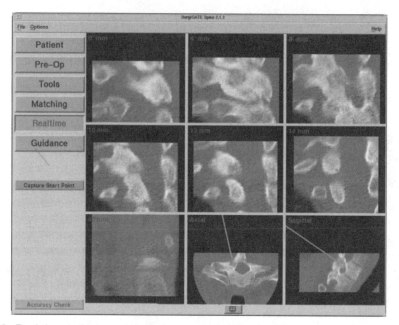

FIG. 29.6. Real-time trajectory view during tumor localization. Seven image sections perpendicular to the axial orientation of the tool are computed and displayed in real time. The first section is immediately at the tip of the tool. Sections 2 through 7 are 4, 8, 10, 12, 18, and 40 mm away from the tip. The eighth and ninth images show sections defined by a plane through the tool axis (quasiaxial and quasisagittal). In sections 8 and 9, the tool is displayed as a line.

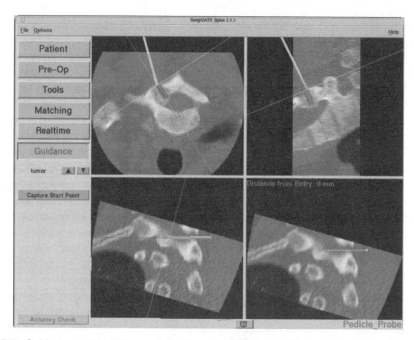

FIG. 29.7. Guidance mode. This module allows for precise guidance toward a preoperatively defined target. The target position is indicated in red, the current tool position in green. The window on the *lower right* indicates the deviation of the tip and the orientation of the instrument with respect to the planning.

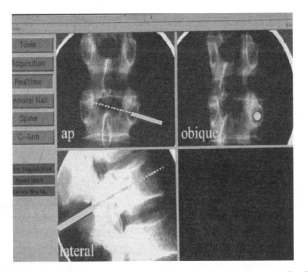

FIG. 29.8. Navigation with fluoroscopic images. The surgical instrument is displayed in multiple fluoroscopic images in real time.

Cross-referencing of the image intensifier with the surgical object allows real-time-image, interactive navigation of surgical tools with one registered radiograph image with no further image updates (Fig. 29.8). This is equivalent to the use of a C-arm unit in constant mode during the intervention, which normally implies considerable radiation exposure for the patient and the surgical staff. Furthermore, the system allows acquisition and real-time use of multiple registered images, which provides advanced multidirectional control during surgical maneuvering. In this way, simultaneous multiplanar guidance is achieved with a single C arm. This is helpful during operations in which multiplanar C-arm images are needed, such as atlantoaxial transarticular fixation and repair of dens fractures. A fluoroscopy-based system can be seen as a complement to the CT-based system. The advantage of instant availability without preoperative CT allows use of the system for several applications in orthopedics and traumatology.

DISCUSSION

The use of posterior cervical spinal fixation has become increasingly popular in recent years (13). The biomechanical advantage of a three-column fixation device, such as a pedicle screw, implanted to secure an unstable cervical spine has proved to be a valuable for spinal surgeon. However, successful placement of pedicle screws in the cervical spine requires sufficient three-dimensional understanding of pedicle structure to allow accurate identification of the ideal screw axis. Not only must the screw's trajectory be correct, but also the proper screw length must be chosen. Most conventional techniques are difficult because it is not easy to replicate a precise angle with only visual guidance, and the anatomic configuration of the cervical pedicle and cervical lateral masses is variable. Computer-assisted image guidance systems can easily be used in the operative protocol of cervical spine surgery and can help in accurate placement of pedicle and lateral mass screws.

Having been used for lumbar spinal surgery, computer-assisted technology is being used more and more frequently in the management of lesions of the cervical spine. CAS is proving more accurate than conventional techniques in placement of pedicle screw and lateral mass screws. Localization of tumors in the lamina and other posterior elements of the cervical spine and determination of safe margins for resection during tumor removal can be accurate with CAS. The computer-assisted technique allows a less invasive approach, because an excessive exposure for visualization purposes can be avoided. Further clinical studies have to prove the clinical benefit or decrease in complications with these new techniques.

In conclusion, image-guided surgery systems can be used accurately in complex operations on the cervical spine. They minimize the risk of potential complications. Computer systems also can be important during diagnosis because they facilitate preoperative planning and can be an informative teaching aid for surgeons and residents.

REFERENCES

1. Bolger C, Wigfield C, Melkent T, et al. Frameless stereotaxy and anterior cervical surgery. *Comput Aided Surg* 1999;4:322–327.
2. Clarke R, Horsley V. On a method for investigating the deep ganglia and tracts of the central nervous system (cerebellum). *Br Med J* 1906;2:1799–800.
3. Foley K, Smith K, Smith M. Frameless stereotactic guidance of cervical spine lateral mass screw placement. In: Nolte L, Ganz R, eds. *Computer assisted orthopaedic surgery.* Bern: Hogreffe & Huber, 1999:89–98.
4. Girardi F, Cammisa F, Sandhu H, et al. The placement of lumbar pedicle screws using computerised stereotactic guidance. *J Bone Joint Surg Br* 1999;81:825–829.
5. Gong J, Bachler R, Sati M, et al. Restricted surface matching: a new approach to registration in computer assisted surgery. In: *Proceedings of the 3rd International Symposium on Medical Robotics and Computer Assisted Surgery (MRCAS).* 1997:597–605.
6. Graham A, Swank M, Kinard R, et al. Posterior cervical arthrodesis and stabilisation with a lateral mass plate: clinical and computed tomographic evaluation of lateral mass screw placement and associated complications. *Spine* 1996;21:323–329.
7. Heller J, Carlson G, Abitbol J, et al. Anatomic comparison of the Roy-Camille and Magerl techniques for screw placement in the lower cervical spine. *Spine* 1991;16:S552–S557.
8. Heller J, Silcox D, Sutterlin C. Complications of posterior cervical plating. *Spine* 1995;20:2442–2448.
9. Klein G, Ludwig S, Vaccaro A, et al. The efficacy of using an image-guided Kerrison punch in performing an anterior cervical foraminotomy. An anatomic analysis. *Spine* 1999;24:1358–1362.
10. Kotani Y, Cunningham B, Abumi K, et al. Biomechanical analysis of cervical stabilization systems: an assessment of transpedicular screw fixation in the cervical spine. *Spine* 1994;19:2529–2539.
11. Laine T, Schlenzka D, Makitalo K, et al. Improved accuracy of pedicle screw insertion with computer assisted surgery: a prospective clinical trial of 30 patients. *Spine* 1997;22:1254–1258.
12. Langlotz F, Stucki M, Bachler R, et al. The first twelve cases of computer assisted periacetabular osteotomy. *Comput Aided Surg* 1997;2:317–326.
13. Ludwig S, Kramer D, Vaccaro A, et al. Transpedicle screw fixation of the cervical spine. *Clin Orthop* 1999;359: 77–88.
14. Merloz P, Tonetti J, Eid A, et al. Computer assisted spine surgery. *Clin Orthop* 1997;337:86–96.
15. Merloz P, Tonetti J, Pittet L, et al. Pedicle screw placement using image guided techniques. *Clin Orthop* 1998; 354:39–48.
16. Nolte L, Zamorano L, Arm E, et al. Image-guided computer-assisted spine surgery: a pilot study on pedicle screw fixation. *Stereotact Funct Neurosurg* 1996;66:108–117.
17. Pettine K, Klassen R. Osteoid-osteoma and osteoblastoma of the spine. *J Bone Joint Surg Am* 1986;64:354–361.
18. Roy-Camille R, Saillant G, Mazel C. Internal fixation of the unstable cervical spine by a posterior osteosynthesis with plates and screws. In: Cervical Spine Research Society, eds. *The cervical spine.* Philadelphia: JB Lippincott, 1989:390–403.
19. Schwarzenbach O, Berlemann U, Jost B, et al. Accuracy of computer-assisted pedicle screw placement: an in vivo computed tomography analysis. *Spine* 1997;22:452–458.
20. Smith M, Anderson P, Grady M. Occipitocervical arthrodesis using contoured plate fixation: an early report on a versatile fixation technique. *Spine* 1993;18:1984–1990.
21. Stanescu S, Ebraheim N, Yeasting R, et al. Morphometric evaluation of the cervicothoracic junction: practical considerations for posterior fixation of the spine. *Spine* 1994;19:2082–2088.
22. Vandevelde D, Leenders T, Mahieu G, et al. Reduction in variability of acetabular cup position using computer assisted surgery. In: Lemke et al., eds. Proceedings of the 14th International Congress CARS 2000. Computer Assisted Radiology and Surgery, San Francisco, June 28–July 1, 2000. Amsterdam: Elsevier 2000:231–235.
23. Visarius H, Gong J, Scheer C, et al. Man-machine interfaces in computer assisted surgery. *Comput Aided Surg* 1997;2:102–107.
24. Welch W, Subach B, Pollack I, et al. Frameless stereotactic guidance for surgery of the upper cervical spine. *Neurosurgery* 1997;40:958–963.

Economic and Ethical Considerations in the Management of Spinal Stenosis

The Degenerative Cervical Spine,
edited by Marek Szpalski and Robert Gunzburg
Lippincott Williams & Wilkins, Philadelphia © 2001.

30

Methodology for Economic Evaluation

Christian Mélot

Department of Intensive Care, Erasme University Hospital, B-1070 Brussels, Belgium

---

MAJOR STUDY DESIGNS FOR ECONOMIC EVALUATION OF HEALTH CARE SERVICES
AN EXAMPLE
  Step 1: Statistical Evaluation of Survival • Step 2: Cost-effectiveness Analysis • Step 3: Cost-benefit Analysis
CONCLUSIONS

To be trained in medicine, nursing or one of the other "sharp end" disciplines and then be faced with some hard-nosed, cold-blooded economist placing money values on human life and suffering is anathema to many.
> G. Mooney, *The Economics of Health and Medicine,* 1992

The essence of economic evaluation is a comparison of the costs and consequences of different health care programs. When no comparison between alternatives are made—that is, one service or program is being evaluated—there is no true evaluation but only a description of the service or of the program. These economic approaches often are labeled *partial economic evaluations* (1,6).

In full economic evaluations, there are a variety of meaningful ways to measure consequences. During the past three decades quality of life measures have been developed that provide a new and relevant approach to assessing the consequences of the use of health care resources. The strategies of combining traditional methods of economic evaluation with the newer techniques of quality of life assessment in which the concept of utility is used have lead to the cost-utility approach to health care. From a health policy perspective, cost-benefit analysis, whereby the consequences are translated into monetary terms, is the most powerful of the techniques of economic evaluation because it can be used to address directly questions of allocative efficiency the other techniques cannot address (7). The major forms of economic evaluation are briefly described and practical considerations of combining these methods are presented.

MAJOR STUDY DESIGNS FOR ECONOMIC EVALUATION OF HEALTH CARE SERVICES

Economic evaluation relies on estimation of the dollar costs of providing alternative forms of health care services, such as surgical versus medical therapy for the same con-

TABLE 30.1. *Major study designs for economic evaluations*

Type of analysis	Compares	With
Cost minimization	Monetary value of resource used	Identical clinical effects produced
Cost-effectiveness	Monetary value of resource used	Different clinical effects produced
Cost to utility	Monetary value of resource used	Quality of life produced by the clinical effects
Cost to benefit	Monetary value of resource used	Monetary value of resources saved or created

dition or one drug regimen versus another. The monetary costs include direct costs (items such as professional fees for service, drugs, hospitalization, diagnostic tests) and indirect costs (earnings of patient forgone as a result of treatment) (1,5,6). The basic study designs for the four major forms of economic evaluation are summarized in Table 30.1. The outcomes or consequences are defined differently for each type of analysis, and costs are uniformly defined in terms of monetary expenditure (1,5,6).

In *cost-minimization* analysis, the treatments to be compared are considered to be equally efficacious on the basis of previous research, and thus only treatment costs are compared. This type of analysis focuses on the differences in total costs associated with the study treatments. The objective of cost-minimization analysis is to identify the most efficient treatment method.

In *cost-effectiveness* analysis, outcomes are measured in natural units of clinical effects. These units are typically the ones used in clinical studies. They may be as narrow as millimeters of mercury for reduction in blood pressure or as broad as life-years gained for reductions in mortality. The key feature of a cost-effectiveness analysis design is that the analyst need not assign a dollar value to the outcome. The analyst can also continue to rely on standard clinical measures.

In *cost-utility* analysis, the measure of clinical effects is adjusted to reflect the quality of life of the outcome. In this approach, life-years are converted into quality-adjusted life-years (QALY). The methods of estimating QALY are discussed elsewhere (1,6,10). As in costs-effectiveness analysis, the analyst is not required to place a dollar value on the outcome. Unlike that approach, however, cost-utility analysis does explicitly incorporate quality of life information in the results.

In *cost-benefit* analysis, costs and consequences are expressed in monetary terms. In the context of health care, however, most analysts have found cost-benefit analysis to be less satisfactory than cost-effectiveness analysis or cost-utility analysis for several reasons. In particular, many analysts are uncomfortable with ethical judgments that appear to accompany assigning dollar values to people's lives and their suffering. The result has been that cost-effectiveness analysis studies have become the dominant study design in health care evaluation.

The following example shows that it is impossible to develop a valuable cost-benefit analysis without first performing a rigorous cost-effectiveness analysis or, less often, a cost-utility or cost-minimization analysis.

AN EXAMPLE

To understand the principle of cost-effectiveness and cost-benefit analyses (2), let us imagine a homogenous population among which a cohort of 1,000 patients have a disease that shortens survival expectation.

Step 1: Statistical Evaluation of Survival

Epidemiologic and statistical studies have shown that a patient with the disease has 6 in 10 to survive 4 years without treatment (survival rate $p = .6$) or 4 in 10 to have a normal life span of 20 years (survival rate $p = .4$). Therefore, with no treatment, the prognosis of a patient's having the disease can be presented as a lottery (10) (Fig. 30.1.).

After the chance nodes (solid circles), both possible outcomes are figured on both branches—either a survival period of 4 years or a survival period of 20 years with the probability (likelihood) of each of them. The mean expected survival time for an individual patient can be calculated as follows:

$$0.6 * 4 + 0.4 * 20 = 10.4 \text{ years}$$

This means that if the 1,000 patients with the disease are not treated, 600 will survive 4 years and 400 will survive 20 years. The total survival time for these 1,000 patients will be $2,400 + 8,000 = 10,400$ years; that is, 1,000 times the mean individual survival time ($1,000 * 10.4$ years).

To improve survival, two treatments are available. Treatment A is of low cost. Using it will cost \$50 per patient. With treatment A, the probability of surviving 20 years improves from 0.4 to 0.54. The lottery associated with treatment A is shown in Fig. 30.2. The mean expected survival time, which was 10.4 years without treatment, becomes

$$0.46 * 4 + 0.54 * 20 = 12.6 \text{ years}$$

Treatment B is more expensive. Using it will cost \$250 per patient. With treatment B, the probability of surviving 20 years improves from 0.4 to 0.7. Moreover, in the less favorable situation, 6 years of survival will be obtained rather than 4 years. The lottery associated with treatment B is shown in Fig. 30.3.

The mean expected survival time with treatment B is

$$0.3 * 6 + 0.7 * 20 = 15.8 \text{ years}$$

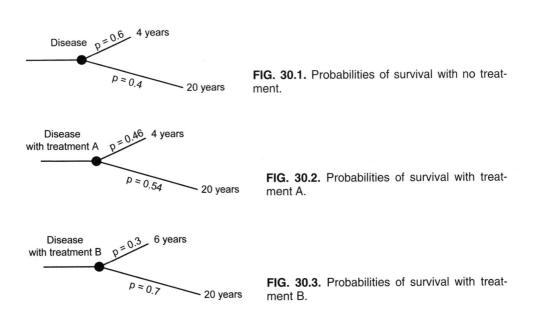

FIG. 30.1. Probabilities of survival with no treatment.

FIG. 30.2. Probabilities of survival with treatment A.

FIG. 30.3. Probabilities of survival with treatment B.

TABLE 30.2. *Cost and expected survival for each treatment option*

Therapeutic option	Cost per patient ($)	Expected individual survival time (yr)
No treatment	0	10.4
Treatment A	50	12.6
Treatment B	250	15.8

The gain of expected survival time attributable to treatment B is 5.4 years (15.8 − 10.4) per treated patient (Table 30.2.)

Step 2: Cost-effectiveness Analysis

Considering these results, we need to answer the following two questions:

1. If the global budget for these 1,000 patients is determined at a fixed level, how can we use this fixed budget to maximize the mean survival from a collective standpoint?
2. If the objective is to maximize collective mean survival, how can we reach this target with a minimal expense?

To answer both questions, we draw a cost-effectiveness plot with cost in monetary terms and effectiveness expressed as the expected survival for the entire group. Each point in Fig. 30.1 is the result obtained for every therapeutic option: *N* for no treatment, *A* for treatment A, and *B* for treatment B. For example, use of treatment B by 1,000 patients leads to a global survival time of 15,800 years for a total cost of $250,000 (Fig. 30.4, point *B*).

To understand the meaning of cost-effectiveness, we must imagine the different ways to obtain a given survival time. For instance, we could get 12,600 years of survival using treatment A for a cost of $50,000 (Fig. 30.5, point *A*) or using treatment B for a cost of $101,800 (Fig. 30.5, point *E*).

Along the line *NB,* cost-effectiveness pairs are obtained when treatment B is used by a fraction of the cohort of 1,000 patients. For example, if we treat 200 patients with treatment B and the remaining 800 patients receive no treatment, the cost is

$$200 * 250 + 800 * 0 = \$50,000$$

and total survival time is

$$200 * 15.8 + 800 * 10.4 = 11,480 \text{ years}$$

which is figured with point *C* in Fig. 30.5.

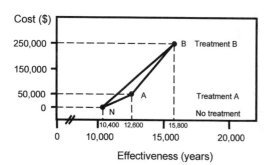

FIG. 30.4. Cost-effectiveness plot for the disease with no treatment (point *N*), with treatment A (point *A*), and treatment B (point *B*).

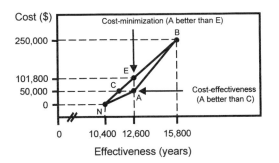

FIG. 30.5. Cost-minimization approach for a mean survival time of 12,600 years and cost-effectiveness approach for a total cost of $50,000.

Even though equity is not achieved, point C is a mixing between strategies N and B applied to the cohort in a proportion of 80% and 20%, respectively. This strategy is not cost-effective because treatment A is more effective for the same cost of $50,000 (cost-effectiveness approach).

We can also try to answer question 2. To obtain a total survival time of 12,600 years with a strategy of administering treatment B to a fraction of the population, we can compute the fraction of the 1,000 patients to be treated:

$$[p * 15.8 + (1 - p) * 10.4] * 1,000 = 12,600$$

The solution is

$$p = 2,200 / 5,400 = .407$$

If we administer treatment B to 407 patients and give no treatment to 593 patients, the total survival time is

$$407 * 15.8 + 593 * 10.4 \approx 12,600 \text{ years}$$

The associated cost is

$$407 * 250 + 593 * 0 \approx \$101,800$$

The result is figured with point E in Fig. 30.5. Solution E is not cost effective because treatment A is less expensive for the same total survival time of 12,600 years. In a cost-minimization approach, we would choose solution A. With a linear programming approach to the problem, it can be shown that cost-effective strategies rely on the segment lines NA and AB. In summary, each point on the graph in Fig. 30.5 can be interpreted in two different but equivalent ways: (a) For a given total survival, we can find the treatment leading to the lowest cost (cost-minimization approach). (b) For a given cost, we can find the highest survival (cost-effectiveness approach).

Along the line segment NA, patients receiving no treatment are combined with patients given treatment A in an increasing proportion from N to A (Fig. 30.6). If 500 patients were to receive no treatment and 500 were given treatment A, we would obtain the point R with a total survival time of

$$500 * 10.4 + 500 * 12.6 = 11,500 \text{ years}$$

and a cost of

$$500 * 0 + 500 * 50 = \$25,000$$

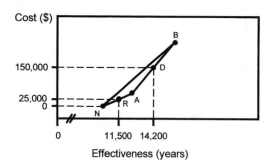

FIG. 30.6. Cost-effectiveness for combination of treatment A with no treatment (point *R*) and combination of treatment A with treatment B (point *D*).

Similarly, along line represent *AB*, patients treated with A and patients treated with B are combined in a variable proportion (Fig. 30.6). If 500 patients were to receive treatment A and 500 treatment B, we would obtain point *D* with total survival time of

$$500 * 12.6 + 500 * 15.8 = 14,200 \text{ years}$$

and a cost of

$$500 * 50 + 500 * 250 = \$150,000$$

To summarize these relations between cost and effectiveness, an average *cost to effectiveness ratio* (C/E) can be defined; that is, cost per year of survival. For example, at point *R*

$$C/E = 25,000/11,500 = \$2.17 \text{ per year}$$

and at point *D*

$$C/E = 150,000/14,200 = \$10.56 \text{ per year}$$

It is clear that the average C/E increases with effectiveness. However, it can be shown that the average C/E gives a biased result. For example, at point *R,* a survival effectiveness of 11,500 years is attributed to treatment A. This effectiveness is obviously overestimated if we recall that no treatment gives a survival time of 10,400 years. The true gain in effectiveness attributable to treatment A is 1,100 years (11,500 − 10,400) for a real cost of $50,000. Therefore, the average C/E is an underestimate of the cost per year gained with treatment A.

The *marginal cost-effectiveness ratio* (ΔC/ΔE) is related to the cost of producing one extra unit of output, that is, one extra year of survival. For example, the marginal cost-effectiveness of treatment A is (Fig. 30.7)

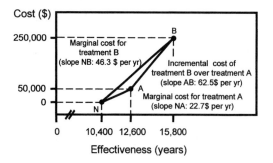

FIG. 30.7. Marginal cost of treatments A and B. Incremental cost for treatment B divided by cost of treatment A.

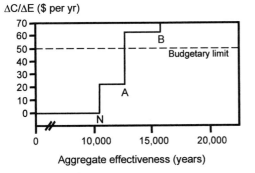

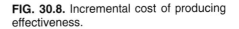

FIG. 30.8. Incremental cost of producing effectiveness.

$$\Delta C/\Delta E = (50,000 - 0)/(12,600 - 10,400) = \$22.7 \text{ per additional year of life}$$

and the marginal cost-effectiveness of treatment B is (Fig. 30.7)

$$\Delta C/\Delta E = (250,000 - 0)/(15,800 - 10,400) = \$46.3 \text{ for each additional year of life}$$

The *incremental cost-effectiveness ratio* ($\Delta C/\Delta E$) is used to refer to the difference, in cost and effect, between the two treatments. So the incremental cost-effectiveness of treatment B over treatment A is (Fig. 30.7):

$$\Delta C/\Delta E = (250,000 - 50,000)/(15,800 - 12,600) = \$62.5 \text{ per additional year of life}$$

Unfortunately, the terms *marginal* and *incremental* often are used interchangeably in the literature. If they both refer to a change in the scale of an activity, strictly speaking they have different meanings in economic evaluation (1,6).

This example can be used to determine how a fixed budget can be spent if the objective is to maximize the number of life years to be gained. Figure 30.8 shows incremental cost-effectiveness ratios, starting with the do-nothing option. We then begin by implementing treatment A with the lowest incremental ratio and add treatment B. The steps in the curve indicate the increases in the incremental cost of producing life-years as successive treatments are added. Each budgetary limit defines a shadow price of life years gained. In Fig. 30.8, the budgetary limit of $50 per year implies that we are not willing to pay more than $50 for a unit of effectiveness.

Step 3: Cost-benefit Analysis

At variance with consumer goods, there is no market price in health care to value the output unit, that is, 1 year of the human life. The collective willingness-to-pay approach can be used to give a monetary value to human life. Methods used to determine the value of one extra year of survival are beyond the scope of this chapter and are described elsewhere (1,4,6,8,9). In most developed countries, health care services are funded and delivered on the basis of insurance (private company) or tax (public social security system) contributions. This reflects an important characteristic of the health care market, which is that illness and the demand for health care are uncertain. The consequence of such insurance or tax arrangements is that persons do not bear the full cost of the service at the point of delivery. Hence it has been argued that willingness-to-pay questions should be framed in a way that incorporates this demand side uncertainty (3). Moreover, in the willingness-to-pay approach, a distinction must be made between an *ex post* perspective or user-based approach (assuming you have the disease, what would you pay out-ofpocket?) and an *ex ante* perspective or insurance-based scenario (assuming you have a 10% chance of contracting the disease, what are you ready to pay for that risk?). The *ex post* scenario usually gives a lower willingness to pay than the *ex ante* scenario, which incorporates the risk aversion into the valuation (8).

With a monetary value attributed to human life, a sensitivity analysis with a cost-benefit approach can be performed to determine the best health care policy from a societal standpoint. For instance, consider a disease with similar epidemiologic characteristic in three different countries (C1, C2, and C3) where the collective willingness to pay for one extra year of survival is $18, $35, and $75, respectively, for cultural, economic or other reasons.

In the allocative economic framework, the worth or value of a thing to a person is determined simply by what a person is willing to pay for it. If a consumer is ready to pay as much as $5 for a good, it may be inferred that it is worth to him or her no less than $5. If the good is priced at $2, the purchase of the good provides the person with a consumer's surplus of $3. This consumer's surplus is the most crucial concept in measurement of social benefits in any social cost-benefit calculation (7). From a societal standpoint, the optimal level of effectiveness of treating a patient for a disease is the level that maximizes the social surplus, that is, the difference between the collective willingness to pay minus the cost to be paid for that level of effectiveness.

Applying the rule to the three countries for treatments A and B administered to 1,000 patients with a disease and comparing the social surpluses obtained without any treatment, the cost-benefit analysis is different in each country (Tables 30.3 through 30.6). The political choice based on a cost-benefit analysis is different in each country, as follows: In country C1, because of the low value of human life, providing no treatment is

TABLE 30.3. *Social surplus for treatment A in three countries with different willingness to pay for 1 extra year of survival*

Country	Benefit related to willingness to pay for 1 extra yr	Treatment A cost ($)	Social surplus ($)
C1	12,600*18	50,000	176,800
C2	12,600*35	50,000	391,000
C3	12,600*75	50,000	895,000

TABLE 30.4. *Social surplus for treatment B in three countries with different willingness to pay for 1 extra year of survival*

Country	Benefit related to WTP for one extra year	Treatment B cost	Social surplus
C1	15,800*18	250,000	34,400
C2	15,800*35	250,000	303,000
C3	15,800*75	250,000	935,000

TABLE 30.5. *Social surplus in the absence of treatment in three countries with different willingness to pay for 1 extra year of survival*

Country	Benefit related to WTP for one extra year	No treatment cost	Social surplus
C1	10,400*18	0	187,200
C2	10,400*35	0	364,000
C3	10,400*75	0	780,000

TABLE 30.6. *Social surplus for the three possible therapeutic options in three countries with different degrees of willingness to pay for 1 extra year of survival*

	Country		
Treatment	C1	C2	C3
None	**187,200**	364,000	780,000
A	176,800	**391,000**	895,000
B	34,400	303,000	**935,000**

Treatment that maximizes social surplus is in bold type.

preferred; in C2, treatment A maximizes the social surplus; and in C2, treatment B is choice (Table 30.6).

In summary, it is impossible to develop a valuable cost-benefit analysis without first performing a rigorous cost-effectiveness analysis. Moreover, the marginal or incremental cost-effectiveness ratio ($\Delta C/\Delta E$) is more informative than the average cost-effectiveness ratio (C/E), which is more popular.

CONCLUSIONS

Cost-benefit analysis is, at least in theory, the most powerful of the techniques of economic evaluation because it can directly address questions of allocative efficiency that the other techniques cannot. But this advantage comes only after the analyst has overcome a number of difficulties associated with assigning a monetary value to program benefits. The different techniques for economic evaluations are embedded together in the sense that it is impossible to develop a valuable cost-benefit analysis without first performing a rigorous cost-effectiveness analysis. The most important disadvantage of the benefit-cost framework is the requirement that human lives and quality of life be valued in monetary units. Many decision makers find this difficult or unethical or do not trust results of analyses that depend on such valuations.

REFERENCES

1. Drummond MF, O'Brien BJ, Stoddart GL, et al., eds. *Methods for the economic evaluation of health care programmes,* 2nd ed. Oxford, UK: Oxford University Press, 1997.
2. Eeckhoudt L, Crott R. Méthodologie des études. In: Annemans L, Crott R, eds. *Aspects socio-économiques des soins de santé en Belgique.* Bruxelles: IBES, 1998:233–255.
3. Gafni A. Using willingness-to-pay as a measure of benefits: what is the relevant question to ask in the context of public decision-making? *Med Care* 1991;29:1246–1252.
4. Grabowski HG, Hansen RW. Economic scales and tests. In: Spilker B, ed. *Quality of life assessments in clinical trials.* New York: Raven Press, 1990:61–69.
5. Mélot C. Principles of cost-benefit analysis. In: Szpalski M, Gunzburg R, Pope MH, eds. *Lumbar segmental instability.* Philadelphia: Lippincott Williams & Wilkins, 1999:259–273.
6. Mélot C. Economic evaluation in health care. In: Gunzburg R, Szpalski M, eds. *Lumbar spinal stenosis.* Philadelphia: Lippincott Williams & Wilkins, 2000:357–365.
7. Mishan EJ. *Cost-benefit analysis,* 4th ed. London: Routledge, 1994:22–37.
8. Neumann P, Johannesson M. The willingness-to-pay for in vitro fertilization: a pilot study using contingent valuation. *Med Care* 1994;32:686–699.
9. Ryan M. Using willingness to pay to assess the benefits of assisted reproductive techniques. *Health Econ* 1996;5:543–558.
10. Sonnenberg FA. Introduction to decision theory and utilities. In: Staquet MJ, Hays RD, Fayers PM, eds. *Quality of life assessment in clinical trials: methods and practice.* Oxford: Oxford University Press, 1998:93–117.

The Degenerative Cervical Spine,
edited by Marek Szpalski and Robert Gunzburg
Lippincott Williams & Wilkins, Philadelphia © 2001.

31

Cost-Utility of Two Anterior Cervical Disc Procedures

Björn Zoëga, Bengt Lind

Department of Orthopedics, Sahlgrenska University Hospital, S-413 45 Göteborg, Sweden

---

MATERIAL AND METHODS
RESULTS
DISCUSSION

Health care cost-effectiveness comparisons are used for two basic purposes—to determine the most efficient way to allocate limited resources among a variety of interventions for different diseases and to choose between two or more therapies for the same disease. To allocate funds, interventions may be ranked from those that return the most benefit per dollar invested to those that return the least. Patient outcome measures must be in the same units for such comparisons (7). Cost-effectiveness comparisons more frequently are used as a way of choosing between two or more competing therapies for the same health problem. Choosing the most cost-effective health intervention appears to be simple. The alternatives are compared, and the one that delivers the most additional benefit for the least additional cost is chosen. Behind this facade of clarity lurk a host of difficulties, including controversial judgments influence the results of the analysis. Because cost-effectiveness is a comparative concept, the ratio of average costs to average patient outcomes for a single treatment tells one little by itself. Without a standard of comparison, it is impossible to know when a ratio crosses the line between efficiency and inefficiency. In health care, the standard for comparison is typically another treatment.

Cost-effectiveness analysis is a general term that covers three different types of comparisons—cost-effectiveness, cost-benefit, and cost-utility. These methods are differentiated according to method used to measure noncost outcomes. A cost-effectiveness analysis may measure patient outcomes in any of a variety of relevant units, such as points on a blood pressure scale, lives saved, or other measures. *Cost-benefit analysis* converts health outcomes to monetary values. For example, they can be used to determine the value of additional work productivity resulting from a health intervention or the amount a person would be willing to pay for a specific improvement in health. *Cost-utility analyses* weight outcomes according to the value that patients place on them. The resulting outcome measure is a combination of actual outcomes adjusted for patients' preferences. Because patients typically consider some outcomes more important than others, the preferred intervention is not necessarily the one that offers the most change but is the one that makes the greatest improvements in the areas the patient thinks is most important.

Quality-adjusted life-years (QALY) gained are the typical measurement unit in cost-utility analysis. QALY gained are constructed by combining life-years gained from an intervention with weighting of the quality of those years. Some authorities define acceptable cost-effectiveness per QALY gained as a range of $20,000 to $100,000 US and others define it more conservatively to $20,000 to $40,000 US (5,9,10).

The use of cost-effectiveness studies has been limited in spine research. Surgery of lumbar disc herniation has in a retrospective study been reported to be $29,200 per QALY (1993 US$) (11). In a study of 55 truck drivers with herniated discs, it was found that first-year charges for surgically and medically treated patients were $20,700 and $9,600 (1989 US$), respectively (15). To our knowledge only one study (18) has been published on the cost-effectiveness of cervical disc herniation. McLaughlin et al. (13), however, reported on the use of a cervical spine locking plate in the management of two-level anterior cervical fusion for radiculopathy. The patients treated with plate fixation had a significantly earlier return to light activities, driving, and unrestricted work than did those treated without plate fixation. The authors concluded that the higher cost of treatment with plate fixation was more than offset by the benefits of earlier mobilization.

MATERIAL AND METHODS

A prospective, randomized study of plate fixation in anterior cervical spinal fusion was performed in the department of orthopedics, Sahlgrenska University Hospital, Sweden, between January 1994 and November 1995. The primary aim of the study was to evaluate the effect of plate fixation on anterior cervical spinal fusion. Forty-six patients were included in the study. The last 24 consecutively registered patients participated in this study and in a separate study the object of which was to evaluate the cost-utility of surgery with and without instrumented fusion. Eight of these 24 patients underwent one-level operations without plate fixation and seven with plate fixation. Nine patients underwent two-level operations, five with plate fixation and four without. Ten of the 24 patients (seven women) related their symptoms to a low velocity motor vehicle accident (whiplash injury).

Before the operation, the patients filled out a questionnaire that included the EuroQol index. They also gave their written consent for inclusion in the study and written permission to collect data on the costs of their sick leave. Register data, such as the patient's sick leave and costs before surgery, were gathered from the files of the local social insurance office. The duration of symptoms and sick-leave period before surgery was recorded. The time from referral of the patient to our hospital and meeting with the surgeon was recorded, as was the waiting time from this visit at until the operation. The costs for the in-hospital care related to the neck problems were taken from the hospital accountant register. All costs during the hospital stay were included. One and 2 years after the operation, the patients filled in the questionnaires once again, including the EuroQol form.

EuroQol is a general health-related quality of life index that includes five subissues: mobility, activities of daily living, usual activities, pain-discomfort, and anxiety-depression. The scale ranges from 1.0 (best possible quality of life) to 0 (dead). Negative values are possible, because some health conditions are regarded "worse than death," such as paralysis in combination with excruciating pain. EuroQol has been validated in several European countries, including Sweden (2,3). The average healthy adult Swede has a score of 0.89 (1).

In the calculation of cost-utility of surgical treatment, the mean value of the preoperative EuroQol score was subtracted from the mean 2-year postoperative EuroQol score. The difference is a measure of the quality of life change. This value multiplied by the duration of the improved quality of life gives a value for utility—the QALY. In this study it was assumed that in case of improved quality of life, this improvement would last for the rest of the patient's life. Each patient's expected remaining lifetime was taken from the National Central Bureau of Statistics in Sweden. The determined total hospital cost divided by the utility value gives a quotient—costs per QALY. The lower the quotient, the more effective is the procedure. The baseline for monetary calculations was the exchange rate on April 30 1998. All monetary values are expressed in U.S. dollars.

RESULTS

The patients reported that they had had symptoms for an average of 20.4 months (SD 12, range 0.5 to 48) before surgery. The mean preoperative sick leave was 270 days (SD 260). The patients waited an average of 3.4 months (SD 1.9) before they were examined by an orthopedic surgeon and 5.6 months (SD 2.7) before surgery. For the total group of 24 patients, the EuroQol had not improved significantly 2 years after surgery, irrespective of type of procedure. Separation of the patients into two groups, those who claimed a previous whiplash injury and those who did not, revealed a significant improvement in EuroQol among the later but not among the former group (Table 31.1) (14).

The costs for the patients are shown in Table 31.2. The mean hospital costs for those who underwent plate fixation and those who did not did not differ significantly. The mean calculated remaining number of years left to live among the patients who did not have whiplash was 33.8 years.

The cost-utility analysis involved only on the patients without whiplash injury, because there was a change in EuroQol score only in this group. The average cost for these patients was $5,141 US. The quality of life improvement (EuroQol change) was 0.30. This gives a cost-utility quotient of 171 at 2 years and a cost-utility of $8,568 US [5,141/(0.3 × 2)] (QALY). If the improvement in quality of life stays the same throughout the patient's remaining life, the cost-utility is $507 US ($406 1990 US$; Table 31.3). Four of 10 patients who related their symptoms to whiplash injury returned to work. Ten of 14 patients who had not sustained such an injury returned to work.

TABLE 31.1. *Mean (SD), Euroqol, for the patients who related their symptoms to a whiplash injury versus those who did not*

	Preoperatively	1 yr postoperatively	2 yr postoperatively	P value[a]
Whiplash injury	0.48 (0.26)	0.29 (0.41)	0.35 (0.36)	P > .30
No whiplash injury	0.38 (0.34)	0.61 (0.33)	0.68 (0.18)	P = .041

[a]Comparing preoperative scores to the ones recorded 2 years postoperatively. Fisher test for pair comparison (14).

TABLE 31.2. *Mean costs in U.S. dollars*

Cost	Whiplash injury	No whiplash injury
Hospital costs	6,580	5,141
Costs of sick leave before surgery	16,902	26,567
Costs of sick leave after surgery	30,406	21,474
Physician costs before surgery	2,137	1,877
Physician costs after surgery	917	944
Physiotherapy costs before surgery	673	545
Physiotherapy costs after surgery	797	913
Total costs	58,412	57,462

TABLE 31.3. *Cost utility of different therapies*

Therapy	Cost utility[a]
Neurosurgical intervention for head injury	405
Anterior fusion for herniated cervical disc, current study	406
Pacemaker implantation	1,850
Hip replacement	1,990
CABG (left main vessel disease, severe angina)	3,520
Kidney transplant	7,930
Heart transplantation	13,200
Discectomy for herniated lumbar disc	24,800
Hospital hemodialysis	37,000
Neurosurgical intervention for malignant intracranial tumor	181,500

[a]US$, 1990.

Data from Malter AD, Larson EB, Urban N, et al. Cost-effectiveness of lumbar discectomy for the treatment of herniated intervertebral disc. *Spine* 1996;21:1048–1054 and Maynard A. Developing the health care market. *Econ J* 1991;101:1277–1286.

DISCUSSION

The patients reported that they had symptoms for 20 months before surgery. This is much longer than the optimal time for a good outcome. Two to three months has been considered sufficient to try conservative treatment, although this has not been verified in prospective, randomized studies (4,16). The pain duration has to be considered in comparisons of the findings with those of earlier studies, in which the time between onset of symptoms and surgery has been much shorter. If the surgery had been performed earlier in our study, the cost to society would probably have been smaller, because the patients would most likely have returned to work earlier. If the waiting time before consultation and the time from consultation to operation can be reduced from 3.5 and 5.6 months, respectively, to a more optimal 1 to 1.5 months, the total waiting time to surgery would be 7.5 months shorter. This would save about $22.140 US per patient (patients without whiplash). More important is that most patients would benefit from a reduction of the period with pain.

The need for detailed cost estimates is obvious in today's climate of cost reduction and health care priorities. The cost for cervical spinal surgery probably varies greatly among different countries depending on different surgical techniques, postoperative treatment, type of reimbursement, and variable methods of calculating. The age of the patients, complication rate, and costs for convalescence are other important factors. Further variations may be due to different health care management systems and different economic incentives and disincentives in health care and social welfare policies. The costs for patients treated with or without plate fixation did not differ significantly. This might be explained by the small number of patients in this study.

How do we know how long the effect of surgery will last? Results of few long-term studies have been reported, but in a study by Gore and Sepic (6), patients who underwent anterior discectomy and fusion were observed for more than 20 years. During these years, about 30% of the patients had a recurrence of symptoms, and about one half of the episodes had undergone reoperation by the time of follow-up evaluations. Patients with radiculopathy or with axial neck pain as the sole symptom were included in the study.

The cost-utility of anterior cervical discectomy and fusion found in this study compares favorably with that of other medical interventions (11,12,17). If the assumption is made that the effect of the treatment will last for the patient's remaining life, this type of surgery is one of the most cost-effective surgical interventions reported (Table 31.3).

Comparisons have to be made with caution, because the methods of measuring cost-utility differ between the authors. Variations may be caused by factors such as year of study and type of operation, country where the study was performed, and discount rate. There are also many ethical considerations in evaluating such data. To be able to use this kind of information as an instrument in allocating health care resources, one has to perform the studies at the same time, in the same country, and use the same quality of life score and the same type of cost evaluation.

The cost-utility quotient for patients without whiplash was 171. This can be compared with the results of a study of hip prostheses conducted with the same methods at our hospital in 1991 (8). In that study the cost-utility quotient for an uncemented hip prosthesis was 213 and for a cemented hip prosthesis was 171. An important consideration is that most patients receiving hip prostheses are elderly and many are retired, whereas most of the patients in the current study were young or middle-aged. It is probably easier to obtain an improved quality of life score among the elderly than it is among younger persons in regard to function. Among retired patients, however, the economic benefits of return to work are absent in most instances. Nevertheless, patients without whiplash in the current study had the same cost-utility quotient patients receiving cemented hip prosthesis and a lower (better) quotient than patients receiving uncemented hip prostheses.

In conclusion, the cost utility of anterior cervical discectomy and fusion in the treatment of patients with radiculopathy and without a history of a whiplash injury is high. Further studies are needed with larger study groups.

REFERENCES

1. Björk S, Norinder A. The weighting exercise for Swedish Version of the EuroQol. *Health Econ* 1999;8:117–126.
2. Brooks RG. *Health status and quality of life measurement: issues and developments.* Lund, Sweden: Institute for Economics in Healthcare, 1991.
3. Brooks RG, EuroQol Group. EuroQol: the current state of play. *Health Policy* 1996;37:53–72.
4. Fellrath RF, Hanley EN. Anterior cervical discectomy and arthrodesis for radiculopathy. In: Clark CR, ed. *The cervical spine,* 3rd ed. Philadelphia: Lippincott-Raven Publishers, 1998:785–798.
5. Goldman L, Gordon DJ, Rifkind BM, et al. Cost and health implications of cholesterol lowering. *Circulation* 1992;85:1960–1968.
6. Gore DR, Sepic SB. Anterior discectomy and fusion for painful cervical disc disease: a report of 50 patients with an average follow-up of 21 years. *Spine* 1998;23:2047–2051.
7. Hadorn DC. Setting health care priorities in Oregon: cost-effectiveness meets the rule of rescue. *JAMA* 1991;265:2218–2225.
8. Hansson E, Axelsson H. *Använding av hälsoekonomisk utvärdering för prioritring inom ortopedisk kirugi* [Swedish]. SPRI rapport U 25856. Förvaltningshögskolan Gothenburg University, 1993.
9. Kaplan RM, Bush JW. Health related quality of life measurement for evaluation research and policy analysis. *Health Psychol* 1982;1:61–80.
10. Laupacis A, Feeny D, Detsky AS, et al. How attractive does a new technology have to be to warrant adoption and utilization? Tentative guidelines for using clinical and economic evaluations. *Can Med Assoc J* 1992; 146:473–481.
11. Malter AD, Larson EB, Urban N, et al. Cost-effectiveness of lumbar discectomy for the treatment of herniated intervertebral disc. *Spine* 1996;21:1048–1054.
12. Maynard A. Developing the health care market. *Econ J* 1991;101:1277–1286.
13. McLaughlin MR, Purighalla V, Pizzi FJ. Cost advantages of two-level anterior cervical fusion with rigid internal fixation for radiculopathy and degenerative disease. *Surg Neurol* 1997;48:560–565.
14. Odén A, Wedel H. Arguments for Fischer's permutation test. *Ann Stat* 1975;3:518–520.
15. Shvartzman L, Weingarten E, Sherry H, et al. Cost-effectiveness analysis of extended conservative therapy versus surgical intervention in the management of herniated lumbar intervertebral disc. *Spine* 1992;17(2):176–182.
16. Smith GW, Robinson RA. The treatment of certain cervical spine disorders by anterior removal of the intervertebral disc and interbody fusion. *J Bone Joint Surg Am* 1958;40:607–623.
17. Williams A. Economics of coronary artery bypass grafting. *Br Med J* 1985;291:326–329.
18. Zoëga B. *Cervical discectomy and fusion with or without plate fixation: a randomized clinical and radiographic study on outcome and cost-utility* [thesis]. Gothenburg, Sweden: University of Gothenburg, 1998.

The Degenerative Cervical Spine,
edited by Marek Szpalski and Robert Gunzburg
Lippincott Williams & Wilkins, Philadelphia © 2001.

32

Fitness for Work and Costs in the Surgical Management of the Cervical Spine

Marc Du Bois, Peter Donceel

*Department of Occupational and Insurance Medicine, School of Public Health,
Katholieke Universiteit Leuven, 3000 Leuven, Belgium*

METHODS
  Fitness for Work • Analysis of Costs • Statistics
RESULTS
  Trends in Surgery Rates • Fitness for Work • Analysis of Costs
DISCUSSION
  Trends in Surgery Rates • Fitness for Work • Analysis of Costs

---

Disease of the cervical spine is primarily degenerative or discogenic and is a major contributor to overall morbidity in developed countries (12). Disorders of the cervical spine are common among the older population (10). As a consequence, the number of patients seeking surgical treatment for cervical disorders is steadily increasing. At any time 1% of the U.S. population is permanently disabled from spine-related disorders and an equal percentage are temporarily disabled (9). Notwithstanding that the prevalence of cervical pain is less than that of back-related disorders, the figure remains significant.

The management of cervical and lumbar radiculopathy due to disc herniation or degenerative osteophyte formation has been the subject of surgical attention for many years (13). To our knowledge, however, no information about surgery rates and outcomes is available for the Belgian population. Herein we attempt to provide some insight into the current costs and outcome of the surgical management of cervical spinal disorders. The goals of the study were fourfold:

1. To delineate the trends in surgery rates for cervical degenerative disorders in Belgium
2. To assess return to work rates 1 year after surgery for cervical degenerative disorders
3. To assess differences in an array of variables between return to work rates during the postoperative year
4. To investigate the costs related to surgery for cervical degenerative disorders

METHODS

The study was conducted with administrative patient record files from the largest Belgian sickness fund. It covered approximately 45% of the population in Belgium, where sickness insurance is legally imposed. Using the Belgian procedure code for medical and surgical procedures, surgical interventions on the cervical spine were selected. The procedure code is a numerically encoded system, which refers to the official description of a surgical intervention for financial reimbursement purposes. The surgeon has to register every intervention performed for cervical disorders in line with this procedure code. Between January 1998 and January 1999, 1,012 enrollees in the Christian Sickness Fund underwent surgical intervention for cervical disorders. Details about diagnosis or clinical or radiologic signs are not included in the database. Patient records were followed until 1 year after surgical intervention.

The official nomenclature descriptions of the selected surgical procedure are *cervical intercorporal fusion with harvesting of the graft* and *surgery for cervical disc herniation.* We also obtained data with respect to surgery for cervical disorders from 1989 till 1998 from Christian Sickness Fund claims files. We calculated surgery rates by dividing the number of treated patients by the year-specific total sickness fund enrollees for 1989 through 1998. Rates were not adjusted for age or sex.

Fitness for Work

Patients were evaluated by medical advisers of social security. Individual medical evaluations took place regularly from about 1 month after surgical intervention until patients were judged fit for resuming work according to the legal criteria in the sickness and invalidity insurance. In the first 6 months of work incapacity, the medical adviser evaluated fitness for work with regard to the patient's last job. After an incapacity period of 6 months, the criterion was extended to all occupations the patient may have access to, according to professional career and education.

We determined patient outcome by reviewing the time between surgery and return to full-duty work on claims files of patients belonging to the working population who were operated on in 1998. There were 191 women and 246 men in the study. The available preoperative features were obtained through a review of the individual files of the claimants. The retrieved information is shown in Table 32.1. Patients who returned to work within 1 year were classified as having a good outcome.

Analysis of Costs

In Belgium, health care and sickness benefits are insured by a social security system financed with contributions from both employees and employers. In the health care in-

TABLE 32.1. *Patient data*

Characteristic	Value
Sex (no. of patients)	
Female	191
Male	264
Age (yr; range)	45 (23–68)
Occupation (no. of patients)	
Self-employed	33
Blue collar worker	274
White collar worker	130
Duration of work incapacity before surgery (no. of patients)	
<1 mo	218
1–6 mo	132
>6 mo	87
No. undergoing instrumented surgery	208

surance, tariff agreements are made between health care providers, government, and sickness funds. In this system, each medical procedure or intervention is valued at a fixed price. A day lump sum is provided for hospitals to finance medical equipment, nursing, lodging, and administration. Patients belonging to the working population are compensated during the recovery period until fitness for work. They receive a daily compensation in accordance with their previous salary level. The expenditures for medical procedures, work incapacity compensation, hospital nursing, lodging, and administration add up to the social insurance costs.

The cost-assessment phase of the study determined the social insurance cost for a follow-up period of 1 postoperative year. In view of the retrospective design of this study, we were not able to rule out medical care costs unrelated to intervention for cervical spinal disorders.

Patients' claims files were broken down into the following cost items: kinesitherapy, anesthesiology, orthopedics, radiography, implants, medication, and nursing and lodging. For the working population, daily sickness fund payments compensating for working time lost after 1 month of working incapacity also were calculated. No information about compensation payments during the first month of sick leave was available (to be paid by the employer in the Belgian social security system). All costs are expressed in 1998 U.S. dollars.

Statistics

Comparisons of outcomes by independent factors such as age, sex, preoperative period of work incapacity and instrumentation were made by means of χ^2 analysis. Kruskal-Wallis one-way analysis of variance was used to identify the continuous factors related to ability to work postoperatively. Logistic regression was performed to identify factors independently associated with return to work status 1 year after intervention. Cost items were retrieved from the Christian Sickness Fund data warehouse (Oracle database management system). Statistical significance was assumed at the 5% level. Computations were made with a commercially available software program, SPSS 9.0. Kaplan-Meier curves, pie charts, and trend figures were drawn with SPSS 9.0 and Excel 7.0 for Windows.

RESULTS

Trends in Surgery Rates

Current rates of surgery (Fig. 32.1) for cervical disorders were obtained from the Christian Sickness Fund claims files. These data are used primarily for reimbursement

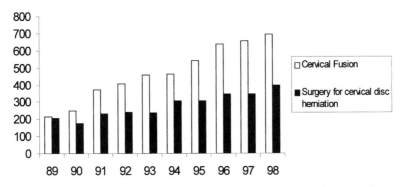

FIG. 32.1. Annual number of operations for cervical disorders in the Christian Sickness Fund population.

purposes and therefore may be vulnerable to erroneous and biased coding. From 1989 to 1998 7,991 cervical operations were performed on Christian Sickness Fund enrollees. The 1998 annual rate of surgery for cervical disorders was 26,04 per 100,000 enrollees. Over the last 10 years, the frequency of fusion of the cervical spine increased more than 300%, whereas the surgery rate for cervical disc herniation doubled. This trend goes along with the international increase in surgery rate in the management of disorders of the lumbar and cervical spine.

Fitness for Work

The working population who underwent intervention for cervical spinal disorders in 1998 consisted of 437 patients (Fig. 32.2). The mean age was 45 years. There were 191 women and 246 men. Twenty-five percent of the study population had a work incapacity period longer than 117 days before intervention; 84.6% of the patients returned to work within 1 year of the operation. There was no statistically significant difference between the median time to return to after cervical fusion (127 days) and time after cervical disc herniation (121 days).

Comparison of the features among the bad and good outcome groups showed that there was no significant statistical difference in working capacity with respect to sex. Professional category had an effect on postoperative working capacity. Self-employed patients resumed work a median of 148 days after the operation and blue collar workers 127 days postoperatively. This was a significantly longer period than that for white collar workers (91 days).

Period of working incapacity before surgical intervention affected postoperative working capacity: 34.4% who were more than 6 months out of work at the time of operation

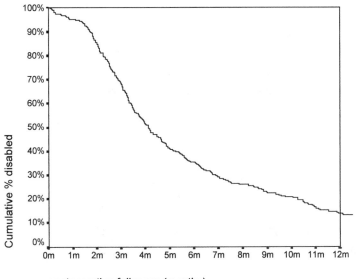

postoperative follow-up (months)

FIG. 32.2. Duration of work incapacity after surgical intervention for cervical spinal disorders in the worker compensation population (n = 437).

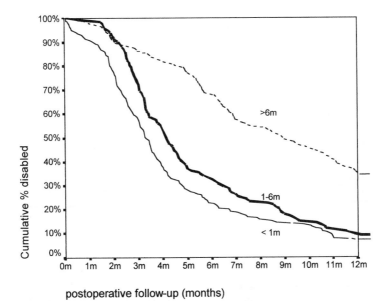

FIG. 32.3. Work incapacity after surgical intervention for cervical disorders. Outflow curves for subgroups with different preoperative work incapacity periods (>6 months, 1 to 6 months, <1 month).

were still unable to return to work after 1 year. For patients less than 1 month out of work for medical reasons, only 7.3% were unable to work 12 months after the operation (Fig. 32.3). Age was not significantly associated with return to work. Eighty-nine of the patients younger than 40 years resumed work, as did 88% of the patients in the older age categories (Fig. 32.4).

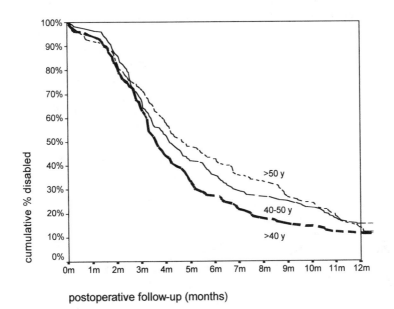

FIG. 32.4. Work incapacity after surgical intervention for cervical disorders. Outflow curves for subgroups in different age groups (older than 50 years, 40 to 50 years, and younger than 40 y).

TABLE 32.2. *Median social security cost per case (U.S. dollars) during a one-year period after surgery for cervical spine disorders (n=1012)*

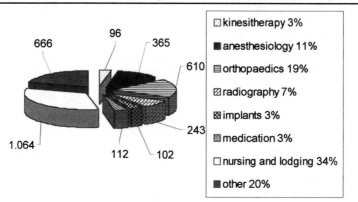

☐ kinesitherapy 3%

■ anesthesiology 11%

▤ orthopaedics 19%

▨ radiography 7%

▨ implants 3%

▨ medication 3%

☐ nursing and lodging 34%

■ other 20%

Patients who underwent surgery with implants did not have a statistically different outcome. In the regression analysis duration of work incapacity before the operation was significantly ($P < .001$) associated with a return to work within 1 year after the operation. A patient who had a work incapacity period longer than 6 months before surgery had a 6 times higher risk of being incapable to resume work 1 year after surgery. This variable explained the variance in return to work (partial correlation coefficient, .30).

Analysis of Costs

The administrative database provides information on costs. The cumulative social security expenses for the 1,012 patients who underwent operations for a cervical disorder in the year after operation was $6,661,925. The median social security costs of surgery for cervical disorders was approximately $4,000 per case for a 1-year period after intervention. The median costs per item are depicted in Table 32.2. Kinesitherapy and implants accounted for approximately 6% of the social security cost during the follow-up period. Instrumentation was used in operations on 51.6% of the patients, and in 66.8% of the cases kinesitherapy was prescribed. The median duration of hospital stay was 7 days.

Patients who have a good outcome entail lesser costs than do patients with a longer period of incapacity. The economic differences of good outcomes lie primarily in the lesser worker compensation payments. For the cervical disc herniation group there was no significantly additional benefit in return to work or postoperative hospital stay for patients who underwent instrumented surgery.

DISCUSSION

This study was retrospective and as such suffers from the shortcomings of all retrospective studies (14). It was therefore impossible to provide information on a variety of diseases of the cervical spine, including disc disease, instability due to trauma, failed fusion, pseudoarthrosis after disc surgery, and cervical spondylosis (1,3,5). Random allocation of patients to groups also was not possible, and the hypotheses being tested were generated after the fact. Therefore we are not making comparisons for choice of surgical technique, nor are we commenting on the criteria to make that decision. Nonetheless some valid conclusions can be drawn from this study.

Trends in Surgery Rates

The rising trend in surgical rates in Belgium illustrates the internationally rising surgery rate in the management of disorders of the spine. Two factors directly related to this phenomenon are the increase in the aging of the Belgian population and the availability of such noninvasive neuroradiologic imaging modalities as magnetic resonance imaging in the early diagnosis and management of osseous lesions of the cervical spine (1,10). The imaging aids combined with the smaller surgical incisions and precise dissection have led to a decrease in postoperative pain, earlier mobilization, and a decrease in hospital stay (13). This improvement in neurosurgical management may also contribute to the growing trend in surgery for cervical disorders because it further bolsters the patient's confidence in returning as soon as possible to daily activities.

Fitness for Work

We found that 15% of all patients were still unable to resume work 1 year postoperatively. The median return to work interval was approximately 4 months. Onimus et al. (8) found an average return to work rate of 3 months after surgical intervention for cervical soft disc herniation. In some studies patients receiving worker compensation returned to work a mean of 7.6 weeks (range 2 to 12 weeks) after the operation (13). These authors also found evidence that patients receiving worker compensation and other patients involved in litigation have poorer outcomes than do patients without a secondary gain influence (12). Because work incapacity benefits are mandatory in the Belgian sickness and invalidity legislation, we can not support that conclusion.

We investigated the role of factors associated with outcome, which include sex, age, instrumented surgery, occupation, and period of work incapacity before surgery. Our data support the finding that sex is unrelated to the outcome of surgery for cervical disorders. Tomaras et al. (13) found that there is no difference in return to work with regard to sex.

In our data the period of work incapacity before the intervention was the strongest factor related to professional outcome. Our finding confirmed the findings of Lee et al. (6), who showed that duration of symptoms for more than 18 months was associated with poorer gait improvement after surgery for nontraumatic cervical spondylosis with myelopathy. In the management of degenerative cervical spinal disorders there has been a lack of prospective, randomized trials comparing surgical and nonsurgical modalities. Therefore the decision to operate often is based on the surgeon's experience (10).

Age at intervention was not related to the prognosis of the patient's ability to return to work after the operation. This finding is in agreement with the results of Razack et al. (10), who studied the results of surgery for cervical myelopathy among geriatric patients (10).

Our study provides evidence that occupation has an effect on postoperative working capability. Nonetheless, the effect of occupation in the univariate analysis was not sustained in the logistic regression procedure. This effect was caused by the statistically significant positive correlation between period of preoperative work incapacity and occupation. Among the blue-collar workers, 51.7% of had a preoperative work incapacity period longer than 6 months; the incapacity period was only 13.8% among the white-collar workers.

Despite dramatic proliferation in the development and use of internal fixation hardware and techniques on the cervical spine, our figures suggest that instrumented cervical surgery is not associated with a better outcome. Instrumentation in surgery undoubtedly adds to the cost of cervical spinal surgery. A large, randomized, multicenter study is needed to assess the economic and medical value of instrumentation (2,11).

Analysis of Costs

An important cost item was accrued work incapacity compensation payments in line with the length of the work incapacity period. It is estimated that on average a benefit for work incapacity amounts to $34 a day. The amount and duration of disability can be lessened by giving patients advice concerning returning to activities as quickly as tolerated and by simply discussing patients' concerns about neck pain. As stated by Rainville et al. (9), successful performance of exercises in the presence of pain can improve patients' confidence about other wellness activities, including work. Many functional restoration programs show that patients with chronic neck pain can improve their functional ability to normal levels (9).

The median hospital stay was 7 days, which was consistent with the findings in the international literature (13). A striking finding in the cost analysis was that instrumented surgery did not alter the 1-year return to work rate in relation to noninstrumented intervention. Instrumented surgery also did not shorten postoperative hospital stay, so cost-effectiveness could not be proved. Neither procedure was superior in the time it took the patient to resume gainful employment. In the atmosphere of restraints on medical expenditures the advantage of reduced hospital stay for instrumented surgery could not be found. This finding does not cast doubt on the cost-effectiveness of some device fusions (1,2,4,7). Moreover, this conclusion must be correctly addressed within the retrospective analysis of an administrative database with missing information on indications for surgery. In that respect it is generally assumed that in the cervical spine most radicular symptoms begin improving within 3 months of the operation. Only if there are substantial persisting signs and symptoms confirmed with abnormal results of imaging studies should surgery be contemplated. The success rates for cervical fusion performed to manage neck pain have not yet been adequately documented.

This retrospective analysis of cervical operations supports the following conclusion: The frequency of surgery for degenerative cervical disorders is increasing. It is reasonable to expect resumption of work within 4 months in the Belgian social security system. Inpatient costs such as nursing, lodging, and surgery are a large portion of the expenditures associated with morbidity and for the health care system. During the recovery phase, outlays for work incapacity benefits grow steadily. Decreasing the duration of disability therefore is a major concern from an economic and a medical point of view.

REFERENCES

1. Bose B. anterior cervical fusion using Caspar plating: analysis of results and review of the literature. *Surg Neurol* 1998;49:25–31.
2. Caspar W, Geisler FH, Pitzen T et al. Anterior cervical plate stabilization in one- and two level degenerative disease: overtreatment or benefit? *J Spinal Disord* 1998;11:1–11.
3. Gore DR, Sepic SB. Anterior discectomy and fusion for painful cervical disc disease: a report of 50 patients with an average follow-up of 21 years. *Spine* 1998;23:2047–2051.
4. Hilibrand AS, Yoo YU, Carlson GD, et al. The success of anterior cervical arthrodesis adjacent to a previous fusion. *Spine* 1997;22:1574–1579.
5. Inoue H, Ohmori K, Ishida Y, et al. Long-term follow-up review of suspension laminotomy for cervical compression myelopathy. *J Neurosurg* 1996;85:817–823.
6. Lee TT, Manzano GR, Green BA. Modified open-door cervical expansive laminoplasty for spondylotic myelopathy: operative technique, outcome, and predictors for gait improvement. *J Neurosurg* 1997;86:64–68.

7. Munoz FLO, Garcia de las Heras B, Lopez VC, et al. Comparison of three techniques of anterior fusion in single-level cervical disc herniation. *Eur Spine J* 1998;7:512–516.

8. Onimus M, Destrumelle N, Gangloff S. Le traitement chirurgical des hernies discales cervicales: abord antérieur ou abord postérieur *Rev Chir Orthop Reparatrice Appar Mot* 1995;81:296–301.

9. Rainville J, Sobel JB, Banco RJ, et al. Low back and cervical spine disorders. *Orthop Clin North Am* 1996;27: 729–746.

10. Razack N, Greenberg J, Green BA. Surgery for cervical myelopathy in geriatric patients. *Spinal Cord* 1998;36: 629–632.

11. Sawin PD, Traynelis VC, Menezes AH. A comparative analysis of fusion rates and donor-site morbidity for autogeneic rib and iliac crest bone grafts in posterior cervical fusions. *J Neurosurg* 1998;88:255–265.

12. Silvers R, Lewis PJ, Suddaby LS, et al. Day surgery for cervical microdiscectomy: is it safe and effective? *J Spinal Disord* 1996;9:287–295.

13. Tomaras CR, Blacklock JB, Parker WD, et al. outpatient surgical treatment of cervical radiculopathy. *J Neurosurg* 1997;87:41–43.

14. Watters WC, Levinthal R. Anterior cervical discectomy with and without fusion: results, complications, and long-term follow-up. *Spine* 1994;19:2343–2347.

The Degenerative Cervical Spine,
edited by Marek Szpalski and Robert Gunzburg
Lippincott Williams & Wilkins, Philadelphia © 2001.

33

Outcome Scores in Degenerative Cervical Disc Surgery

Bengt Lind, Björn Zoëga

Department of Orthopedics, Sahlgrenska University Hospital, S-413 45 Göteborg, Sweden

DISEASE-SPECIFIC OUTCOME SCORES FOR THE CERVICAL SPINE
NON–DISEASE-SPECIFIC OR GENERIC SCORES
OUTCOME STUDY ON CERVICAL DISC SURGERY
CONCLUSIONS

The definition of patient outcome is observation of a patient over time, often associated with an intervention, such as an operation or administration of a new drug. The outcome can be measured with different kinds of scores, which facilitates comparisons of different treatments and comparisons of outcome between institutions. The value of outcome measures has become evident over the last years in medical society (1–10, 13–19). The reason for this is an increased interest among clinicians but also an increased interest among health authorities, economists, and politicians in different countries. With increased costs and new treatment methods but with scarce resources, and with the introduction in many countries of managed competition in health care, health authorities may now require health providers to deliver efficient and effective care. With unreliable or wrongly selected outcome measures, erroneous conclusions can be drawn that may affect allocation of resources. It is therefore important that there exist measuring tools that are reliable and suitable for the variables and the disorder studied.

Any outcome measure should, according to Deyo et al. (2), entail the following criteria: reliability, validity, responsiveness, practicality, and comprehensiveness. *Reliability* means reproducibility between raters and by one rater from one administration to another. *Validity* is the ability of the instrument to measure what it is supposed to measure. *Responsiveness* is the sensitivity of the instrument to detect clinically important changes. Also important is that the score be understood by all patients regardless of age and social or educational status. An internationally used score should after translation be tested for these basic criteria in the current language. Very few measures used meet all these criteria. There are many fewer methods of assessing outcome of treatment of the cervical spine than there are for treatment of the lumbar spine. Only recently have outcome measures for the neck been developed and validated (16,19).

There exist different kinds of measures. Some are disease specific, such as instruments for rheumatoid arthritis, hip disease, and lumbar spinal disorders (5,10,16). Non–disease-specific or generic instruments measure general health and quality of life (1,4,7,17,18).

The latter scores are gaining popularity, and some of them can be used in cost-effectiveness analysis. Yet other scores are used to measure a specific symptom, such as pain or anxiety (9,10,20).

DISEASE-SPECIFIC OUTCOME SCORES FOR THE CERVICAL SPINE

Problems related to degeneration of the cervical spine often are self-limited. However, for some patients these problems might necessitate surgery, the most predominant symptoms being pain and neurologic deficit. Outcome after this surgery usually is relief of pain. The instrument most commonly used to measure this change is the criteria defined by Odom et al. (12) (Table 33.1). This is mainly a subjective rating scale, and outcome may vary depending on the rater. Thus results when this scale are used are unreliable and make conclusions or comparisons of one study with other similar studies difficult. The outcome rating is excellent and good to fair and poor.

Cervical myelopathy is more common in Japan than elsewhere owing to the high prevalence of ossification of the posterior longitudinal ligament. The Japanese Orthopedic Association therefore designed a score (8) to follow the course and response to treatment of this condition. This score comprises assessments of how disturbance of function in the upper and lower extremities affects activities of daily living. The score is useful in the study of myelopathy but not of impairment due to radiculopathy and neck pain.

The Neck Disability Index (NDI) (16) was introduced in 1991 and is a modification of the Oswestry Disability Index (5) used for low back pain. The NDI was designed to assess chronic disability after soft-tissue injury to the cervical spine. It comprises five scales from the original Oswestry Index and five new scales. The NDI has been validated and found to have a high degree of reliability and internal consistency. Most of the questions relate to how the neck pain affects activities of daily living, but there also are questions about pain intensity and headache.

The Neck Pain and Disability Index (NPAD) (19) is the most recently published instrument for measuring neck pain and disability. The NPAD index also is derived from a lumbar spinal measure and was designed with the Million visual analog scale (VAS) (11) as a template. The 20 items in the scale measure intensity of pain and its effect on vocational, recreational, social, and functional aspects of living. The NPAD also takes in account the presence of emotional factors. The face validity has been established, and like the NDI, the NPAD has been found to have a high degree of internal consistency.

Pain is the most important item in all of the measures described. It is multidimensional and an unpleasant personal experience. Therefore pain is difficult to measure and to define. There is no objective correlate, and one has to rely on patients' reports and memory of pain. Pain memory, however, is unreliable because one often remembers more pain than the baseline ratings show. A number of one-dimensional rating scales have been designed to quantify pain or pain relief, such as categorical verbal rating or ordinal scales. Probably the most

TABLE 33.1. *Outcome according to Odom criteria*

Outcome	Criteria
Excellent	All preoperative symptoms relieved. Abnormal findings alleviated.
Good	Minimal persistence of preoperative symptoms. Abnormal findings unchanged or alleviated.
Fair	Definite relief of some preoperative symptoms. Other symptoms unchanged or slightly alleviated.
Poor	Symptoms and signs unchanged or worse.

commonly used is a VAS (9). These scales entail lines on which the patient is asked to indicate the pain. The lines are either vertical or horizontal, marked at the end points with extreme descriptions of pain, and they sometimes are graded. The advantage of these scales is that they are easy to administer and quick to score. The disadvantages are that they require careful instruction and more concentration than the categorical scales. A VAS is not suited for very old or young patients. Quality of pain is best assessed with pain questionnaires, of which the McGill Pain Questionnaire (10) probably is used most often. This is a multidimensional measure reflects three dimensions—sensory, affective, and evaluative. The McGill Pain Questionnaire is reliable but time consuming. A combination of a quantitative and a qualitative measure seems to be the most complete in assessing pain.

NON–DISEASE-SPECIFIC OR GENERIC SCORES

The great advantages with generic measures are that they can be used to compare outcomes across different populations and after medical interventions and that they can be used for cost-effectiveness analysis. They measure quality of life, of which general health is the most important. Several available instruments measure general health, some of which are extensive questionnaires. Others are short and more suited for long-term follow-up evaluation in the daily practice of an outcome clinic.

The 36-item short-form questionnaire (SF-36) (1,7,17) is probably the most commonly used instrument in orthopedic research. It has been extensively validated and translated and used in many countries. It is a shortened form of 149 health-related questions that have been validated in a large study of medical outcome in the United States. The SF-36 measures three aspects of health—functional ability, well-being, and overall health. These are further subdivided into eight multiple-item scales, four of which are related to physical health and four to mental health. The scales are ranked from 0 (worst possible health) to 100 (best health). One criticism is that the questionnaire is too long to be used in a large-scale study. Another is that it is good for studying changes in a group of patients but not for monitoring an individual patient.

A shortened version of SF-36 has been constructed and validated—the 12-item short-form questionnaire (SF-12) (18). Twelve items were identified after a forward step-regression analysis of the SF-36 physical and mental health questions. These 12 items were found to reproduce more than 90% of the variance in the SF-36 questions and to reproduce the average scores for the two summary measures of SF-36. The SF-12 is completed in one-fifth the time used to complete SF-36. However, the SF-36 defines more levels of health and better represents the content of health measures, which makes it more suitable than the SF-12 in studies with a small sample size.

Another popular validated quality of life instrument is the EuroQol (4). This index includes five scales representing mobility, activities of daily living, usual activities, pain-discomfort, and anxiety. The scales range from 0 (dead) to 1.0 (best health), but negative values are possible because some health conditions are regarded as worse than death. The measure is short and easily completed within a couple of minutes.

The preferred strategy for spine research in the future should be to combine two validated instruments—one disease-specific (lumbar or cervical) and one generic.

OUTCOME STUDY ON CERVICAL DISC SURGERY

An outcome study was performed with 46 consecutive patients referred to the department of orthopedics, Sahlgren University Hospital, Sweden, with cervical disc herniations at one or two levels. The patients were randomized between anterior cervical discectomy and Smith-Robinson fusion with or without plate fixation (CSLP, Synthes). All patients were unable to work before the operation. The mean duration of symptoms was 32 months. Seventeen patients had a history of involvement in a low-velocity motor vehicle accident. Before the operation the patients completed a questionnaire that included a modified Million index and an Oswestry disability index. They also recorded neck and arm pain on a VAS. Two years postoperatively the patients were administered the same questionnaire by mail. They completed the questionnaire a third time at a follow-up visit 1 week after completing the mail questionnaire (test-retest). A neurologist examined the patients before the operation. The same neurologist performed the 2-year follow-up examinations unaware of which group the patients belonged to. He also graded the patients according to the Odom criteria.

The Wilcoxon signed rank test was used to analyze the results. A Bonferroni correction was applied because of the small sample size and the multiple comparisons made. A logistic regression was performed to identify any variables (sex, age, pain duration, type of injury, type of operation, preoperative score, and pain registration) that might influence the outcome.

Reproducibility was found to be good for the questionnaire with a significant correlation ($P < .0001$) between test and retest for the scores used. There was no significant improvement in any of the scores among patients who underwent operations on one level, even though 81% said they were satisfied with the outcome. All patients who underwent operations on two levels were satisfied with the outcome, but only patients who did not have plates inserted had significant improvement in Million index ($P < .05$) and in Oswestry index ($P < .05$) (Table 33.2). However, the patients with plate fixation had a more pronounced decrease in arm pain ($P < .05$) recorded on the VAS (Table 33.3). There was no difference between the two groups in outcome according to the Odom criteria regardless of number of levels treated (Table 33.2). In the regression analysis, none of the variables was found to have any influence on outcome. In a comparison of the less sophisticated but more commonly used Odom score with the composite Million and Oswestry scores, it was found that patients with an excellent or good result had a significantly lower score (better result) on both these measures ($P < .0005$).

TABLE 33.2. *Outcome on Million and Oswestry index and grading according to the Odom criteria*

Index or criterion	Plate		No plate	
	One level	Two levels	One level	Two levels
Million index (median and range)				
Preoperative score	5.6 (0.6–8.3)	7.0 (4.2–8.7)	5.0 (2.0–7.1)	6.5 (4.2–7.7)
Score 2 yr postoperatively	4.9 (1.5–8.2)	3.8 (0.3–8.5)	4.8 (0.2–7.6)	4.2 (0.3–7.0)
P value[a]	>.3	.056	>.3	.026
Oswestry index (median and range)				
Preoperative score	42 (14–68)	52 (30–64)	36 (6–64)	48 (24–74)
Score 2 yr postoperatively	48 (8–76)	30 (0–66)	38 (0–64)	33 (0–62)
P value[a]	>.3	.075	>.3	.016
Odom criteria (no. of patients)				
Excellent/good	11	8	8	7
Fair/poor	4	1	4	3

[a]The *P* values for the difference between the preoperative and 2-year follow-up values are given. Wilcoxon rank sum test with Bonferroni correction was used.

TABLE 33.3. *Visual analog scale values for arm and neck pain*

Type of value	Plate		No plate	
	One level	Two levels	One level	Two levels
Arm pain				
Preoperative score	4.0 (1.0–9.5)	5.1 (3.1–8.6)	6.3 (2.9–8.6)	5.8 (3.7–7.8)
Score 2 yr postoperatively	4.5 (0.3–8.0)	0.5 (0–3.7)	5.9 (0–7.8)	3.0 (0.6–5.7)
P value[a]	>.3	.016	.046	.034
Neck pain				
Preoperative score	5.4 (3.1–8.8)	6.4 (3.7–8.3)	6.3 (4.4–9.1)	6.3 (3.3–9.9)
Score 2 yr postoperatively	5.8 (1.7–8.8)	2.7 (0–6.6)	5.6 (0–8.2)	3.6 (0.5–7.1)
P value[a]	>.3	.024	>.3	.034

Values other than *P* value are median and range.
[a]The *P* values for the difference between the preoperative and 2-year follow-up values are given.
Wilcoxon rank sum test with Bonferroni correction was used.

The results in this study do not support the use of a plate as an adjunct to surgery on one disc. However, plate fixation when two discs are excised and fused seems to be better at reducing arm pain. This hypothesis has to be further evaluated for a larger series of patients. We are aware that the statistical power of this study is weak owing to the small sample sizes. Bonferroni corrections were used in an effort to overcome the lack of power. None of the neck-specific measures was available when the study was initiated. Some authors have proposed that the low back questionnaires may be applicable to the cervical spine. The results of this study are in accordance with that view. The results registered with the Odom criteria, however, seem to agree with the results obtained with other scores, even if statistical significance was not reached. Nevertheless, we are of the strong opinion that the neck-specific instruments now available should be further evaluated and used in future studies. They should be used instead of the Odom criteria, which are subjected to too many biases.

CONCLUSIONS

Future studies of cervical disc degeneration should be conducted only with valid and reliable measures. These studies should include a neck-specific measure such as the NDI or NPAD (16,19) in combination with a generic measure, such as SF-36, SF-12, or EuroQol (1,4,17,18). Patients expectations perhaps also should be evaluated with a single question about patient satisfaction (3). Only by using such measures can a reliable comparison be made between different studies from all over the world.

REFERENCES

1. Brazier JE, Harper R, Jones NMB, et al. Validating the SF-36 health survey questionnaire: new outcome measure for primary care. *Br Med J* 1992;305:160–164.
2. Deyo RA, Andersson G, Bombarider C, et al. Outcome measures for studying patients with low back pain. *Spine* 1994;19[Suppl]:S2032–S2036.
3. Deyo RA, Battie M, Beurskens AJHM, et al. Outcome measures for low back pain outcome: a proposal for standardized use. *Spine* 1998;23:2003–2013.
4. EuroQol Group. EuroQol: a new facility for the measurement of health-related quality-of-life. *Health Policy* 1990;16:199–208.
5. Fairbanks JCT, Coupier J, Davies JB, et al. The Oswestry Low Back Disability Questionnaire *Physiotherapy* 1980;66:271–273.
6. Greenough CG, Fraser RD. Assessment of outcome in patients with low-back pain. *Spine* 1992;17:1:36–41.
7. Grevitt M, Khazim R, Webb J, et al. The short form-36 health survey questionnaire in spine surgery. *J Bone Joint Surg Br* 1997;79:48–52.

8. Hirabayashi K, Miyakawa J, Satomi K, et al. Operative results and postoperative progression of ossification among patients with ossification of cervical posterior longitudinal ligament. *Spine* 1981;6:354–364.
9. Huskisson EC. Measurement of pain. *Lancet* 1974;9:1127–1131.
10. Melzack R. The McGill Pain Questionnaire: major properties and scoring methods. *Pain* 1975;1:277–299.
11. Million R, Hall W, Haavik Nilsen K, et al. Assessment of the progress of the back-pain patient. *Spine* 1982; 7:3:204–212.
12. Odom GL, Finney W, Woodhall B, et al. Cervical disk lesions. *JAMA* 1958;166:1:23–28.
13. Ruta DA, Garratt AM, Wardlaw D, et al. Developing a valid and reliable measure of health outcome of patients with low back pain. *Spine* 1994;19:1887–1896.
14. Streiner DL, Norman GR. *Health measurements scales: a practical guide to their development and use.* Oxford, UK: Oxford University Press, 1989.
15. Turk DC, Rudy TE. Spine up-date: methods for evaluating treatment outcomes—ways to overcome potential obstacles. *Spine* 1994;19:1759–1763.
16. Vernon H, Mior S. The neck disability index: a study of reliability and validity. *J Manipulative Physiol Ther* 1991;14:7:409–415.
17. Ware JE, Sherbourne C. The MOS 36-item short-form survey (SF-36), I: conceptual framework and item selection. *Med Care* 1992;30:473–483.
18. Ware JE, Snow KK, Kosinski M, et al. *SF-36 health survey: manual and interpretation guide.* Boston: The Health Institute, New England Medical Center, 1993.
19. Wheeler AH, Goolkasian P, Baird AC, et al. Development of the neck pain and disability scale: item analysis, face, and criterion-related validity. *Spine* 1999;24:13:1290–1294.
20. Zung WWK. A self-rating depression scale. *Arch Gen Psychiatry* 1965;12:63–70.

The Degenerative Cervical Spine,
edited by Marek Szpalski and Robert Gunzburg
Lippincott Williams & Wilkins, Philadelphia © 2001.

34

Diagnosis and Treatment in Evidence Based Health Care Systems

Charles G. Greenough

*Department of Orthopaedics, Middlebrough General Hospital, Middlesbrough
TS5 5AZ, United Kingdom*

DIAGNOSIS
  Tumor and Infection • Myelopathy • Radiculopathy • Combined Myelopathy and Radiculopathy • Mechanical Neck Pain
TREATMENT

Increasingly in western societies, the cost of health care is outstripping the means to pay for it. The response of governments and health care purchasers has been to consider restricting the clinical freedom of practitioners. One method used is to construct algorithms based on evidence-based practice. This trend will certainly continue. The first question, therefore, is what constitutes evidence? In the investigation and management of conditions of the cervical spine, there is no shortage of literature. Unfortunately, however, when subjected to impartial scrutiny, the evidence for many treatments is limited. For the purpose of this discussion, the definition of evidence used by the Canadian Task Force (1990) may be considered.

Level 1. At least one randomized, controlled trial.
Level 2-I. Well-designed controlled trial.
Level 2-II. Well designed cohort or case-controlled study.
Level 2-III. Comparisons between times or places.
Level 3. Opinions of respected authorities or committees.

Surgical treatment poses difficulties in this regard. Many practical difficulties are encountered if attempts are made to randomize patients between operative and non-operative treatments. Evidence for surgical therapy often is found only in level 2 or level 3 (5).

The Cochrane collaboration was initiated to provide practitioners with systematic reviews of the literature on a topic basis. Systemic searches through the literature are combined with detailed assessment of methodologic quality of studies to provide a summary of the available evidence for the efficacy and efficiency of treatments. These reviews are available to health care practitioners and to health care purchasers. To construct an algorithm for the investigation and management of cervical disorders, several resources can be called upon.

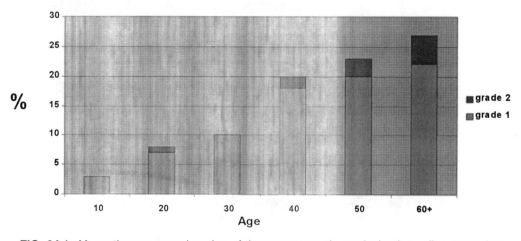

FIG. 34.1. Magnetic resonance imaging of the asymptomatic cervical spine—disc protrusion (497 patients). (Adapted from Matsumoto M, Fujimura Y, Suzuki N, et al. MRI of cervical inter-vertebral discs in asymptomatic subjects. *J Bone Joint Surg Br* 1998;80:19–24.)

The purpose of investigation is to inform prognosis and treatment. There is increasing interest in the specificity and sensitivity of investigations performed. Investigation that does not lead to a decision on management is of questionable value. It may use unnecessary resources. False-positive results cause unnecessary distress and may precipitate incorrect therapy. False-negative results may leave patients untreated for correctable pathologic conditions. The quality of detail of the anatomic features produced by modern magnetic resonance imaging (MRI) is far beyond what might have been imaged only a few years before. Clinicians' difficulty now is not seeing what is going on but understanding what it means.

Many studies have shown a significant incidence of anatomic abnormalities in asymptomatic cervical spines. In 1987 Teresi et al. (6) performed MRI of the cervical

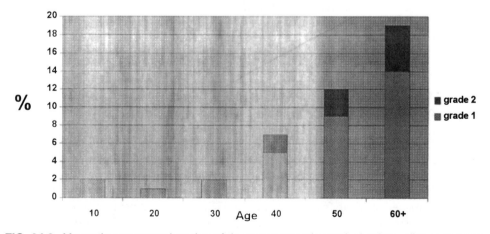

FIG. 34.2. Magnetic resonance imaging of the asymptomatic cervical spine—disc space narrowing. (Adapted from Matsumoto M, Fujimura Y, Suzuki N, et al. MRI of cervical intervertebral discs in asymptomatic subjects. *J Bone Joint Surg Br* 1998;80:19–24.)

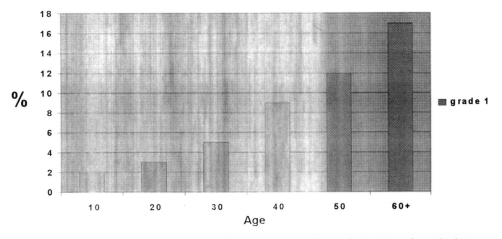

FIG. 34.3. Magnetic resonance images of the asymptomatic cervical spine—foraminal stenosis. (Adapted from Matsumoto M, Fujimura Y, Suzuki N, et al. MRI of cervical intervertebral discs in asymptomatic subjects. *J Bone Joint Surg Br* 1998;80:19–24.)

spine on 100 persons without symptoms. They found a disc bulge or disc herniation in 20% of the subjects between 45 and 54 years of age and in 57% of subjects 65 years or older. Posterolateral disc protrusion impinging on the nerve root was present in 10% of patients, most of whom were 65 years or older. Cord impingement was present in 16% of patients younger than 65 years and 26% of those 65 years or older. Seven percent of patients had cord compression, although none had more than 16% decompression.

In a more recent study, Matsumoto et al. (4) examined 497 volunteers who did not have symptoms. Overall a significant incidence of disc protrusion was found: 67% of subjects

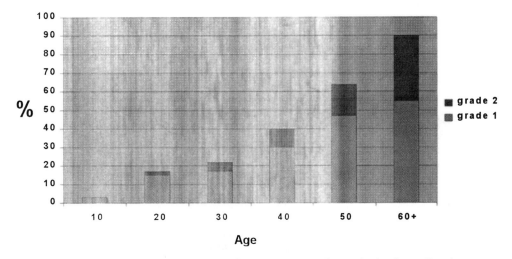

FIG. 34.4. Magnetic resonance images of the asymptomatic cervical spine—disc degeneration (497 patients). (Adapted from Matsumoto M, Fujimura Y, Suzuki N, et al. MRI of cervical intervertebral discs in asymptomatic subjects. *J Bone Joint Surg Br* 1998;80:19–24.)

Cancer

	Sensitivity	Specificity
Age >= 50	77	71
Previous Cancer	31	98
Unexplained weight loss	15	94
Failure to improve 1/12	31	90
No relief in bed	>90	46

Cancer

	Sensitivity	Specificity
Patients >= 50		
Previous cancer OR unexplained weight loss OR failure to improve	100	60

Infection

	Sensitivity	Specificity
I.V. drug abuse OR urinary infection OR skin infection OR HIV	40	N/A

A,B,C

FIG. 34.5. A, B, C: Lumbar red flags.

The Investigation of Cervical Disorders

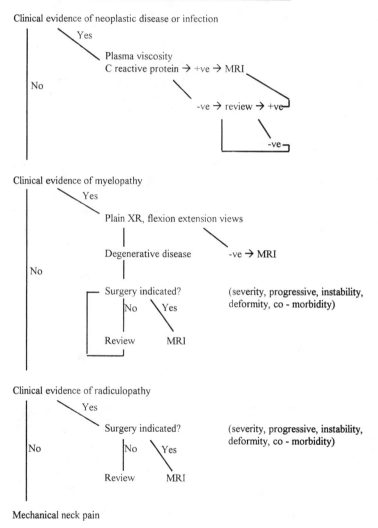

Clinical evidence of neoplastic disease or infection
— Yes → Plasma viscosity / C reactive protein → +ve → MRI
— -ve → review → +ve
— -ve
— No

Clinical evidence of myelopathy
— Yes → Plain XR, flexion extension views
  Degenerative disease   -ve → MRI
  Surgery indicated?   (severity, progressive, instability, deformity, co - morbidity)
  No / Yes
  Review   MRI
— No

Clinical evidence of radiculopathy
— Yes → Surgery indicated?   (severity, progressive, instability, deformity, co - morbidity)
  No / Yes
  Review   MRI
— No

Mechanical neck pain

Plain films not routinely indicated
MRI contra indicated

FIG. 34.6. Investigation of cervical disorders.

had moderate disc bulge, 26% had paramedian protrusion, and 7% had lateral protrusion. Cord compression was present in 7.6% of the subjects, mainly those older than 40 years. The investigators also found a high incidence of other abnormalities, including disc degeneration, disc space narrowing, disc protrusion, and foraminal stenosis (Figs. 34.1 through 34.4). The illustrations show that abnormalities are common and increase considerably with age. It is quite clear, therefore, that considerable care is needed in the interpretation of these images and that "the presence of an imaging study abnormality does not automatically imply causality" (3).

Just as imaging can provide positive findings than can be merely a reflection of age, it is important to examine the value of clinical history and examination in the accurate identification of more serious pathologic findings. One reason advanced for undertaking imaging is to "rule out" the possibility of tumor or infection. Studies of the lumbar spine have clarified the sensitivity and specificity of some commonly used features of the history and examination in predicting metastatic disease (Fig. 34.5A). With a combination of these factors, a high level of sensitivity can be achieved (Fig. 34.5B). The sensitivity of clinical features in the correction of an infective lesion in the lumbar spine is less satisfactory (Fig. 34.5C).

DIAGNOSIS

After the history and clinical features are considered, an algorithm for the investigation of cervical disorders can be proposed (Fig. 34.6).

Tumor and Infection

Investigation of suspected tumor or infection rests with hematologic indices such as plasma viscosity (erythrocyte sedimentation rate in some centers), measurement of C-reactive protein, and blood cultures. Radiologic investigations include plain radiographs, bone scanning, and MRI.

As far as the hematologic indices are concerned, plasma viscosity is likely to be the most sensitive. Infective changes of osteomyelitis can produce positive images on bone scans at 7 days. Infective discitis does not produce systemic or radiologic changes until a loss of integrity of the disc itself has occurred. In animal models, MRI provides enough information for a diagnosis of infective discitis 6 days after infection begins (6). Plain radiographs take longer to depict abnormalities, and changes may be apparent between only 2 to 6 weeks after the onset of infection. In suspected metastasis or infection, MRI is the imaging method of choice.

Myelopathy

Myelopathy is essentially a clinical diagnosis. The principal features in the history include unsteadiness of gait and a feeling of heaviness in the legs. Upper limb symptoms include loss of dexterity and loss of hand sensation. Examination findings include hyperreflexia with spasticity, extensor plantars, and a positive Lhermitte sign.

Evaluation for myelopathy of the cervical spine is concerned with several potential causes. The first, compression from tumor or an extrinsic neoplastic process, is considered earlier in the algorithm. Other causes include intrinsic neoplastic process, persistent mechanical instability, disorders such as multiple sclerosis, and the most common cause—degenerative changes in the discs.

Plain radiographs in flexion and extension should be obtained. If the findings are normal, MRI should be considered with a view to making a diagnosis of intrinsic neoplastic process, multiple sclerosis, or another condition. If substantial degenerate changes are seen on plain radiographs, the function MRI is to clarify the level or levels involved and the extent of involvement as an aid to surgical treatment. It follows, therefore, that if surgical treatment is not being contemplated, MRI scan can be considered of less value.

Whether surgical treatment is indicated depends on a number of considerations. The severity of the myelopathy and whether it is progressive are of primary importance. Demonstration of marked instability or progressive deformity can be a strong indication for surgery and imaging. Patients with degenerative cervical disease often are in the age group in which comorbidity is common. Comorbidity increases the risk of surgery and represents a relative contraindication to surgery and, therefore, possibly a contraindication to MRI. If surgery is not indicated, careful documentation of the history and examination findings with careful follow-up evaluation may be the optimum course of action.

Radiculopathy

The essential clinical features of radicular compression are pain and sensory changes that occur in a dermatomal pattern. Motor deficits based on a nerve root are confirmatory. In the absence of clinical indication of a more serious pathologic condition, such as infection or neoplastic disease, the purpose of imaging is primarily to inform the surgeon about the surgical anatomic features. It follows, therefore, that imaging in the evaluation of radiculopathy is not indicated if surgery is not indicated. The same surgical considerations may be taken into account as in myelopathy. Duration and severity of the symptoms and signs are of prime importance. Careful notice should be made whether the lesion is progressing or resolving. Serious comorbidity again is a relative contraindication to surgery. If surgery is indicated, MRI is the imaging modality of choice. If surgery is not indicated, the value of imaging is greatly reduced.

Combined Myelopathy and Radiculopathy

Patients may have both myelopathic features and radiculopathy. In the presence of degenerative disc disease, careful consideration should be given to whether surgery is indicated. If surgery is indicated, imaging informs the surgeon. If surgery is not indicated, the value of imaging again is greatly reduced.

Mechanical Neck Pain

There has been little evidence to suggest that degenerative changes in the cervical spine are correlated with symptoms. Radiographs of the cervical spine for neck pain alone in the absence of clinical suspicion or other evidence of serious pathologic changes are therefore likely to be noncontributory and are not indicated (5). Changes on MR images are extremely common among the population without symptoms. It is likely, therefore, that any changes seen on MR images of a patient with neck pain are not related to the pain. There is no doubt, however, of the serious implications of telling a patient that he or she has "a crumbling disc," which is of itself associated with serious iatrogenic chronicity. MRI is contraindicated in the evaluation of simple neck pain.

TREATMENT

Treatment here is restricted to the consideration of neck pain without evidence of myelopathy or radiculopathy. Many therapies have been used in the management of simple neck pain. The Cochrane collaboration has produced a review of patient education for mechanical neck disorders (1). Three randomized, controlled trials of sufficient methodologic quality were found. These did not support the value of the education in the management of simple neck pain. Other management techniques were examined in a second review for the Cochrane collaboration on physical medicine modalities for mechanical neck disorders (2).

Electromagnetic therapy was supported for short-term use by results of two randomized, controlled trials. The data are somewhat weakened by the fact that both trials were performed by the same investigators. Although results were statistically significant, insufficient information was available to determine whether the treatment was clinically valuable. Laser therapy was demonstrated to be ineffective in three randomized, controlled trials. Spray and stretch, traction, and the use of transcutaneous electrical stimulation (TENS) machines were not supported in a number of small randomized, controlled trials. The power of these studies was not high. For acupuncture and for exercise regimes, there was some evidence of beneficial effect in randomized, controlled trials, but these studies were hampered by methodologic weaknesses.

In summary, there is little evidence of benefit of many physical therapies commonly used in the management of simple neck pain. For some therapies, there is evidence that they are ineffective; for others treatments may be effective, but the power of the studies was insufficient to demonstrate an effect. Algorithms such as the one presented or others are being used increasingly by health care purchasers to inform their decision making when funding investigations and treatment. As health care practitioners, it is vital that we base these decisions on the best evidence so that our patients may continue to benefit from effective treatments. It is incumbent on health care practitioners to promote accurate and methodologically sound research.

REFERENCES

1. Gross AR, Aker PD, Goldsmith CH, et al. Patient education for mechanical neck disorders. Cochrane Review. Cochrane Library Issue 4, Oxford Update Software 1999.
2. Gross AR, Aker PD, Goldsmith CH, et al. Physical medicine modalities for mechanical neck disorders. Cochrane Review. Cochrane Library Issue 4, Oxford Update Software, 1999.
3. Kaiser JA, Holland BA. Imaging of the cervical spine. *Spine* 1998;23:2701–2712.
4. Matsumoto M, Fujimura Y, Suzuki N, et al. MRI of cervical intervertebral discs in asymptomatic subjects. *J Bone Joint Surg Br* 1998;80:19–24.
5. Royal College of Radiologists. *Guidelines for doctors.* London: Royal College of Radiologists, 1998.
6. Teresi LM, Lukfin RB, Reicher MA, et al. Asymptomatic degenerative disc disease and spondylosis of the cervical spine: MR imaging. *Radiology* 1987;164:83–88.

Subject Index

Page numbers followed by the letter f refer to figures; those with the letter t refer to tabular material.